中文翻译版

肺癌诊治新进展

New Therapeutic Strategies in Lung Cancers

原　著　Solange Peters
　　　　Benjamin Besse
主　译　胡　坚
副主译　汪路明　包飞潮
译　者　（以姓氏笔画为序）
　　　　包飞潮　闫茂慧　许亚萍　何哲浩
　　　　汪路明　林　钢　袁小帅　顾飞英
　　　　蒋晨雪　程　钧　曾理平

科学出版社
北　京

图字:01-2017-2105 号

内 容 简 介

肺癌是目前全球死亡率最高的恶性肿瘤,其诊治涉及胸外科、肿瘤科、放疗科、放射科等多个学科,原先的单一学科治疗肺癌的模式已经难以适应新时代肺癌的诊治要求,目前必须通过多学科诊治方能提高治疗效果。本书主要内容共分为五个部分,即诊断新进展、早期非小细胞肺癌治疗新进展、局部晚期非小细胞肺癌治疗新进展、分子治疗进展、特定类型转移性非小细胞肺癌诊治进展,参考了最新发表的关于肺癌外科微创治疗、放射治疗、化学治疗、靶向治疗、免疫治疗等领域相关文献及有突破意义的临床研究,观点新颖,内容科学,力求全面展现肺癌诊治的最新面貌,符合肺癌专科医生的实际需求,是一本不可多得的专著。

图书在版编目(CIP)数据

肺癌诊治新进展/(瑞士)索兰格·彼得斯(Solange Peters),(法)本杰明·贝西(Benjamin Besse)著;胡坚主译. —北京:科学出版社,2017.4
书名原文: New Therapeutic Strategies in Lung Cancers
ISBN 978-7-03-052499-7

Ⅰ.①肺… Ⅱ.①索… ②本… ③胡… Ⅲ.①肺癌-诊疗 Ⅳ.①R734.2

中国版本图书馆 CIP 数据核字(2017)第 073620 号

责任编辑:王灵芳 / 责任校对:高明虎
责任印制:赵 博 / 封面设计:龙 岩

Translation from the English language edition:
New Therapeutic Strategies in Lung Cancers
Edited by Solange Peters and Benjamin Besse
Copyright ©SPRINGER International Publishing Switzerland 2015
This Springer imprint is published by Springer Nature
The registered company is Springer International Publishing AG
All Rights Reserved

科学出版社 出版
北京东黄城根北街 16 号
邮政编码:100717
http://www.sciencep.com

中国科学院印刷厂 印刷
科学出版社发行 各地新华书店经销
*

2017 年 4 月第 一 版 开本:720×1000 1/16
2017 年 4 月第一次印刷 印张:14 3/4 彩插 3
字数:284 000

定价:78.00 元
(如有印装质量问题,我社负责调换)

译者前言

肺癌是目前全球死亡率最高的恶性肿瘤,其诊治涉及胸外科、肿瘤科、放疗科、放射科等多个学科,所以原先的单一学科治疗肺癌的模式已经难以适应新时代肺癌的诊治要求,目前肺癌的诊治必须通过多学科诊治方能提高治疗效果。

本书主要内容共分为五个部分,即诊断、早期肺癌治疗、局部晚期肺癌治疗、分子靶向治疗、特殊转移性肺癌治疗。本书参考了最新发表的关于肺癌外科微创治疗、放射治疗、化学治疗、靶向治疗、免疫治疗等领域相关文献及有突破意义的临床研究,观点新颖,内容科学,全面展现了肺癌诊治的最新面貌,符合肺癌专科医生的实际需求,是一本不可多得的专著。

译者所在科室是国内重要的胸部肿瘤诊治中心,已主译多部胸外科著作,在此也希望本书可以开阔肺癌专科医生的视野,使其具有多学科综合诊治的视野。

译 者

原著序言

晚期非小细胞肺癌的传统治疗方式为单一化疗，化疗方式往往也缺乏效果，而目前，根据特定的标准对患者进行放疗，适当限制部分晚期患者的手术适应证，提高了肺癌的治疗水平。本书涉及目前肺癌的关键性进展，可以为临床医生提供专业的相关知识。所有章节均由各个领域，如流行病学、病理学、呼吸科、胸外科、放射肿瘤学以及临床肿瘤学等的专业人士撰写。内容包括病理学、肺癌早期诊断及筛查、肺癌的治疗选择等多个方面。另外，本书特别关注了各个单一治疗方式的进展，以及是否可以通过多学科联合治疗方式进一步提高肺癌的治疗效果。

在此，我特别感谢所有同事和朋友在本书撰写过程中付出的努力，本书通过肺癌专科医生的共同努力撰写编辑，旨在为所有该领域的医生提供最新的相关进展。在此感谢本书的所有作者在本书撰写过程的辛勤劳动。

瑞士洛桑　Solange Peters
法国维莱特　Benjamin Besse

原著前言

胸部肿瘤学目前进展很快,肺癌是发达国家死亡率最高的肿瘤。在比利时,肺癌居男性恶性肿瘤死亡率首位,女性肺癌发病率也在迅速升高。针对肺癌,人们已经在诸多方面做了很多工作以减少其对人群健康的影响,而在烟草控制(一级预防),高风险患者早期发现(二级预防),利用现代影像和活检技术获得准确的病理分期诊断、分子诊断、多学科诊治以及新型药物的研发等方面的研究对肺癌诊治产生了积极的影响。

本书题为《肺癌诊治新进展》,由 Solange Peters 和 Benjamin Besse 等学者主编,两位主编在肺癌研究领域有诸多贡献,可为我们提供肺癌领域的新进展。肺癌在工业化国家的主要病因是烟草,因此肺癌一级预防主要依靠国家立法限制公共场所吸烟,禁止烟草相关广告,提高烟草产品税收,这些措施可有效降低肺癌死亡率,统计表明,2012 年欧盟国家男性肺癌死亡率较 2007 年下降约 10%[1],而 1975~2000 年,美国通过烟草控制减少了 550 000 例男性肺癌死亡患者和 250 000 例女性肺癌死亡患者[2]。而女性肺癌发病率则依然在增长。根据 2013 年欧洲肿瘤死亡率预测数据,女性肺癌死亡率与乳腺癌死亡率相近[3]。肺癌的二级预防主要在于早期发现,最近的大型随机对照试验表明胸部 CT 可疑用于筛查肺癌高危患者,但仍需进一步研究如何确定哪些患者是肺癌高危患者。第 2 章介绍了目前肺癌诊断的新进展,主要涉及 PET/CT 和超声内镜活检诊断两个方面,可帮助提高分期的准确性[4,5]。

此外,本书还由各个领域的专家介绍了局限性肺癌的根治性治疗方法,如微创手术、体外立体定向放射治疗、个体化围术期化疗、局部晚期肿瘤放化疗联合手术治疗等。越来越多的早期肺癌,尤其是Ⅰ期肺癌,采用微创手术治疗。而局部晚期肺癌可通过化疗提高根治率,另有多种新型药物正在进行相关的试验。Ⅲ期肺癌可通过放疗联合铂类为基础的化疗达到 20%~30% 的治愈率,部分Ⅲ期肺癌也可通过手术方式达到治愈。

本书剩余章节介绍了转移性肺癌,即Ⅳ期肺癌的治疗方法,分为个体化化疗、特定分子突变患者的靶向治疗、免疫治疗以及特定类型转移性肺癌的治疗等四部分。自 1970 年开始,肺癌分为对化疗敏感的小细胞肺癌,以及其他非小细胞肺癌,标志着肺癌个体化治疗的开始,而目前肺癌个体化治疗不仅要考虑组织学类型,如腺癌、鳞癌等,还需考虑是否合并特定类型分子突变,是否可行个体化的分子靶向治疗。截止目前,根据分子类型指导化疗的模式效果未达到使其可以临床推广的程度,仍是临床研究的一大热点。合并特定类型分子突变肺癌患者,如 EGFR 突变、ALK 基因重排等通过靶向治疗取得了较好的效果,可以明显提高患者无疾病生存期以及肿瘤缓解率。靶向治疗已经作为肺癌的常规治疗选择手段,尽管除了远东地区,其他地区患者 EGFR 突变率很低。还有许多肺癌分子突变类型被逐渐发现,也正在开发相关的靶向药物。本书有一章节介绍了免疫治疗进展,经过数十年的研究,肿瘤免疫机制的理解也逐渐加深,最近临床试验表明多种免疫药物可以有较好的肺癌治疗效果。本书最后数章为肺癌寡转移、肺癌脑转移患者的诊治,提出局部治疗方式可以有效去除病灶,甚至达到根治效果。

  肺癌的诊治是极其复杂的,必须通过多学科诊治方能获得最佳效果[6]。欧美国家正在形成一门新兴学科,胸部肿瘤学,以全面评估肺癌诊治质量及整合各个国家的优势资源[7]。本书可为肺癌相关医生提供了肺癌诊治的最新进展信息。

Jean-Paul Sculier

References

1. Malvezzi M, Bertuccio P, Levi F, La VC, Negri E. European cancer mortality predictions for the year 2012. Ann Oncol. 2012;23(4):1044-52.
2. Moolgavkar SH, Holford TR, Levy DT, Kong CY, Foy M, Clarke L, et al. Impact of reduced tobacco smoking on lung cancer mortality in the United States during 1975-2000. J Natl Cancer Inst. 2012;104(7):541-8.
3. Malvezzi M, Bertuccio P, Levi F, La VC, Negri E. European cancer mortality predictions for the year 2013. Ann Oncol. 2013;24(3):792-800.
4. Giroux DJ, Rami-Porta R, Chansky K, Crowley JJ, Groome PA, Postmus PE, et al. The IASLC Lung Cancer Staging Project: data elements for the prospective project. J Thorac Oncol. 2009;4(6):679-83.
5. Travis WD, Brambilla E, Noguchi M, Nicholson AG, Geisinger KR, Yatabe Y, et al. International Association for the Study of Lung Cancer/American Thoracic Society/European Respiratory Society international multidisciplinary classification of lung adenocarcinoma. J Thorac Oncol. 2011;6(2):244-85.
6. Blum TG, Rich A, Baldwin D, Beckett P, De RD, Faivre-Finn C, et al. The European initiative for quality management in lung cancer care. Eur Respir J. 2014;43(5):1254-77.
7. Gamarra F, Boffetta P, De RD, Felip E, Gaga M, Grigoriu B, et al. Thoracic Oncology HERMES syllabus: setting the basis for thoracic oncology training in Europe. Eur Respir J. 2013;42(3):568-71.

目 录

第1章　肺癌筛查 …………………………………………………… (1)

第一部分　诊断新进展 …………………………………………… (13)
　第2章　PET/CT 与 EBUS/EUS …………………………………… (13)

第二部分　早期非小细胞肺癌治疗新进展 ……………………… (21)
　第3章　早期非小细胞肺癌的微创治疗 …………………………… (21)
　第4章　Ⅰ期非小细胞肺癌的体部立体定向放射治疗 …………… (26)
　第5章　早期非小细胞肺癌围术期个体化化疗 …………………… (42)

第三部分　局部晚期非小细胞肺癌治疗新进展 ………………… (61)
　第6章　局部晚期 NSCLC 的放射治疗进展 ……………………… (61)
　第7章　局部晚期非小细胞肺癌外科治疗 ………………………… (84)
　第8章　Ⅳ期非小细胞肺癌个体化化疗 …………………………… (102)

第四部分　分子治疗进展 ………………………………………… (113)
　第9章　EGFR 突变肺癌治疗策略 ………………………………… (113)
　第10章　ALK 重排肺癌治疗策略 ………………………………… (126)
　第11章　KRAS 突变肺癌治疗策略 ……………………………… (135)
　第12章　其他分子类型突变肺癌治疗策略 ……………………… (165)
　第13章　肺癌免疫治疗 …………………………………………… (181)

第五部分　特定类型转移性非小细胞肺癌诊治进展 …………… (193)
　第14章　肺癌寡转移 ……………………………………………… (193)
　第15章　骨转移 …………………………………………………… (197)
　第16章　脑转移肿瘤 ……………………………………………… (215)

第1章
肺癌筛查

作者:John K. Field
译者:袁小帅

背景

全世界范围内,肺癌的死亡率为诸类癌症之最。1996年,Peto等[1]曾对44个发达国家的吸烟人群做了评估,他们认为由于吸烟导致的总死亡人数在将2020年以后超过1000万。最近数十年来,全球肺癌死亡率并无显著变化,其中2008年的肺癌死亡人数约为140万[2],其中中国的肺癌死亡人数增长速度特别值得关注[3]。这与筛查及治疗方面已得到长足发展的癌症(颈部癌、乳腺癌、前列腺癌以及结直肠癌等)的情况有很大差异。肺癌发生率在已实施有效烟草控制的国家有明显下降,这表明肺癌发病率从政策介入开始到发病率下降需要约20年的时间来完成。然而,高龄前烟民中很大一部分均属于潜发肺癌的人群。当肺癌在有症状表现的情况下得到诊断时则预后很差,其总5年生存率在美国为16%;而在英国更低,男性甚至仅有7.8%,而女性则为9.1%。

根据国际肺癌研究学会(International Association for the Study of Lung Cancer,IASLC)肺癌分期项目的大量试验研究[4]结果表明,疾病分期是总生存率的最佳预测指标,pT1aN0期患者5年生存率可达77%,pT4Nx期患者则为22%,而pT4-期伴有恶性胸腔积液及多发结节的患者则低至为2%。

肺癌最主要的病因学因素为烟草使用,烟草的人群归因分值(population attributable fraction,PEF)为86%,英国约34 600例患者可归因于烟草(源自2010年数据)[5]。肺癌患者中约15%从未吸烟,这可能归因于环境暴露、遗传因素及二手烟等[4]。国际癌症研究署(International Agency for Research on Cancer,IARC)列出一部分肺癌的诱发因素,其中包括电离辐射、职业性暴露(例如:石棉、二氧化硅)等[6]。肺癌在有肺癌疾病家族史的人群中高发,特别是同胞[7]或既往呼吸系统疾病史(COPD、慢性支气管炎、肺气肿、肺结核、肺炎等)[8,9]的情况。

在NLST试验结果发表之前,尚未有肺癌筛查可降低死亡率的明确证据[10]。然而,2011年美国国立肺癌筛查试验(National Lung Screening Trial,NLST)数据显示肺癌死亡率下降了20.0%,而所有死因死亡率亦下降了6.7%[11]。该试验分别比较了低剂量CT(low dose CT,LDCT)与胸部X线摄影在基线水平、1年和2年后的变化。受试者纳入标准为:55~74岁,吸烟史大于等于30包/年,并在近15年内一直吸烟。在美国,符合NLST入围标准及其他补充条件的受试者将进入数家指定的专业机构[12-16]以及美国预防医学工作组(US Preventive Service Task Force,USPSTF)[17]进行筛查。然而,这将潜在导致大量获益可能较小的受试者纳入,降低了CT筛查的费用效益比。"前列腺、肺、结直肠、大肠、卵巢"(Prostate,Lung Colorectal and Ovarian,PLCO)肺癌风险预测模型的应用也有力支持这一论点[18]。NLST的研究者们并未公布费用效益的数据,但由NLST模拟的数据预估可知,不同数据的费用效益在每生活质量调整寿命年(QALY)下在19 000美元到126 000~169 000美元[19,20]。费用效益是各个国家,包括英国在内,实施肺癌筛查项目决定中需要解决的最主要问题,同时在未来也将继续作为其重大影响因素之一。

近年来,由于一些尚未得到合理解决的问题,关于是否有足够证据支持肺癌筛查项目的实施这一问题在国际上存在广泛争论。2011年IASLC制定了共识声明,概述了肺癌筛查中尚需进一步研究的一些重要问题,包括:更为有效的风险评估和合适风险人群选择,诊断算法与烟草控制措施的进一步整合,等等[21]。

肺癌筛查的依据

对存在风险人群的3年期低剂量CT筛查是否真的可降低肺癌相关死亡率,NLST已经回答了这一最主要的问题。高风险人群定义为:55~74岁,具有30包/年吸烟史的吸烟者或既往吸烟者;其中过往吸烟者戒烟时间应不超过15年。与试者应具备无症状、适合手术、无既往侵袭性肿瘤病史、且在纳入试验前18个月内并未进行胸部CT扫描。NLST报道三年度回合的胸部低剂量CT相较X线片筛查的肺癌相关死亡率下降了20%[11]。同时,PLCO试验结果证实,相比常规护理,胸部X线片的年度筛查并不能显著降低肺癌死亡率[22],但这并不能消除胸部X线片其他的优势。

目前在欧洲范围内进行中的是否应做肺癌CT筛查的临床随机试验项目有8个:MILD(意大利多中心肺癌筛查项目)[23],DANTE(新型影像及分子检测技术检测早期肺癌项目)[24],Depiscan(法国随机对照试验比较低剂量螺旋CT与X线筛查肺癌)[25],ITALUNG(意大利CT筛查肺癌项目)[26],NELSON(荷兰-比利时项目)[27],DLCST(丹麦肺癌筛查项目)[28],LUSI(德国肺癌筛查干预项目)[29]以及UKLS(英国肺癌筛查项目)[30]。

其中有三项研究已经公布了结果,证实肺癌CT筛查并无显著的死亡率获益[28,31,32]。然而,一篇NLST包含在内的meta分析提出相反意见,研究者认为肺癌 CT 筛查可使总死亡率下降 19%（RR=0.81，95% CI 0.70~0.92），这与 NLST 单独的研究结果相符[33]。NELSON 试验[27]是肺癌 CT 筛查在欧洲最大的临床试验，预计将于 2015 年发布研究结果，紧接着是欧洲 RCT 数据关于死亡率和成本效益数据的汇总[34]。这些或将有可能支持着欧洲筛查工作数据的证据。

肺癌筛查的国际回顾主要是由国际肺癌研究学会（International Association for the Study of Lung Cancer，IASLC）牵头召集的研究组开展的[21]，在 NLST 试验结果发布之后 6 个月也公布了其研究结果[11]。IASLC 研究组制定了 6 个建议：①高危人群的识别以进行肺癌 CT 筛查项目；②发展中国家筛查项目中放射性指南的制订；③经由 CT 筛查项目发现的不定性结节临床诊断指南的制订；④肺癌 CT 筛查项目中结节病理报告的指南；⑤经由肺癌 CT 筛查项目发现可疑结节的外科治疗干预的建议；⑥戒烟实践整合入未来的国家肺癌 CT 筛查项目。

以国家卫生保健系统建立起最有效的肺癌 CT 筛查项目这一过程中尚有几个主要问题亟待解决。虽然问题的最佳解决办法尚未落实，但现已有一些方案被提出。例如，筛查的放射学和诊断学检查已在 NLST、NELSON 及其他欧洲临床试验中得到应用。一旦必要的死亡率和成本效益的数据成为可用，在 CT 筛查被推广实施前便应完全解决所有 IASLC 出版物概述的建议，这种规定将是很不现实的。

我们期待着 2015/2016 年 NELSON 试验死亡率结果以及汇总的欧盟 CT 筛查成本效益试验数据的公布。同时，要被提及的主要问题有：合适的高风险患病人群的选择；包括不定性结节体积分析等的放射性方案；依赖项目设计和死亡率预防回报的筛查方案可能存在的负担；以及 CT 筛查到的小结节是否进行手术切除的选择，等等。这些方面对应的则是在实施肺癌筛查前应考虑的突出问题，如图 1.1。

肺癌风险预测模型

现如今，国内外学者探究出大量风险预测模型以图预测个体发生肺癌的可能性[35]。诸如此类的模型可帮助我们筛选出那些相对高风险的人群[36]。大部分此类风险模型均主要依据为年龄和吸烟，其中包括 Bach[37]，Spitz[38]，LLP[39]，Tammemagi[18]，Kovalchik[40]等。

然而，伴随着其他流行病学危险因素的增加，肺癌风险模型的准确度需要提高[41]。PLCO 肿瘤筛查试验肺癌风险模型[42]是基于目前为止最大的数据组建立的一个肺癌风险预测模型。此模型的一个修订版已被应用到 NLST 数据库中，从该数据库中成功筛选出 81 人进行进一步检查，减少了 12 例死亡[18]。

Kovalchik 等[40]将患者风险分为 5 级，进一步比较 NLST 试验 CT 筛查组和

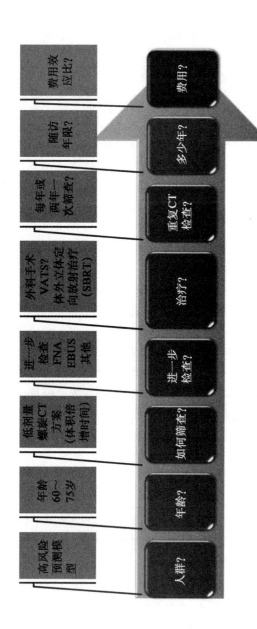

图1.1 肺癌筛查项目应用前需考虑的不确定因素

胸部 X 线片对照组的 10 000 人/年的肺癌死亡数，发现随着患者风险分级增加，CT 筛查减少的患者死亡数也明显增加，第 1 级减少 0.2 例，第 2 级减少 3.5 例，第 3 级减少 5.1 例，第 4 级减少 11.0 例，第 5 级减少 12.0 例。NLST 试验中 60% 的肺癌高风险（第 3～5 级）受试者，占肺癌死亡数的 88%，而其中 20% 的低风险（第 1 级）受试者仅占肺癌死亡者中的 1%。因此，对高风险人群筛查可以有效减少肺癌死亡风险。

利物浦肺计划（Livepool Lung Project，LLP）风险模型是以一项同名的大型研究为基础建立的[39,43]。LLP 风险预测模型结合了年龄、性别、肺癌家族史、吸烟时长、其他肿瘤个人史、非恶性呼吸系统疾病以及石棉的职业暴露等各项因素[39,43]。LLP 风险模型已在两个国际实验-对照研究（Harvard 和 EUELC）和一项独立的队列研究（LLP 7500）[44]中被证实为一项稳定的研究。LLP 风险模型具备独特优势：首先，所有预测变量均被明确定义同时易于从患者基本情况中获得；其次，患者可仅依据之前的信息被分配到适合的不同风险等级中去。风险模型尤其是 LLP 风险模型的利用近期得到了国立癌症研究所（National Cancer Institute，NCI）的高度关注[45]。LLP（第二版）风险模型[46]在 UKLS 试验中被应用来选择试验样本，这是在 RCT CT 筛查试验中首次应用了一个具体的风险模型。5 年期内可进展为肺癌的绝对风险值不低于 5% 的个体被筛选并纳入 UKLS 试点筛选试验。截至当前，UKLS 已证明以此为基线的肺癌患病率为 1.7%，这相较 NLST 和 NELSON 试验均有显著提升[47]。

肺癌筛查有利有弊，故而选择具备充分风险的人群以最大化利益风险平衡是急需解决的问题。

CT 筛查肺癌敏感性

CT 筛查肺癌具有高度敏感性，但特异性欠佳。NELSON 和 UKLS 试验使用 CT 鉴别结节良恶性以最大程度降低假阳性结果的不良影响。不确定结果指的是恶性肿瘤的概率较低，可以考虑不行活检，通过考 3 或 12 个月后再次进行 CT 扫描，计算结节的体积倍增时间（volume doubling time，VDT）。体积增长的定义应与简单的直径定义相区分。例如，一个直径 25% 的增长（8～10mm），其体积变化则从 268mm^3 变为 524mm^3，几乎是增倍（95%）。而同样的 25% 体积增长（80～100mm^3），考虑到 CT 直径测量的标准偏差，其直径变化则仅为 8%（5.35～5.78mm）[48,49]。

NLST 试验中，直径 4mm 是结节是否需要进一步影像学检查及观察抑或手术切除的临界值。尽管绝大多数此类受试者均通过各类影像技术随访，但还是导致了很多假阳性结果的出现。

NELSON 试验结论的解释则是基于结节体积进行的。小于 50mm^3 的结节被认为是阴性,大于 500mm³ 的结节则被认为是阳性,而 50～500mm³ 的结节则被认为是不定性的[27]。不定性结节则需 3 个月的 LDCT 随访以观察增长情况（通过 VDT[50]区别是阳性或阴性筛查,VDT 小于 400 且符合额外诊断策略为阳性）。NELSON 报道的筛查敏感度为 94.6%,阴性预测值为 99%。试验中的所有快速增长的肺部恶性结节指的是以基线肺癌筛查标准下经由 3 个月随访 CT 后 VDT 不多于 232 天。综上,降低 VDT 阈值可减少假阳性,而不减少肺癌检出的敏感性。

综上,三维体积可通过全面测量整个结节,准确性和可重复性均优于二维测量,尤其是对于非球形或不对称生长的结节生长比较有着重要的诊断价值。

如何界定缓慢生长肺部结节,其阈值的判定有一定的争议,大多数研究都采用 ELCAP 研究提出的 400 天阈值[51]。GGO 的 VDT 阈值目前尚不确定[52],有文献报道使用 769 天的 VDT 阈值[53]。

肺部结节的直径和体积是否对早期肺癌的检测率,治疗并发症发生率,死亡率,放疗剂量选择和治疗费用等方面存在影响有待后续研究。另外,两种不同检测方法的副作用,如重复 CT、介入性手段、及其他诊断工作和转诊等,在两者的比较中也需要纳入一并考虑。在不远的未来,相信会有很多国际性筛查项目在不定性结节的管理上采用体积分析的方法。

筛查间隔

USPSTF 建议 55～80 岁的人群应每年进行筛查[17]。然而截至目前,仅有 NLST 试验包含 3 年期的年度筛查数据。为期 25 年的年度筛查其对被筛查者死亡率、成本效益和社会心理效应等长期效应尚未得知。UKLS 近期数据表明,基于 LLP(第二版)风险模型,最佳筛查年龄应为 60～75 岁[46]。

两项临床试验开展了两年期筛查,分别是 NELSON(终筛法)和 MILD 计划[32]。尽管 MILD 试验中并无死亡率获益,但该研究中有更多的肿瘤是年度筛查,而该研究为我们提供了延长筛查间隔对间期肿瘤检测的影响这一全新角度。NELSON 试验中采用了体积 50mm³(直径 5mm)的手术切除标准。基线筛查阴性后 CT 平扫发现肺癌的概率,1 年期为 0.1%,2 年期为 0.3%;基准肿瘤检出率为 0.9%,而第二年的年度筛查中检出率则为 0.7%。因此,延长筛查间隔至 2 年或许将有一定概率导致延误肿瘤发现,哪怕进一步筛查的标准仅为 50mm³。

在预防肿瘤发生和实施年度筛查需要的费用之间需要找到一个平衡点。NLST 试验的成本效益数据尚未公布,但是基于 NLST 模型的模拟推算知,QALY 约为19 000美元到126 000～169 000 美元[19,20]。然而在提供可负担的两年期筛查(仍可拯救很多生命)或无筛查项目之间必须做出决断。筛查的绝对影响主要依赖于之前提及的风险预测模型的基线风险。在未来,针对不同与试者风险的筛查间隔和结节检测阈值或许应当个体化。这就对未来下一代基于 VDT 基线断层特征的风险预测模型的发展提出要求。

可由年度筛查到2年期筛查的变化来计算死亡率的上升,这已于近期被UKLS研究组建模并发表了相应的研究成果[54]。不同潜在情景下的预估证实年度筛查较2年期筛查可使额外20%～40%的人群获得救治[54]。研究结果显示,2年期筛查尽管在绝对数值上相较年度筛查而言效率较低,但却可能具备同样甚至更高的成本效益[54]。

筛查相关风险

在高风险人群中,肺癌CT筛查的效益远大于风险。和肺癌筛查相关的风险主要有:辐射暴露和结节的鉴别结果虽为良性但带来的个体焦虑以及有创检查。

对照实验已证实了肺癌筛查的心理和行为影响[55-59],结果显示筛查造成的不良心理后果在长期随访过程中将不复存在,同时不太可能成为筛查项目引入的问题。

筛查项目与戒烟

肺癌CT筛查试验会提供一个戒烟"大讲堂",内容涉及戒烟所致的所有吸烟相关疾病的有益健康效益。戒烟是一项成本有效干预。NELSON试验中,与人口背景6%～7%戒烟率相比,筛查组和对照组戒烟率分别为14.5%和19.1%[57]。

结论

NLST试验显示,相较于传统X线筛查,CT筛查组可进一步减少20%的死亡率,充分证实了CT在肺癌高危人群筛查中的价值。美国现已建议在55～80岁人群中采用NLST准入标准以开展年度CT肺癌筛查。但是此项建议并未在其他国家进行推广。在欧洲,我们期待NELSON试验的研究成果在近期能发表,以及2016年欧洲各大临床试验结果的汇总。很显然,美国和欧洲国家的保健制度存在较大差别,这也受到进行中临床试验的成本效益数据所影响。目前在欧洲尚存在一系列不确定因素(图1.1),因此建立一套全球通用的肺癌筛查标准尚需时间。

参考文献

1. Peto R, Lopez AD, Boreham J, Thun M, Heath Jr C, Doll R. Mortality from smoking worldwide. Br Med Bull. 1996;52:12-21.
2. IACR, UICC, CRUK. World cancer factsheet. 2012. http://infocancerresearchuk.org/cancerstats/mortality/.
3. Zhao P, Dai M, Chen W, Li N. Cancer trends in China. Jpn J Clin Oncol. 2010;40:281-5.
4. Rami-Porta R, Ball D, Crowley J, et al. The IASLC Lung Cancer Staging Project:proposals for the revision of the T descriptors in the forthcoming (seventh) edition of the TNM classi

fication for lung cancer. J Thorac Oncol. 2007;2:593-602.
5. Parkin DM. 2. Tobacco-attributable cancer burden in the UK in 2010. Br J Cancer. 2011;105 Suppl 2:S6-13.
6. Cogliano VJ, Baan R, Straif K, et al. Preventable exposures associated with human cancers. J Natl Cancer Inst. 2011;103:1827-39.
7. Cote ML, Liu M, Bonassi S, et al. Increased risk of lung cancer in individuals with a family history of the disease:a pooled analysis from the International Lung Cancer Consortium. Eur J Cancer. 2012;48:1957-68.
8. Brenner DR, McLaughlin JR, Hung RJ. Previous lung diseases and lung cancer risk:a systematic review and meta-analysis. PLoS One. 2011;6:e17479.
9. Brenner DR,Boffetta P, Duell EJ, et al. Previous lung diseases and lung cancer risk:a pooled analysis from the International Lung Cancer Consortium. Am J Epidemiol. 2012;176:573-85.
10. Field JK,Duffy SW. Lung cancer screening:the way forward. Br J Cancer. 2008;99:557-62.
11. National Lung Screening Trial Research Team,Aberle DR, Adams AM, et al. Reduced lung-cancer mortality with low-dose computed tomographic screening. N Engl J Med. 2011;365(5):395-409.
12. American Lung Association. Providing Guidance on Lung Cancer Screening to Patients and Physicians. 2012. http:// www. lung. org/lung-disease/lung-cancer/lung-cancer-screening-guidelines/lung-cancer-screening. pdf.
13. Jacobson FL, Austin JH, Field JK, et al. Development of The American Association for Thoracic Surgery guidelines for low-dose computed tomography scans to screen for lung cancer in North America:recommendations of The American Association for Thoracic Surgery Task Force for Lung Cancer Screening and Surveillance. J Thorac Cardiovasc Surg. 2012;144:25-32.
14. Jaklitsch MT, Jacobson FL, Austin JH, et al. The American Association for Thoracic Surgery guidelines for lung cancer screening using low-dose computed tomography scans for lung cancer survivors and other high-risk groups. J Thorac Cardiovasc Surg. 2012;144:33-8.
15. National Comprehensive Cancer Network. NCCN Guidelines V1. 2013 Lung cancer Screening. 2013. http://www. nccn. org/professionals/physician_gls/pdf/lung_screening. pdf.
16. Wender R, Fontham ET, Barrera Jr E, et al. American Cancer Society lung cancer screening guidelines. CA Cancer J Clin. 2013;63:106-17.
17. Humphrey LL,Deffebach M, Pappas M, et al. Screening for lung cancer with low-dose computed tomography:a systematic review to update the U. S. Preventive services task force recommendation. Ann Intern Med. 2013;159:411-20.
18. Tammemagi MC, Katki HA, Hocking WG, et al. Selection criteria for lung-cancer screening. N Engl J Med. 2013;368:728-36.
19. Pyenson BS, Sander MS, Jiang Y, Kahn H, Mulshine JL. An actuarial analysis shows that offering lung cancer screening as an insurance benefi t would save lives at relatively low cost. Health Aff (Millwood). 2012;31:770-9.

20. McMahon PM, Kong CY, Bouzan C, et al. Cost-effectiveness of computed tomography screening for lung cancer in the United States. J Thorac Oncol. 2011;6:1841-8.
21. Field JK, Smith RA, Aberle DR, et al. International Association for the Study of Lung Cancer Computed Tomography Screening Workshop 2011 Report. J Thorac Oncol. 2012;7:10-9.
22. Oken MM, Hocking WG, Kvale PA, et al. Screening by chest radiograph and lung cancer mortality:the Prostate, Lung, Colorectal, and Ovarian (PLCO) randomized trial. JAMA. 2011;306:1865-73.
23. Pastorino U, Bellomi M, Landoni C, et al. Early lung-cancer detection with spiral CT and positron emission tomography in heavy smokers:2-year results. Lancet. 2003;362:593-7.
24. Infante M, Lutman FR, Cavuto S, et al. Lung cancer screening with spiral CT Baseline results of the randomized DANTE trial. Lung Cancer. 2008;59(3):355-63.
25. Blanchon T, Brechot JM, Grenier PA, et al. Baseline results of the Depiscan study:a French randomized pilot trial of lung cancer screening comparing low dose CT scan (LDCT) and chest X-ray (CXR). Lung Cancer. 2007;58:50-8.
26. LopesPegna A, Picozzi G, Mascalchi M, et al. Design, recruitment and baseline results of the ITA-LUNG trial for lung cancer screening with low-dose CT. Lung Cancer. 2009;64:34-40.
27. van Klaveren RJ, Oudkerk M, Prokop M, et al. Management of lung nodules detected by volume CT scanning. N Engl J Med. 2009;361:2221-9.
28. Pedersen J, Ashraf H, Dirksen A, et al. The Danish randomized lung cancer CT screening trial-overall design and results of the prevalence round. J Thorac Oncol. 2009;5:608-14.
29. Becker N, Motsch E, Gross ML, et al. Randomized study on early detection of lung cancer with MSCT in Germany:study design and results of the first screening round. J Cancer Res Clin Oncol. 2012;138:1475-86.
30. Baldwin DR, Duffy SW, Wald NJ, Page R, Hansell DM, Field JK. UK Lung Screen (UKLS) nodule management protocol:modelling of a single screen randomised controlled trial of lowdose CT screening for lung cancer. Thorax. 2011;66:308-13.
31. Infante M, Cavuto S, Lutman F, et al. A randomized study of lung cancer screening with spiral computed tomography:three-year results from the DANTE trial. Am J Respir Crit Care Med. 2009;180:445-53.
32. Pastorino U, Rossi M, Rosato V, et al. Annual or biennial CT screening versus observation in heavy smokers:5-year results of the MILD trial. Eur J Cancer Prev. 2012;21:308-15.
33. Field JK, Hansell DM, Duffy SW, Baldwin DR. CT screening for lung cancer:countdown to implementation. Lancet Oncol. 2013;14:e591-600.
34. Field J, van Klaveren R, Pedersen J, et al. European Randomised lung cancer screening trials:Post NLST. J Surg Oncol. 2013;108(5):280-6.
35. Field JK, Chen Y, Marcus MW, McRonald FE, Raji OY, Duffy SW. The contribution of risk prediction models to early detection of lung cancer. J Surg Oncol. 2013;108:304-11.
36. van Klaveren RJ, de Koning HJ, Mulshine J, Hirsch FR. Lung cancer screening by spiral CT. What is the optimal target population for screening trials? Lung Cancer. 2002;38:243-52.

37. Bach PB, Kattan MW, Thornquist MD, et al. Variations in lung cancer risk among smokers. J Natl Cancer Inst. 2003;95:470-8.
38. Spitz MR, Etzel CJ, Dong Q, et al. An expanded risk prediction model for lung cancer. Cancer Prev Res (Phila). 2008;1:250-4.
39. Cassidy A, Myles JP, van Tongeren M, et al. The LLP risk model:an individual risk prediction model for lung cancer. Br J Cancer. 2008;98:270-6.
40. Kovalchik SA, Tammemagi M, Berg CD, et al. Targeting of low-dose CT screening according to the risk of lung-cancer death. N Engl J Med. 2013;369:245-54.
41. Spitz MR, Hong WK, Amos CI, et al. A risk model for prediction of lung cancer. J Natl Cancer Inst. 2007;99:715-26.
42. Tammemagi CM, Pinsky PF, Caporaso NE, et al. Lung cancer risk prediction:prostate, lung, colorectal and ovarian cancer screening trial models and validation. J Natl Cancer Inst. 2011;103:1058-68.
43. Cassidy A, Myles JP, Liloglou T, Duffy SW, Field JK. Defining high-risk individuals in a population- based molecular-epidemiological study of lung cancer. Int J Oncol. 2006;28:1295-301.
44. Raji OY, Duffy SW, Agbaje OF, et al. Predictive accuracy of the Liverpool lung project risk model for stratifying patients for computed tomography screening for lung cancer:a case-control and cohort validation study. Ann Intern Med. 2012;157:242-50.
45. Peres J. Lung cancer screening gets risk-specific. J Natl Cancer Inst. 2013;105:1-2.
46. McRonald FE, Yadegarfar G, Baldwin DR, et al. The UK Lung Screen (UKLS):demographic profile of first 88,897 approaches provides recommendations for population screening. Cancer Prev Res (Phila). 2014;7(3):362-71.
47. Field JK, Devaraj A, Baldwin DR, et al. UK lung Cancer Screening trial (UKLS):prevalence data at baseline. Lung Cancer. 2014;83:S24-5.
48. Xie X, Zhao Y, Snijder RA, et al. Sensitivity and accuracy of volumetry of pulmonary nodules on low-dose 16- and 64-row multi-detector CT:an anthropomorphic phantom study. Eur Radiol. 2013;23:139-47.
49. Field JK, Oudkerk M, Pedersen JH, Duffy SW. Prospects for population screening and diagnosis of lung cancer. Lancet. 2013;382:732-41.
50. Heuvelmans MA, Oudkerk M, de Bock GH, et al. Optimisation of volume-doubling time cutoff for fast-growing lung nodules in CT lung cancer screening reduces false-positive referrals. Eur Radiol. 2013;23:1836-45.
51. Henschke CI, Yip R, Yankelevitz DF, Smith JP. Definition of a positive test result in computed tomography screening for lung cancer:a cohort study. Ann Intern Med. 2013;158:246-52.
52. Centers for Disease Control and Prevention. Cigarette smoking among adults -United States, 2006. MMWR Morb Mortal Wkly Rep. 2007;56:1157-61.
53. Chang B, Hwang J, Choi Y, et al. Natural history of pure ground-glass opacity lung nodules detected by low-dose CT scan. Chest. 2013;143:172-8.

54. Duffy SW, Field JK, Allgood PC, Seigneurin A. Translation of research results to simple estimates of the likely effect of a lung cancer screening programme in the United Kingdom. Br J Cancer. 2014;110(7):1834-40.
55. Taylor KL, Shelby R,Gelmann E, McGuire C. Quality of life and trial adherence among participants in the prostate, lung, colorectal, and ovarian cancer screening trial. J Natl Cancer Inst. 2004;96:1083-94.
56. Byrne MM, Weissfeld J, Roberts MS. Anxiety, fear of cancer, and perceived risk of cancer following lung cancer screening. Med Decis Making. 2008;28:917-25.
57. van der Aalst CM, van den Bergh KA, Willemsen MC, de Koning HJ, van Klaveren RJ. Lung cancer screening and smoking abstinence:2 year follow-up data from the Dutch-Belgian randomised controlled lung cancer screening trial. Thorax. 2010;65:600-5.
58. van derAalst CM, van Klaveren RJ, van den Bergh KA, Willemsen MC, de Koning HJ. The impact of a lung cancer computed tomography screening result on smoking abstinence. Eur Respir J. 2011;37:1466-73.
59. Aggestrup LM, Hestbech MS, Siersma V, Pedersen JH, Brodersen J. Psychosocial consequences of allocation to lung cancer screening: a randomised controlled trial. BMJ Open. 2012;2:e000663.

第一部分
诊断新进展

第2章
PET/CT 与 EBUS/EUS

作者：Christophe Dooms，Christophe Deroose
译者：程　钧

技术原理

PET/CT

全身正电子发射断层扫描（PET）结合氟-18脱氧葡萄糖（FDG）是一项无创伤性检查。PET摄像机通过观测患者体内放射性示踪剂分布产生三维图像。目前PET扫描的空间分辨率大概为4mm，因此可以精确观察到大于8mm的病灶。而葡萄糖类似物的FDG是目前临床肿瘤成像使用最多的代谢示踪剂。

PET扫描可以集合计算机断层成像（CT）技术或者磁共振（MR）技术[1]。目前PET/CT扫描使用最为广泛，而PET/MR是一项新兴技术。联合使用PET扫描与CT或MRI有三项最主要的优势：①CT含有衰减矫正（AC）功能，可以矫正病人本身信号的干扰；②可以提高占位的精度，形态特征的关联性，减少单一PET不能明确的信号占位；③增强报告医生的信心。除非患者已有可用的增强CT，而PET/CT联合高剂量增强CT，能比单独的低剂量CT，更好地提供准确的TNM分期诊断信息[2]。

超声内镜检查：EBUS与EUS

超声支气管镜引导下经支气管穿刺活检（EBUS-TBNA）和超声食管内镜引导下细针穿刺活检是常用的内镜穿刺技术。超声探头安置在内镜的顶部，内镜可以经此扫描中央气道或者食管深层结构，内镜连接超声系统，更好地分辨实质与血管结构。内镜附有专用针道,用于内镜超声下实时引导穿刺。超声内镜可以穿刺活检部分肺内占位、肺门或纵隔淋巴结。EBUS可穿刺第2R/2L、4R/4L、7组纵隔淋巴结,以及第10、11组甚至第12组淋巴结[3]。EUS则用于上纵隔第4L组淋巴结,以及下纵隔的第7、8、9组淋巴结穿刺[3]。EUS还能穿刺活检左侧肾上腺、肝左叶以及腹腔淋巴结。因此,EUS-FNA能够用于活检其他手段(如EBUS-TBNA、纵隔镜)所不能取到的淋巴结(如第8、9组淋巴结)。有些中心可使用EUS-FNA穿刺活检第5、6组淋巴结,但是由于目前研究数据仍有限,我们不建议常规使用EUS-FNA穿刺活检第5、6组淋巴结[4]。对于为明确诊断的患者,穿刺的目标是获得尽量多的组织,提高诊断阳性率,而对于为明确纵隔淋巴结分期的患者,穿刺应至少探查第4R、4L及7组淋巴结,并且对于大于5mm直径的淋巴结活检。为了避免穿刺针污染所致分期假阳性,淋巴结活检应当自N3淋巴结开始,随后按顺序活检N2、N1淋巴结。

诊断

PET/CT和孤立性肺结节(SPN)

胸部CT检查常可发现非钙化孤立性肺结节(SPNs),低剂量螺旋CT筛查早期肺癌项目发现了许多孤立性肺结节。有研究提出,SPN行PET检查SUV值大于2.5可作为恶性肿瘤的诊断标准,以此为标准,有综述发现SPN大于10mm的PET检查的敏感性、特异性、阳性预测值、阴性预测值和阴性似然比分别为0.95、0.81、0.90、0.90、0.06[5]。而该综述同时提出,根据患者影像学分析评估结节的良恶性,敏感性和阴性似然比分别为0.98和0.02[5]。SUV值小于2.5就排除恶性肿瘤的结论目前广受争议,一项大型前瞻性研究指出,小于25mm的SPN,24%仍为恶性肿瘤[6]。另外,CT提示小于10mm的或亚实型的磨玻璃结节,或者低代谢的结节(如类癌)也存在恶性的可能。因此,任何的PET上FDG高摄取的结节都应该进行临床上的综合评估,而不是基于SUV最大值简单的界定划分。结节的综合评估包括临床特征(吸烟史、年龄),影像学特征以及结节的生长方式,综合评估可明显提高PET预测SPN的恶性可能性的准确性。

美国胸科医师学会(ACCP)研究指出,预计恶性程度小于10%的大于8mm实性孤立肺结节,小于8mm的实性孤立肺结节或者实性部分小于8mm亚实性肺结节,均不建议行PET/CT检查[9]。大于8mm实性孤立肺结节或者实性部分大于8mm亚实性结节预计恶性程度达到10%~60%时,行PET/CT检查可以帮助确定患者是行进一步病理学检查明确还是保守观察治疗。实性或亚实性孤立肺结节预计恶性程度达到60%以上时,患者应行组织病理学诊断以及PET/CT检查明确TNM分期[9]。

超声内镜及组织学分型

由于细针穿刺活检有可能是唯一可获得肿块的组织学分型以及肺癌的基因分

型的方式,近期专家共识建议细针穿刺活检应取尽可能多的组织[10]。已证实可使用小组织样本通过现代病理学的取样切片测定及免疫组化的方式明确非小细胞肺癌分型,并且可使非小细胞肺癌不确定型(NOS)维持在20%以下[10-13]。免疫组化提高了非小细胞肺癌分型的准确度,也提升了病理医生诊断的信心[14]。细针穿刺标本行分子生物学分析是另一个需要关注的方面,有研究证实可使用细针穿刺的活检标本或涂片中提取DNA样本,从而明确肿瘤存在的基因突变类型[13,15,16]。

TNM 分期

PET/CT

已有部分研究评估 PET/CT 作为肿瘤分期的标准检查的价值[17-19,20],共四项研究使用标准检查以及 PET/CT 进行肿瘤分期,其中三项研究以准确的 TNM 分期为主要研究(表2.1),而另一项研究以"无益胸腔手术"率(良性疾病,开胸探查,病理学分期ⅢA-N2/ⅢB,或者在12月内复发、死亡)为终点,PET/CT 组"无益胸腔手术"率显著降低[17]。PET/CT 的使用可指导患者治疗方案选择,如选择根治性治疗还是姑息性治疗,选择化疗还是其他治疗方法,PET/CT 可增加4%~11%的Ⅳ期患者检出率[17-19]。Maziak 等研究发现 PET/CT 可提高可切除的Ⅰ~Ⅲ期非小细胞肺癌分期的准确性。另一项加拿大的研究,纳入不可切除Ⅲ期非小细胞肺癌患者,140例患者行 PET/CT 检查,发现21例(15%)患者分期上调,而149例行 CT 检查的患者仅4例(2.7%)分期上调,两组患者差异具有显著性($P=0.0002$)[19]。目前所有的证据都认为,PET/CT 相比于传统检查分期可明显提高准确率,从而使患者治疗方案选择优化,以及可能的生存获益[21]。有随机对照研究评估全身1.5T MRI/PET 与 PET/CT 联合头颅 MRI 对于Ⅰ~Ⅲ期肺癌分期的准确性,结果显示相对于单独使用肺部 CT 扫描,两种方法可上调20%患者分期,相比于 PET/CT,1.5T MRI/PET 检查可导致更多的不必要的创伤性检查,且在评估胸腔外远处转移没有优势[22]。

表2.1 PET/CT 评估 TNM 分期的随机对照研究列表

研究者	患者数量	患者分期	评价指标	比较分组	结果	P 值
Fischer	189	可切除Ⅰ~Ⅲ期非小细胞肺癌	无益胸腔手术	传统检查 PET/CT	52% 35%	0.05
Maziak	337	可切除Ⅰ~Ⅲ期非小细胞肺癌	分期上调率	传统检查 PET/CT	7% 14%	0.046
Ung	310	不可切除Ⅰ~Ⅲ期非小细胞肺癌	分期上调率	传统检查 PET/CT	3% 15%	0.0002
Chin Yi	330	可切除Ⅰ~Ⅲ期非小细胞肺癌	分期上调率	传统检查 PET/MRI	22% 26%	0.43

增强 CT 可以明确肿瘤与纵隔、胸膜或者胸壁组织的界限,确定肿瘤临床 T 分期,指导手术切除范围。PET/CT 可准确区分肿瘤与肿瘤周围的炎症和肺不张[23]。对于 N 分期,Meta 分析指出,PET/CT 相对于单独的 CT 对于淋巴结分期准确性更高,敏感度为 76%,特异度为 88%[24],阴性似然比为 0.28,阳性似然比为 6.4,提示 PET/CT 纵隔淋巴结阴性不能完全排除纵隔淋巴结转移,而 PET/CT 纵隔淋巴结阳性同样不能确定存在淋巴结转移。由于 PET/CT 诊断纵隔淋巴结转移的阴性预测值(NPV)较高,因此对于 PET/CT 提示纵隔淋巴结阴性,原发肿瘤小于 3cm 的患者可不行有创性的淋巴结分期检查,PET/CT 还可以帮主确定可疑淋巴结的位置,为 EBUS-TBNA,EUS-FNA 或纵隔镜定位。对于 M 分期,PET/CT 明显优于单独使用 CT,但是由于脑部正常组织的糖摄取量较高,因此 PET/CT 评估颅内转移灶敏感性较低。PET 评估骨转移较 ^{99m}TcMDP 骨扫描准确性更高。对于肾上腺转移,PET 诊断肾上腺转移敏感性高,因此 CT 提示肾上腺占位,而 PET 提示代谢低则转移可能性低。PET 也能帮助确定常规检查中诊断不明的肝脏占位。PET 还能显示常见转移部位以外的占位,如软组织占位、腹膜后淋巴结、锁骨上淋巴结、无痛骨占位等。PET/CT 诊断多发转移灶的价值无可替代,但由于存在假阳性或第二原发肿瘤可能,PET 检查发现的孤立性转移灶仍需其他进一步的检查或病理学活检已明确,是当 PET/CT 检出可疑的孤立占位时,需要其他的检查或者组织学活检经行确定,因为存在假阳性或者第二原发肿瘤的可能性。

超声内镜纵隔淋巴结分期(N 分期)

纵隔镜检查曾被作为纵隔淋巴结分期检查的金标准,但目前正在受到 EBUS 和 EUS 的挑战。多篇 Meta 分析研究显示,EUS-FNA、EBUS-FNA 及 EUS-FNA+EBUS-TBNA 的诊断敏感度为 83%~94%[25-29]。目前已有 3 项对照研究结果发表,其中两项在 2007 年 ESTS 指南中提及,比较了 EUS-FNA、EBUS-FNA、EUS-FNA+EBUS-TBNA、纵隔镜、超声内镜+纵隔镜检查诊断纵隔淋巴结分期的准确性,结果见图 2.1[30,31],EUS-FNA+EBUS-TBNA 检查敏感度为 0.94(95% CI 0.85~0.98),明显高于单纯经颈部纵隔镜检查(0.79,95% CI 0.66~0.88,$P=0.02$)[31]。最近有 Meta 分析结果显示超声内镜阴性似然比为 0.15,提示超声内镜检查淋巴结阴性的患者中,有 15% 的患者可能有纵隔淋巴结转移[29],这个比例依然偏高,导致很多患者不能行解剖性根治性切除,因此对于超声内镜检查提示淋巴结阴性的患者仍需行外科手术已明确淋巴结分期。另有一项随机对照研究纳入 153 例 Ⅰ~Ⅲ 期肺癌患者,比较超声内镜和纵隔镜评估淋巴结分期的价值,结果显示两者敏感度及阴性似然比均无显著性差异,需要指出的是,该研究中患者纵隔淋巴结转移率低于其他研究,EBUS-TBNA 对 29% 的纵隔淋巴结取样不够充分,纵隔镜及 EBUS-TBNA 的敏感度分别为 0.79(95% CI 0.62~0.87),0.81 (95% CI 0.68~0.90),阴性预测值分别为 0.90 (95% CI 0.83~0.95),0.91 (95% CI

0.84～0.95),EBUS-TBNA 及纵隔镜联合检查的敏感度为 0.92 (95% CI 0.81～0.98),阴性预测值为 0.96 (95% CI 0.90～0.99)[32]。最近的一项研究比较了2种超声内镜方式(EBUS、EUS)的区别,发现两者没有显著差异[33],但 EUS 联合 EBUS 可以明显提高诊断分期的准确性和敏感性,该研究建议可将 EBUS 作为初始诊断方法,而后可使用 EUS 进一步诊断。

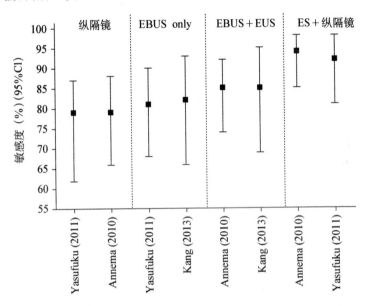

图 2.1 多项临床试验比较纵隔镜、EBUS-TBNA、EBUS＋EUS、ES＋纵隔镜应用于可切除 Ⅰ～Ⅲ 期肺癌纵隔淋巴结分期的敏感性结果。ES:EBUS＋EUS。Yasufuku 等[32],Annema 等[31],Kang 等[33]

超声内镜下穿刺活检对于诊断评估 Ⅰ～Ⅲ 期肺癌纵隔淋巴结分期有效可减少 50% 以上的外科有创性淋巴结分期检查的使用[31-34],EBUS-TBNA 联合 EUS-FNA 检查安全,并发症发生率小于 1%[25,26,35]。

参考文献

1. DeWever W, Stroobants S, Verschakelen JA. Integrated PET/CT in lung cancer imaging: history and technical aspects. JBR-BTR. 2007;90:112-9.
2. Pfannenberg AC, Aschoff P, Brechtel K, et al. Low dose non-enhanced CT versus standard dose contrast-enhanced CT in combined PET/CT protocols for staging and therapy planning in non-small cell lung cancer. Eur J Nucl Med Mol Imaging. 2007;34:36-44.
3. Rusch VW, Asamura H, Watanabe H, et al. The IASLC lung cancer staging project: a proposal for a new international lymph node map in the forthcoming seventh edition of the TNM classification for lung cancer. J Thorac Oncol. 2009;4:568-77.

4. von Bartheld MB, Rabe KF, Annema JT. Transaortic EUS-guided FNA in the diagnosis of lung tumors and lymph nodes. Gastrointest Endosc. 2009;69:345-9.
5. Fischer B, Mortensen J, Hojgaard L. Positron emission tomography in the diagnosis and staging of lung cancer: a systematic, quantitative review. Lancet Oncol. 2001;2:659-66.
6. Bryant AS, Cerfolio RJ. The maximum standardized uptake values on integrated FDG-PET/CT is useful in differentiating benign from malignant pulmonary nodules. Ann Thorac Surg. 2006;82:1016-20.
7. Swensen SJ, Silverstein MD, Ilstrup DM, et al. The probability of malignancy in solitary pulmonary nodules. Application to small radiologically indeterminate nodules. Arch Intern Med. 1997;157:849-55.
8. Herder GJ, Van Tinteren H, Golding RP, et al. Clinical prediction model to characterize pulmonary nodules: validation and added value of 18F-fluorodeoxyglucose positron emission tomography. Chest. 2005;128:2490-6.
9. Patel V, Naik S, Naidlich D, et al. A practical algorithmic approach to the diagnosis and management of solitary pulmonary nodules. Chest. 2013;143:840-6.
10. Thunnissen E, Kerr KM, Herth FJ, et al. The challenge of NSCLC diagnosis and predictive analysis on small samples. Practical approach of a working group. Lung Cancer. 2012; 76:1-18.
11. Nicholson A, Gonzalez D, Shah P, et al. Refining the diagnosis and EGFR status of non-small cell lung carcinoma in biopsy and cytologic material, using a panel of mucin staining, TTF-1, cytokeratin 5/6, and p63, and EGFR mutation analysis. JThorac Oncol. 2010;5:436-41.
12. Tournoy K, Caprieaux M, Deschepper E, et al. Are EUS-FNA and EBUS-TBNA specimens reliable for subtyping non-small cell lung cancer? Lung Cancer. 2012;76:46-50.
13. Navani N, Brown J, Nankivell M, et al. Suitability of endobronchial ultrasound-guided transbronchial needle aspiration specimens for subtyping and genotyping of non-small cell lung cancer. A multicenter study of 774 patients. Am J Respir Crit Care Med. 2012;185:1316-22.
14. Steinfort D, Russell P, Tsui A, et al. Interobserver agreement in determining non-small cell lung cancer subtype in specimens acquired by EBUS-TBNA. Eur Respir J. 2012;40:699-705.
15. Arcila M, Oxnard G, Nafa K, et al. Rebiopsy of lung cancer patients with acquired resistance to EGFR inhibitors and enhanced detection of the T790M mutation using a locked nucleic acid-based assay. Clin Cancer Res. 2011;17:1196.
16. van Eijk R, Licht J, Schrumpf M, et al. Rapid KRAS, EGFR, BRAF and PIK3CA mutation analysis of fine needle aspirates from non-small-cell lung cancer using allele-specific qPCR. PLoS One. 2011;6:e17791.
17. Fischer B, Lassen U, Mortensen J, et al. Preoperative staging of lung cancer with combined PET-CT. N Engl J Med. 2009;361:32-9.
18. Maziak DE, Darling GE, Inculet RI, et al. Positron emission tomography in staging early lung cancer: a randomized trial. Ann Intern Med. 2009;151:221-8.
19. Ung Y, Sun A, Macrae R, et al. Impact of positron emission tomography (PET) in stage Ⅲ non-small cell lung cancer: a prospective randomized trial. J Clin Oncol. 2009;27S:a7548.

20. Dinan MA, Curtis LH, Carpenter WR, et al. Stage migration, selection bias, and survival associated with the adoption of positron emission tomography among medicare beneficiaries with non-small cell lung cancer, 1998-2003. J Clin Oncol. 2012;30:2725-30.
21. Wauters I, Stroobants S, De Leyn P, et al. Impact of FDG-PET induced treatment choices on long-term outcome in NSCLC. Respiration. 2010;79:97-104.
22. Yi C, Lee K, Lee H, et al. Coregistered whole body magnetic resonance imaging-positron (MRI-PET) versus PET-computed tomography plus brain MRI in staging resectable lung cancer. Cancer. 2013;119:1784-91.
23. Lardinois D, Weder W, Hany TF, et al. Staging of non-small cell lung cancer with integrated positron-emission tomography and computed tomography. N Engl J Med. 2003;348:2500-7.
24. Lv Y, Yuan D, Wang K, et al. Diagnostic performance of integrated positron emission tomography/computed tomography for mediastinal lymph node staging in non-small cell lung cancer. A bivariate systematic review and meta-analysis. J Thorac Oncol. 2011;6:1350-8.
25. Micames C, McCrory D, Pavey D, et al. Endoscopic ultrasound-guided fine-needle aspiration for non-small cell lung cancer staging:a systematic review and meta-analysis. Chest. 2007;131:539-48.
26. Gu P, Zhao YZ, Jiang LY, Zhang W, Xin Y, Han BH. Endobronchial ultrasound-guided transbronchial needle aspiration for staging of lung cancer:a systematic review and meta-analysis. Eur J Cancer. 2009;45:1389-96.
27. Adams K, Shah PL, Edmonds L, Lim E. Test performance of endobronchial ultrasound and transbronchial needle aspiration biopsy for mediastinal staging in patients with lung cancer: systematic review and meta-analysis. Thorax. 2009;64:757-62.
28. Chandra S, Nehra M, Agarwal D, Mohan A. Diagnostic accuracy of endobronchial ultrasound- guided transbronchial needle biopsy in mediastinal lymphadenopathy:a systematic review and meta-analysis. Respir Care. 2012;57:384-91.
29. Zhang R, Ying K, Shi L, et al. Combined endobronchial and endoscopic ultrasound-guided fine needle aspiration for mediastinal lymph node staging of lung cancer:a meta-analysis. Eur J Cancer. 2013;49:1860-7.
30. De Leyn P, Lardinois D, Van Schil PE, et al. ESTS guidelines for preoperative lymph node staging for non-small cell lung cancer. Eur J Cardiothorac Surg. 2007;32(1):1-8.
31. Annema JT, van Meerbeeck JP, Rintoul RC, et al. Mediastinoscopy vs endosonography for mediastinal nodal staging of lung cancer:a randomized trial. JAMA. 2010;304(20):2245-52.
32. Yasufuku K, Pierre A, Darling G, et al. A prospective controlled trial of endobronchial ultrasound-guided transbronchial needle aspiration compared with mediastinoscopy for mediastinal lymph node staging of lung cancer. J Thorac Cardiovasc Surg. 2011;142:1393-400.
33. Kang H, Hwangbo B, Lee G, et al. EBUS-centered versus EUS-centered mediastinal staging in lung cancer:a randomised controlled trial. Thorax. 2014;69(3):261-8. doi:10.1136/thoraxjnl-2013-203881.
34. Tournoy KG, De Ryck F, Vanwalleghem LR, et al. Endoscopic ultrasound reduces surgical

mediastinal staging in lung cancer:a randomized trial. Am J Respir Crit Care Med. 2008;177: 531-5.
35. Varela-Lema L, Fernández-Villar A, Ruano-Ravina A. Effectiveness and safety of endo bronchial ultrasound-transbronchial needle aspiration:a systematic review. Eur Respir J. 2009;33: 1156-64.

第二部分
早期非小细胞肺癌治疗新进展

第3章
早期非小细胞肺癌的微创治疗

作者：Brian E. Louie，Eric Vallières
译者：包飞潮

前言

在过去20年中，微创手术在早期非小细胞肺癌也得到了长足的发展和推广，这在一定程度上是由肺癌的疾病谱变化所导致，由于CT应用的广泛，无症状性的早期肺癌检出增多，外周型肺腺癌逐渐取代中央型鳞癌，成为肺癌的主要类型，而随着CT筛查项目的开展，这种趋势也将更加显著。

本章将介绍胸外科微创手术的定义和类型，同时根据现有临床证据分析其术式、肿瘤学效果方面的优缺点。

胸外科微创手术

1912年，瑞典医生Jacobeus首次使用腔镜行胸膜腔活检[1]。经过半个多世纪的发展，电视成像，以及内镜用直线型缝合器的诞生促成了腔镜技术新时期的飞速发展，时至今日，绝大多数的胸外科手术，如肺癌肺叶切除等都能够在胸腔镜下完成[2]。

微创解剖性肺切除的特点是使用约5cm的主操作孔，若干个小切口（<1cm），不使用肋骨撑开，经腔镜显示器图像操作完成，现阶段主要有三种方式：

1. 电视辅助胸腔镜（VATS）：包括主操作孔在内一般使用2~4个孔。
2. 机器人辅助胸外科手术（RATS）：该方式由3个副操作孔和1个主操作孔

完成,或者;或在人孔 CO_2 气胸的情况下使用 4 个操作孔,在取出标本时延长其中一个操作孔。

3. 单孔电视辅助胸腔镜(uVATS):镜头和操作器械均经单一操作孔置入,不经肋骨撑开。

根据胸外科协会(STS)最新数据显示,北美 50% 以上的解剖性肺切除经上述三种微创方式完成,其中绝大部分为肺叶切除,但肺段切除数量增加较快,目前已达微创解剖性肺切除的 40%[3,4]。

微创肺切除的优势

围术期效果

微创手术由于其创伤小,理应可提高患者围术期效果。仅有的两个随机对照试验为 20 世纪 90 年代的两个小样本试验,对比了 VATS 肺叶切除和开胸肺叶切除的效果,显示可减少围术期并发症,但在其他方面并无差异[5,6]。尽管近年来 VATS 技术和开胸技术均有明显提高,但尚缺乏随机对照试验评估两种方式的围术期效果差异。

而非随机对照试验结果显示,微创术式可减轻患者术后疼痛,减少术后肺功能不全,从而减少患者住院时间,更便于患者短期内恢复正常生活[7,8],尤其是高龄虚弱患者,可减少患者术后止痛药物使用,使围术期并发症减少[9-11]。对于肺功能不全(FEV1 或 DLCO<60%)的患者,微创手术可减少术后呼吸系统并发症,如急性呼吸窘迫综合征(ARDS)、肺炎、机械通气等[12]。有研究显示微创肺切除可减少术后新发房性心律失常[7]。另外 VATS 肺叶切除可加快患者术后康复,使患者更易耐受化疗[13],但近期有研究对此持反对意见[14]。

手术死亡率

同历史数据相比,肺叶切除的手术死亡率已明显下降,这可能与微创手术相关。STS 数据显示,肺癌的手术死亡率为 2%[15],而根据美国住院患者数据(NIS)报道,开胸手术的死亡率为 3.7%,而 VATS 的手术死亡率为 3.4%[16]。Ken 等于 2014 年报道 VATS 肺叶切除的手术死亡率为 1.1%,而机器人辅助肺叶切除的手术死亡率则仅为 0.2%[3]。中国 4312 例肺癌患者手术死亡率为 1%,其中 VATS 为 0.8%,而开胸手术为 1.1%[17]。丹麦 1513 例肺癌患者手术死亡率为 2%,其中 VATS 为 1.1%,开胸手术为 2.9%[18]。

肿瘤学效果

多个临床试验对比了 VATS 和开胸肺叶切除治疗肺癌的长期生存和复发情况,其中多数为临床Ⅰ期肺癌患者,目前尚缺乏Ⅱ、Ⅲ期肺癌的对比数据。2009 年,一篇 Meta 分析通过纳入 21 项研究的 2641 例患者,结果显示 VATS 治疗早期肺癌可减少全身复发和 5 年死亡率[19]。而 Gopaldas 等于 2013 年通过多中心的倾向匹配性分析 4312 例患者生存状况,显示两种手术方式的 5 年生存率均为 62%[17]。另有两个小样本研究显示两者长期生存无显著性差异[18,20]。

淋巴结清扫的彻底性一直是微创胸外科手术广受争议的焦点。近期 STS 的数据显示临床Ⅰ期,淋巴结分期阴性患者,行开胸肺叶切除者术后病理提示淋巴结分期阳性的比例较 VATS 组高[4],但进一步的分析显示,如限定为经验丰富的外科医生行两种术式,则两者在术后淋巴结阳性率方面无显著性差异,提示外科医生的操作经验对此的影响显著。

理论上,临床早期,淋巴结分期阴性肺癌,术后淋巴结分期阳性率降低可引起肿瘤局部复发率增高,从而使患者全身复发率增高,降低 5 年生存率,但实际上,多数研究认为 VATS 可提高临床Ⅰ期肺癌的远期生存,有学者认为这是因为 VATS 可减轻手术创伤,减少术后部分细胞因子的生成,从而以减少术后免疫抑制,利用免疫作用对抗肿瘤[21,22],另有几种解释,如上述 meta 分析研究的潜在误差,患者和肿瘤生物学类型在非随机对照试验中存在差异性。

VATS,RATS,uVATS 对比结果

目前尚缺乏随机对照试验评估三种不同微创胸外科手术(VATS,RATS,uVATS)的效果差异,由于均不需肋骨撑开,理论上三者在围术期效果、住院时间、手术时间均接近。有学者认为 RATS 有固有技术优势,因此理论上应有更好的效果,研究显示 RATS 治疗早期肺癌术后淋巴结分期阳性率与开胸术式相当,明显高于 VATS[24],但 RATS 是否可提高长期生存率目前尚未明确,而两者在围术期效果上无显著性差异[8,23]。

近年来,单孔 VATS 由于其切口少,美观效果好逐渐受推崇,尤其是在欧洲和亚洲地区,但目前尚缺乏单孔 VATS 与其他微创胸外科术式的对比研究结果。

结论

心肺功能良好的早期非小细胞肺癌患者可行微创手术切除作为标准治疗方式。目前的非手术方式需与微创手术行对比分析。

参考文献

1. Jacobeus H. Uber laparo and thorakoscopic. Beitr Klin Tuberk. 1912;25:185.
2. Kirby TJ, Mack MJ, Landreneau RJ, Rice TW. Initial experience with video-assisted thoracoscopic lobectomy. AnnThorac Surg. 1993;56(6):1248-53.
3. Kent M, Wang T, Whyte R, Curran T, Flores R, Gangadharan S. Open, video-assisted thoracic surgery, and robotic lobectomy:review of a national database. Ann Thorac Surg. 2014;97(1):236-42; discussion 242-4.
4. Boffa DJ, Kosinski AS, Paul S, Mitchell JD, Onaitis M. Lymph node evaluation by open or video-assisted approaches in 11,500 anatomic lung cancer resections. AnnThorac Surg.2012;

94(2):347-53; discussion 353.

5. Kirby TJ, Mack MJ, Landreneau RJ, Rice TW. Lobectomy-video-assisted thoracic surgery versus muscle-sparing thoracotomy. A randomized trial. JThorac Cardiovasc Surg. 1995; 109(5):997-1001; discussion 1001-2.

6. Sugi K, Kaneda Y, Esato K. Video-assisted thoracoscopic lobectomy achieves a satisfactory long-term prognosis in patients with clinical stage IA lung cancer. World JSurg. 2000;24(1): 27-30; discussion 30-1.

7. Paul S, Altorki NK, Sheng S, Lee PC, Harpole DH, Onaitis MW, et al. Thoracoscopic lobectomy is associated with lower morbidity than open lobectomy: a propensity-matched analysis from the STS database. J Thorac Cardiovasc Surg. 2010;139(2):366-78.

8. Louie BE, Farivar AS, Aye RW, Vallières E. Early experience with robotic lung resection results in similar operative outcomes and morbidity when compared with matched videoassisted thoracoscopic surgery cases. Ann Thorac Surg. 2012;93(5):1598-605.

9. Port JL, Mirza FM, Lee PC, Paul S, Stiles BM, Altorki NK. Lobectomy in octogenarians with non-small cell lung cancer: ramifications of increasing life expectancy and the benefits of minimally invasive surgery. Ann Thorac Surg. 2011;92(6):1951-7.

10. Demmy TL, Curtis JJ. Minimally invasive lobectomy directed toward frail and high-risk patients. Ann Thorac Surg. 1999;68(1):194-200.

11. Jaklitsch MT, Bueno R, Swanson SJ, Mentzer SJ, Lukanich JM, Sugarbaker DJ. New surgical options for elderly lung cancer patients. Chest. 1999;116(6 Suppl):480S-5.

12. Ceppa DP, Kosinski AS, Berry MF, Tong BC, Harpole DH, Mitchell JD, et al. Thoracoscopic lobectomy has increasing benefit in patients with poor pulmonary function: a Society of Thoracic Surgeons Database analysis. AnnSurg. 2012;256(3):487-93.

13. Lee PC, Mirza FM, Port JL, Stiles BM, Paul S, Christos P, et al. Predictors of recurrence and disease-free survival in patients with completely resected esophageal carcinoma. J Thorac Cardiovasc Surg. 2011;141(5):1196-206.

14. Licht PB, Schytte T, Jakobsen E. A national study of adjuvant chemotherapy after thoracoscopic vs open lobectomy. STSAbstr 2014.

15. Boffa DJ, Allen MS, Grab JD, Gaissert HA, Harpole DH, Wright CD. Data from the Society of Thoracic Surgeons General Thoracic Surgery database: the surgical management of primary lung tumors. J Thorac Cardiovasc Surg. 2008;135(2):247-54.

16. Gopaldas RR, Bakaeen FG, Dao TK, Walsh GL, Swisher SG, Chu D. Video-assisted thoracoscopic versus open thoracotomy lobectomy in a cohort of 13,619 patients. Ann Thorac Surg. 2010;89(5):1563-70.

17. Cao C, Zhu Z-H, Yan TD, Wang Q, Jiang G, Liu L, et al. Video-assisted thoracic surgery versus open thoracotomy for non-small-cell lung cancer: a propensity score analysis based on a multi-institutional registry. Eur J Cardiothoracic Surg. 2013;44(5):849-54.

18. Licht PB, Jørgensen OD, Ladegaard L, Jakobsen E. A national study of nodal upstaging after thoracoscopic versus open lobectomy for clinical stage I lung cancer. Ann Thorac Surg. 2013;

96(3):943-50.
19. Yan TD, Black D, Bannon PG, McCaughan BC. Systematic review and meta-analysis of randomized and nonrandomized trials on safety and efficacy of video-assisted thoracic surgery lobectomy for early-stage non-small-cell lung cancer. J ClinOncol. 2009;27(15):2553-62.
20. Lee PC, Nasar A, Port JL, Paul S, Stiles B, Chiu Y-L, et al. Long-term survival after lobectomy for non-small cell lung cancer by video-assisted thoracic surgery versus thoracotomy. Ann Thorac Surg. 2013;96(3):951-60; discussion 960-1.
21. Yim AP, Wan S, Lee TW, Arifi AA. VATS lobectomy reduces cytokine responses compared with conventional surgery. Ann Thorac Surg. 2000;70(1):243-7.
22. Whitson BA, D'Cunha J, Andrade RS, Kelly RF, Groth SS, Wu B, et al. Thoracoscopic versus thoracotomy approaches to lobectomy: differential impairment of cellular immunity. Ann Thorac Surg. 2008;86(6):1735-44.
23. Jang H-J, Lee H-S, Park SY, Zo JI. Comparison of the early robot-assisted lobectomy experience to video-assisted thoracic surgery lobectomy for lung cancer. Innovations (Phila).2011; 6(5):305-10.
24. Wilson JL, Louie BE, Cerfolio RJ, Park BJ, Vallieres E, Aye RW, et al. The prevalence of nodal upstaging during robotic lung resection in early stage non-small cell lung cancer. AnnThorac Surg. 2014;97(6):1901-7.

第4章
Ⅰ期非小细胞肺癌的体部立体定向放射治疗

作者:Matthias Guckenberger
译者:许亚萍　蒋晨雪　顾飞英

体部立体定向放射治疗(Stereotactic body radiotherapy,SBRT)的原理

肺癌已成为全球男性癌症的第一位死因,女性癌症的第二位死因。非小细胞肺癌(NSCLC)早期诊断才能获得较高的治愈率,但是早期肺癌往往因缺乏症状等原因不易发现,仅占所有分期肺癌的1/4左右。由于人口老龄化和CT筛查项目的开展,Ⅰ期NSCLC患者数量尤其是老年患者数量将大幅上升[1,2]。

治疗早期老年NSCLC患者对肺癌治疗相关学科是一重大挑战。肺叶切除和系统性淋巴结清扫术一直被认为是肺癌治疗的金标准,目前正在接受各方面的挑战,接受外科治疗的早期肺癌患者比例正在逐年下降,早期的统计数据显示,80%以上Ⅰ期患者接受了手术切除[3],但是在西方老年人群中,由于存在伴发疾病以及手术死亡和并发症相关风险的增加,手术治疗的患者比例在下降[4]。从1998~2007年,美国大于65岁的患者进行开放或腔镜手术的比例从75.2%下降到了67.3%[5],而来自荷兰的数据显示,75岁以上患者接受手术的比例下降到了40%以下[6]。

以上数据说明对于合并有伴发疾病的Ⅰ期老年NSCLC患者需要有一种安全有效的非外科治疗方式。有学者认为可对存在合并症的老年患者行最佳支持治疗,而不行根治性治疗,其依据是该类患者预期寿命较短,不足以来评估一个存在潜在不良反应的根治性治疗手段的优劣。加利福尼亚癌症中心的登记数据显示,7%的Ⅰ期NSCLC患者只进行最佳支持治疗[3],而在大于75岁的老年患者中,这个比例增加到了30%[6,7],而未经根治性治疗患者的5年肿瘤特异性生存率(cancer specifi survival,CSS)不到20%,提示根治性治疗对这类患者有潜在价值。

常规分割放疗是不能耐受手术的Ⅰ期NSCLC患者的根治性治疗方法。"常规"放疗是指放疗的技术和分割方法:由于肿瘤浸润范围和肿瘤靶区的不确定性,

照射往往需要较大的安全边界,从而导致大量正常组织受照射。放疗通过多次小分割进行,一般每天 2 Gy(常规分割),总剂量至 60~66 Gy,治疗时间 6~7 周。这种治疗方式成为不能耐受手术患者的标准治疗方式,3 年总体生存率(overall survival, OS)和 CSS 分别为 30% 和 50%,优于最佳支持治疗[8]。肿瘤局部复发是常规放疗失败的最主要原因,回顾性研究显示肿瘤局控率和疾病特异性生存与放疗剂量相关[9-11],照射剂量越高,局控率越高,进而可改善患者生存[8,12]。这些研究结果表明需要既安全又有强度的放疗方法来治疗早期肺癌患者。

SBRT 背景和定义

20 世纪 90 年代中期,颅内立体定向放射治疗/放射外科、体部立体定向放射治疗在瑞典卡罗林斯卡医院首先施行,之后很快被日本[13]和德国[14,15]采用并发展。一些国家和国际机构[16-19]定义 SBRT 为通过单分割或低分割精确给予高放射治疗剂量至颅外病灶的一种外照射治疗技术。

SBRT 可通过配有图像引导技术的传统直线加速器或 SBRT 专用加速器结合专门的治疗系统实施,该原理也适用于光子和粒子治疗。SBRT 的整个工作流程、技术全面优化、质量保证是至关重要的。SBRT 是一个多专业团队合作的工作,涉及放射肿瘤学家、医学物理学家和放射技术人员。其中,针对肿瘤的图像引导技术是最重要的,既要避免漏照,又要避免对肿瘤周围重要正常器官进行高剂量照射,高精确性使得在给予与常规根治性剂量相当的照射剂量时,依然能够保证其安全性。SBRT 总的照射剂量通过数次分割给予,通常治疗 3~10 次,需要根据肿瘤大小和位置来调整单次分割的剂量和总剂量。

早期 NSCLC SBRT 研究结果

老年患者 SBRT 治疗与最佳支持治疗比较

基于荷兰[6,7]和美国[20]人群的研究结果显示,对Ⅰ期老年 NSCLC 患者进行 SBRT 治疗可以改善生存。SBRT 是一种非侵袭性的治疗手段,可以在门诊进行,治疗周期短,只需 1~2 周时间,提高了患者接受根治性治疗的机会和治疗的依从性,对于老年患者来说相当有吸引力。

荷兰一项研究发现,从 1999~2007 年,由于 SBRT 技术的使用,年龄大于 75 岁患者的中位生存时间从 16 个月提高到了 21 个月[7]。SBRT 效果显而易见,所以接受最佳支持治疗的患者比例从 38% 下降到了 28%,而进行根治性放疗的比例从 26% 增加至 42%。在这期间,进行手术治疗患者的比例保持不变。

美国一项研究纳入 SEER 数据库中年龄大于 65 岁的所有Ⅰ期 NSCLC 患者,对最佳支持治疗、常规放疗、SBRT 治疗、亚肺叶切除术和肺叶切除术五种不同治疗手段进行了比较[20]。在 SBRT 和非 SBRT 治疗之间进行了倾向评分匹配,用以纠正种族、性别、教育水平、收入、并存疾病、组织学、肿瘤分级、肿瘤大小以及淋巴结取样情况各方面的不平衡,结果显示,与最佳支持治疗和常规放疗相比,SBRT治疗改善了患者OS,而与亚肺叶切除术和肺叶切除术相比,则没有明显差别。在安全性方面,老年人群中SBRT治疗30天和90天死亡率分别为0和0.8%,而亚肺叶切除术和肺叶切除术90天死亡率为4.1%。

有两项研究报道了SBRT治疗年龄大于80岁患者中的安全性和有效性。一项是日本的研究,入组了109例患者,中位年龄83岁(最大年龄91岁),3年OS为53.7%[21],其中1例患者发生了5级放射性肺炎,该患者因同时患有间质性肺炎和抗中性粒细胞胞质抗体相关性血管炎而无法行手术治疗。另一项是Sandhu等的研究,应用SBRT治疗24例中位年龄为85岁的患者,中位剂量48 Gy,4~5次分割,2年OS为74%,没有患者发生3级以上毒副反应。荷兰有研究用SBRT治疗193例年龄大于75岁(中位年龄79岁)的患者[22],其中,192例患者完成了治疗,3年OS为45%,没有观察到4级及以上毒副反应。以上数据提示,即使患者中位年龄在79~85岁,SBRT治疗也是安全的,326例患者中,只有1例治疗相关死亡及少数患者发生3~4级毒副反应。在80~89岁的患者中,手术的死亡率有10%~15%,而术后并发症的发生率报道大于20%,SBRT与此相比具有明显的优势[23]。

SBRT在肺功能差的患者中是否安全是另一个关注点。Palma等对176例患有慢性阻塞性肺病(COPD)的肺癌患者进行了SBRT治疗,这些患者肺功能的GOLD分级均达到了Ⅲ/Ⅳ级[24],所有患者接受了60 Gy的放疗,3~8次分割,结果3年OS为47%,没有患者发生Ⅳ级以上肺部毒副反应。Guckenberger等分析了5个中心270例患者SBRT治疗前后肺功能的变化[25]。SBRT治疗前肺功能较差(FEV1小于40%)的患者,治疗后2年内肺功能均稳定,说明即使在患有严重肺部合并症的高风险患者人群中SBRT也是安全的。另有一些研究报道SBRT治疗后肺功能没有变化或者只有轻度下降[26-29],这可能因为肺结构相对特殊,高剂量的SBRT多集中在很小区域内。

根治性SBRT可能无法使生存期有限的合并有严重伴发疾病的患者获益,但由于目前尚缺乏筛选这类患者的标准,因此我们认为,除了无法配合SBRT的患者,不论高龄还是伴有肺部合并症的患者,都应推荐使用SBRT。

SBRT与常规分割放疗治疗不可耐受手术患者比较

多项前瞻性Ⅱ期临床试验报道SBRT治疗不可耐受手术的Ⅰ期NSCLC患者中的局控率在84%~98%[30-35],明显高于常规放疗[8];一项Meta分析[36]和一项风险人群分析[20]显示,局控率的改善可以进而转化为OS的提高,SBRT治疗后3年OS接近50%,而治疗前是否存在伴发疾病是显著预后影响因子[37]。

大型的单中心和多中心研究证实了上述前瞻性研究的结果,尽管SBRT方法各异,但是得到的结果高度一致(表4.1)。一项研究对在德国和奥地利13个研究中心进行SBRT治疗的582例患者进行了分析[38],结果发现肿瘤局部控制率和OS独立于不同时期和不同中心应用的SBRT技术,没有观察到学习曲线效应或是过程数量效应,这再次证实了SBRT技术的稳定性。

表4.1 SBRT治疗Ⅰ期NSCLC患者前瞻性和大型回顾性研究结果

研究	年份	病例数	OS(2~3年)(%)	LC(2~3年)(%)
Nagata 等[30]	2005	45	75	98
Baumann 等[31]	2009	57	60	92
Fakiris 等[32]	2009	70	43	88
Ricardi 等[33]	2010	62	57	88
Timmerman 等[34]	2010	55	56	98
Bral 等[35]	2011	40	52	84
前瞻性研究		329	56.2	91.2
Senthi 等[70]	2012	676	55	95
Guckenberger 等[38]	2013	582	47	80
		164[a]	62[a]	93[a]
Grills	2013	859	51.5	94
回顾性研究		2049	51.3	91

a:患者BED剂量大于106Gy

基于以上研究结果,2013年第一版NCCN指南[39]以及ESMO临床实践指南[40]均认为SBRT治疗优于常规放射治疗,应作为不能耐受手术治疗患者标准治疗。

SBRT与射频消融治疗不能耐受手术患者比较

射频消融治疗(radiofrequency ablation,RFA)是Ⅰ期NSCLC患者一种微创的治疗选择。目前缺乏研究直接比较SBRT和RFA的疗效,但最近的一项文献回顾性报道显示,与RFA相比,SBRT治疗后的患者在肿瘤局部控制率、肿瘤特异性生存率和总生存方面均得到了改善[41]。此外,SBRT治疗的不良反应和30天死亡率更低[42],因此,对于高危NSCLC患者,SBRT应作为非手术治疗的首选治疗方式。

SBRT治疗与外科手术治疗可手术患者比较

肺叶切除术是可手术Ⅰ期NSCLC的标准治疗手段,一项随机试验显示,与楔形切除术相比,肺叶切除术提高了肿瘤局部控制率和总体生存率[43]。肺段切除术与肺叶切除术疗效是否相当存在争议[44],有研究认为对于ⅠA期患者中,肺段切除术与肺叶切除术治疗效果相当[45]。

鉴于SBRT在不能耐受手术的患者中所取得的良好结果,研究者启动了三项比较SBRT与手术的随机试验,分别是ROSEL研究、STAR研究和ACOSOG Z4099/RTOG 1021研究,其中前两项比较SBRT与肺叶切除术,RTOG 1021研究比较SBRT与亚肺叶切除术,但是由于缺乏Ⅰ级证据,只有2.8%(68/2410)的患者入组,这三项研究均因入组率低而提前终止。

由于缺乏Ⅰ级证据,一些研究运用匹配配对分析、倾向评分匹配等统计学方法来纠正SBRT患者和手术患者之间特征的不平衡。Grills等进行了一项比较SBRT与楔形切除术的单中心研究,发现SBRT组的肿瘤局部控制率优于楔形切除术,在肿瘤特异性生存方面两者没有区别,而手术组的总生存更好些,可能原因是SBRT组的患者年龄较大,相对来说伴发疾病更多[46]。基于美国人群的一项分析显示,SBRT与亚肺叶切除术或肺叶切除术相比,在OS和CSS方面均没有差异[20]。Puri等的研究结果也显示SBRT与手术患者(80%的患者接受了肺叶切除术)的CSS相当[47],而在OS方面,手术组相对较好,但缺乏显著统计学差异,研究者认为原因是SBRT组的患者肺部合并症较多,在倾向评分匹配的时候没有予以纠正。Verstegen等对性别、年龄、临床肿瘤分期、肿瘤直径、肿瘤部位、肿瘤组织学类型、肺功能(FEV1%)、Charlson合并症评分以及WHO体能评分进行倾向评分匹配后,比较了128例SBRT和胸腔镜辅助下肺叶切除术患者的疗效[48]。结果发现SBRT组的局部控制率优于手术组,两组的无进展生存和总生存相似。

对于适合手术治疗但拒绝手术的患者进行SBRT治疗的结果也有一些报道。日本的研究数据显示5年生存率为70%($n=87$)[49],荷兰的研究3年生存率达到了85%($n=177$)[50],此结果与肺叶切除术后的OS相当。

因此,如患者拒绝行肺叶切除术,SBRT可作为一种备用治疗手段,由于SBRT与亚肺叶切除术疗效相当,两者均可作为治疗的选择,但需向患者说明各种方法的利弊。

肺癌SBRT治疗不良反应和生活质量

SBRT治疗的大部分患者存在严重的肺部合并症,不能耐受手术治疗,因此,肺毒性是SBRT治疗关注的一个主要方面。周围型肿块小于5cm时,SBRT引起的有症状的放射性肺炎的发生率小于10%,较高的肺部照射平均剂量,大范围的低剂量传播照射是放射性肺炎的发生的危险因素[51,52]。有研究显示,SBRT治疗患者肺功能稳定,治疗2年后FEV1和DLCO仅下降约10%[25]。治疗前肺功能很差的患者[25]以及GOLD分级Ⅲ~Ⅳ级的COPD患者[53],SBRT治疗肺毒性也没有增加,但如果患者治疗前存在肺纤维化,放射性肺炎的发生风险则显著增加。

另外,肿瘤位置靠近胸壁正常组织时可能出现相应的胸壁损伤,例如肌炎、神经痛、肋骨骨折、软组织纤维化和皮肤溃疡等。胸壁照射剂量若大于30Gy,以上不良反应风险明显增加,制订治疗计划时应考虑尽量减少正常胸壁的照射剂量[54-56]。

有报道SBRT可以引起严重的臂丛炎(神经性疼痛、肌力减退或者感觉改变)、大支气管损伤(狭窄伴肺不张)和食管损伤(溃疡、穿孔、瘘),但非常罕见。SBRT分割3~4次时,限制臂丛的剂量小于26Gy,可使臂丛毒性降到最低[57]。靠近食管和大支气管的中央型肿块进行SBRT治疗的情况会在下文进一步讨论。

目前研究认为SBRT并不损害患者生活质量(quality-of-life,QoL)[58-60]。所有研究均认为患者生活质量包括呼吸困难、咳嗽在SBRT治疗后处于稳定状态,一项研究还发现SBRT治疗明显改善了患者精神状态[58]。

早期NSCLC SBRT临床实践

肺癌SBRT治疗涉及多个学科,包括了肺癌诊断和治疗的各个学科。在放疗科,SBRT的实施和执行需要专业团队来完成,包括放射肿瘤学家、医学物理学家和放射技师,所有成员都要经过SBRT的专门培训。书面方案制定是保证SBRT质量的重要步骤。

NSCLC的任何治疗都需要多学科综合治疗协作组讨论,SBRT治疗也不例外。仔细评估患者的体能状况有利于制定更合理的治疗方案。患者围术期并发症与高龄和伴发疾病有关[4,61],因此,在估计手术风险和根据患者个体情况调整治疗方案前,推荐对患者的肺功能、心脏以及体能状况等进行临床综合评估。

下文,我们将对Ⅰ期NSCLC SBRT治疗的临床和技术问题进行探讨。

病理未确诊的肺肿块SBRT治疗

在NSCLC治疗前需要明确组织病理学诊断,经支气管穿刺活检或经胸针吸活检是获取病理诊断的主要方法。但有部分患者由于存在肺部或其他合并症,或者因进行穿刺等操作风险较大,而无法活检明确病理,在这种情况下,应该参考恶性肿瘤的放射学诊断标准。Swensen等[62]建立了一个用临床和放射学特征来评估肺部孤立性结节恶性概率的预测模型。参考FDG-PET图像可进一步提高预测模型的准确性[63,64]。根据以上标准,如果恶性可能性大,即使没有病理证据,也可行SBRT治疗[65],外科治疗也常基于此标准[66]。对于处于良恶性边缘的肿块可通过定期复查评估其生长方式,但存在疾病进展的风险[67]。

肿瘤分期

SBRT只对原发病灶进行高剂量照射,往往不行淋巴结照射,因此,所有患者需行全身PET检查以排除淋巴结转移。CT检查淋巴结转移的阴性预测率为90%,PET可以提高诊断准确性[68,69]。从PET检查明确分期到治疗之间的间隔时间不应大于6周,以避免在这期间肿瘤发生进展。对于纵隔淋巴结FDG病理性摄取的情况,必须进一步行EBUS、EUS等检查进行评估。如果仍不明确,可行纵隔镜检查。PET诊断淋巴结转移存在假阴性,PET排除淋巴结转移的患者仍有10%的患者发现存在淋巴结转移[70]。

SBRT方案设计与实施

由于呼吸运动可使肺肿瘤存在几厘米的位移,因此,需要制订一个运动控制方案[71],肿瘤的运动可通过四维 CT(4DCT)也称作呼吸相关 CT 来评估[72,73],4DCT 还可减少由于不典型呼吸位置的捕获所引起的运动伪影和系统误差[74,75]。目前,多种运动控制技术已在临床实践中应用,例如门控技术、实时跟踪技术、屏气照射、内靶区的概念等,各有优缺点[76]。呼吸运动评估需融入到 SBRT 方案设计和实施的各个步骤中,尤其是图像引导过程。尽管运动控制技术被强烈推荐应用于 SBRT,但对于肿瘤活动幅度小于 10~15 mm 的大部分患者,门控、实时跟踪技术等先进的运动控制技术并不能使患者获益[76,77]。

SBRT 可以通过三维适形放疗(3D-conformal radiotherapy,3D-CRT),调强放疗(Intensity-modulated radiotherapy,IMRT)或者容积调强拉弧放疗(Volumetric modulated arc therapy,VMAT)实施。目前,所有公布的前瞻性研究运用的都是 3D-CRT 技术,而 IMRT 和 VMAT 技术在增加剂量适形性和均质性及减少治疗时间方面有明显优势[78]。B 型算法可以实现准确的剂量计算,尤其是在肺组织和软组织交界处的剂量,因此该算法被强烈推荐[79]。蒙特卡罗剂量计算法虽可以获得准确结果,但是与串卷积剂量计算方法的差异较小。

肺肿瘤的位置时时都在变化,在方案涉及和治疗实施时都可能存在变化。这种变化不是由于摆位误差所致,而是肺内肿瘤的相对运动引起,变化幅度平均为 5~7 mm,个别患者可达到数厘米[80,81]。为避免漏照肿瘤进而引起肿瘤局控率下降,有必要引入图像引导放射治疗(Image-guidance radiotherapy,IGRT)[77]。图像引导放疗技术大致可以分为平面成像和立体成像两种,平面成像的主要优点是在治疗实施过程中可以重复验证,但是,需要植入定位标记物使得软组织肿瘤清晰可见,存在气胸风险。立体成像的主要优点是不仅可以验证肿瘤位置,还可以验证肿瘤周围重要器官的位置,如脊髓等。

SBRT 照射剂量和分割

不同研究之间的单次分割剂量存在很大的差别,所以比较物理剂量没有太大的意义,需要将物理剂量转换为生物等效剂量(biological effective doses,BED)来评估分割效应[82]。多项研究均显示肿瘤局控率和剂量明显相关[83-86],当 PTV 的 BED 大于 100 Gy 时,肿瘤局控率超过 90%,这种剂量依赖的局控率的提高可以转化为 OS 的延长[83,87]。近期一项 Meta 分析显示,SBRT 高剂量组(BED 为 83.2~146 Gy)获得了最好的生存,但 BED 大于 146 Gy 组的 OS 不如普通高剂量组,说明过高的治疗剂量可能带来不利影响[88]。

100 Gy 的生物等效剂量一般通过 1~10 次分割给予,但是在美国,由于受医疗报销制度的影响,通常使用 5 次或者更少的分割。最常使用的分割方案是 18 Gy×3 次,以此作为 PTV 的处方剂量[89]。该单次剂量和总剂量在治疗小于 5cm 的周围型肿瘤中是安全的,但是如果是治疗靠近重要危及器官如食管、大支气管等的中央型肿瘤,严重不良反应的发生率很高[90,91]。而中央型肿瘤行 SBRT 治疗时,若分割数增加(5～10次),单次分割剂量下降,则治疗安全[92],这是一个风险分割的概念。中央型肿瘤一般使用每次7.5 Gy,一共8次的分割方案,该方案目前被认为是最佳治疗方案[93]。

治疗评估和随访

推荐2～3年内每3～6个月复查胸部CT,之后每年复查,以便及早发现第二原发肺肿瘤和局部复发,从而可以有机会行挽救性治疗。在CT随访时,无症状的局部急性肺炎和晚期肺纤维化改变很常见,影像学改变可维持数年[94]。随访评估医生应了解SBRT治疗后正常组织的反应,避免误解为肿瘤复发。有学者提出了随访时肿瘤局部复发的高危CT形态学特征,包括以下特征:原发灶部位阴影扩大、持续扩大的肺部阴影、治疗12个月后阴影扩大、阴影处可见膨胀的边缘、线状边缘消失及空气支气管征消失[95],对出现这些复发高风险CT特征的患者,需行PET检查,若SUVmax≥5,则提示肿瘤局部复发。

孤立病灶局部复发的挽救性手术治疗或SBRT治疗报道较少,有5例[96]和7例[97]患者接受了SBRT后挽救性手术治疗,术中没有发现与SBRT治疗相关的明显粘连,手术安全。再次SBRT治疗目前只限用于周围型肿瘤[98]。

总结

目前的循证医学证据提示,对于Ⅰ期NSCLC患者,SBRT是一种可选择的治疗方式。前瞻性研究和回顾性研究结果一致提示:对于Ⅰ期NSCLC,SBRT的肿瘤局部控制率超过90%,总生存率主要受到患者是否伴有合并疾病的影响。出于SBRT的技术安全和质量控制考虑,要求必须由经验丰富以及训练有素的多学科综合治疗团队完成,同时需要有图像引导的放射治疗技术指导。患者是否适合行SBRT治疗需要肿瘤多学科综合治疗组讨论决定,应充分考虑围术期风险及患者个人意愿。

参考文献

1. Smith BD, Smith GL, Hurria A, Hortobagyi GN, Buchholz TA. Future of cancer incidence in the United States: burdens upon an aging, changing nation. J Clin Oncol. 2009;27(17): 2758-65.
2. National Lung Screening Trial Research Team, Aberle DR, Adams AM, Berg CD, Black WC, Clapp JD, Fagerstrom RM, Gareen IF, Gatsonis C, Marcus PM, et al. Reduced lung-cancer mortality with low-dose computed tomographic screening. N Engl J Med. 2011; 365(5):395-409.
3. Raz DJ, Zell JA, Ou SH, Gandara DR, Anton-Culver H, Jablons DM. Natural history of stage I non-small cell lung cancer: implications for early detection. Chest. 2007;132(1):193-9.
4. de Perrot M, Licker M, Reymond MA, Robert J, Spiliopoulos A. Influence of age on opera-

tive mortality and long-term survival after lung resection for bronchogenic carcinoma. Eur Respir J. 1999;14(2):419-22.

5. Vest MT, Herrin J, Soulos PR, Decker RH, Tanoue L, Michaud G, Kim AW, Detterbeck F, Morgensztern D, Gross CP. Use of new treatment modalities for non-small cell lung cancer care in the Medicare population. Chest. 2013;143(2):429-35.

6. Haasbeek CJ, Palma D, Visser O, Lagerwaard FJ, Slotman B, Senan S. Early-stage lung cancer in elderly patients: a population-based study of changes in treatment patterns and survival in the Netherlands. Ann Oncol. 2012;23(10):2743-7.

7. Palma D, Visser O, Lagerwaard FJ, Belderbos J, Slotman BJ, Senan S. Impact of introducing stereotactic lung radiotherapy for elderly patients with stage I non-small-cell lung cancer: a population-based time-trend analysis. J Clin Oncol. 2010;28(35):5153-9.

8. Rowell NP, Williams CJ. Radical radiotherapy for stage I/II non-small cell lung cancer in patients not sufficiently fit for or declining surgery (medically inoperable). Cochrane Database Syst Rev. 2001;(2):CD002935.

9. Martel MK, Ten Haken RK, Hazuka MB, Kessler ML, Strawderman M, Turrisi AT, Lawrence TS, Fraass BA, Lichter AS. Estimation of tumor control probability model parameters from 3-D dose distributions of non-small cell lung cancer patients. Lung Cancer. 1999;24(1):31-7.

10. Willner J, Baier K, Caragiani E, Tschammler A, Flentje M. Dose, volume, and tumor control prediction in primary radiotherapy of non-small-cell lung cancer. Int J Radiat Oncol Biol Phys. 2002;52(2):382-9.

11. Partridge M, Ramos M, Sardaro A, Brada M. Dose escalation for non-small cell lung cancer: analysis and modelling of published literature. Radiother Oncol. 2011;99(1):6-11.

12. Sibley GS, Jamieson TA, Marks LB, Anscher MS, Prosnitz LR. Radiotherapy alone for medically inoperable stage I non-small-cell lung cancer: the Duke experience. Int J Radiat Oncol Biol Phys. 1998;40(1):149-54.

13. Uematsu M, Shioda A, Tahara K, Fukui T, Yamamoto F, Tsumatori G, Ozeki Y, Aoki T, Watanabe M, Kusano S. Focal, high dose, and fractionated modified stereotactic radiation therapy for lung carcinoma patients: a preliminary experience. Cancer. 1998;82(6):1062-70.

14. Wulf J, Hadinger U, Oppitz U, Olshausen B, Flentje M. Stereotactic radiotherapy of extracranial targets: CT-simulation and accuracy of treatment in the stereotactic body frame. Radiother Oncol. 2000;57(2):225-36.

15. Herfarth KK, Debus J, Lohr F, Bahner ML, Fritz P, Hoss A, Schlegel W, Wannenmacher MF. Extracranial stereotactic radiation therapy: set-up accuracy of patients treated for liver metastases. Int J Radiat Oncol Biol Phys. 2000;46(2):329-35.

16. Benedict SH, Yenice KM, Followill D, Galvin JM, Hinson W, Kavanagh B, Keall P, Lovelock M, Meeks S, Papiez L, et al. Stereotactic body radiation therapy: the report of AAPM Task Group 101. Med Phys. 2010;37(8):4078-101.

17. Potters L, Kavanagh B, Galvin JM, Hevezi JM, Janjan NA, Larson DA, Mehta MP, Ryu S,

Steinberg M, Timmerman R, et al. American Society for Therapeutic Radiology and Oncology (ASTRO) and American College of Radiology (ACR) practice guideline for the performance of stereotactic body radiation therapy. Int J Radiat Oncol Biol Phys. 2010;76(2):326-32.
18. Kirkbride P, Cooper T. Stereotactic body radiotherapy. Guidelines for commissioners, providers and clinicians:a national report. Clin Oncol. 2011;23(3):163-4.
19. Sahgal A, Roberge D, Schellenberg D, Purdie TG, Swaminath A, Pantarotto J, Filion E, Gabos Z, Butler J, Letourneau D, et al. The Canadian Association of Radiation Oncology scope of practice guidelines for lung, liver and spine stereotactic body radiotherapy. Clin Oncol. 2012;24(9):629-39.
20. Shirvani SM, Jiang J, Chang JY, Welsh JW, Gomez DR, Swisher S, Buchholz TA, Smith BD. Comparative effectiveness of 5 treatment strategies for early-stage non-small cell lung cancer in the elderly. Int J Radiat Oncol Biol Phys. 2012;84(5):1060-70.
21. Takeda A,Sanuki N, Eriguchi T, Kaneko T, Morita S, Handa H, Aoki Y, Oku Y, Kunieda E. Stereotactic ablative body radiation therapy for octogenarians with non-small cell lung cancer. Int J Radiat Oncol Biol Phys. 2013;86(2):257-63.
22. Haasbeek CJ, Lagerwaard FJ, Antonisse ME, Slotman BJ, Senan S. Stage I nonsmall cell lung cancer in patients aged>or = 75 years:outcomes after stereotactic radiotherapy. Cancer. 2010;116(2):406-14.
23. Saha SP, Bender M, Ferraris VA, Davenport DL. Surgical treatment of lung cancer in octogenarians. South Med J. 2013;106(6):356-61.
24. Palma D,Lagerwaard F, Rodrigues G, Haasbeek C, Senan S. Curative treatment of stage I non- small-cell lung cancer in patients with severe COPD:stereotactic radiotherapy outcomes and systematic review. Int J Radiat Oncol Biol Phys. 2012;82(3):1149-56.
25. Guckenberger M, Kestin LL, Hope AJ, Belderbos J, Werner-Wasik M, Yan D, Sonke JJ, Bissonnette JP, Wilbert J, Xiao Y, et al. Is there a lower limit of pretreatment pulmonary function for safe and effective stereotactic body radiotherapy for early-stage non-small cell lung cancer? J Thorac Oncol. 2012;7(3):542-51.
26. Stephans KL, Djemil T, Reddy CA, Gajdos SM, Kolar M, Machuzak M, Mazzone P, Videtic GM. Comprehensive analysis of pulmonary function Test (PFT) changes after stereotactic body radiotherapy (SBRT) for stage I lung cancer in medically inoperable patients. J Thorac Oncol. 2009;4(7):838-44.
27. Takeda A,Enomoto T, Sanuki N, Handa H, Aoki Y, Oku Y, Kunieda E. Reassessment of declines in pulmonary function>/=1 year after stereotactic body radiotherapy. Chest. 2013; 143(1):130-7.
28. Bishawi M, Kim B, Moore WH, Bilfinger TV. Pulmonary function testing after stereotactic body radiotherapy to the lung. Int J Radiat Oncol Biol Phys. 2012;82(1):e107-10.
29. Henderson M,McGarry R, Yiannoutsos C, Fakiris A, Hoopes D, Williams M, Timmerman R. Baseline pulmonary function as a predictor for survival and decline in pulmonary function over time in patients undergoing stereotactic body radiotherapy for the treatment of stage I

non-small-cell lung cancer. Int J Radiat Oncol Biol Phys. 2008;72(2):404-9.
30. Nagata Y, Takayama K, Matsuo Y, Norihisa Y, Mizowaki T, Sakamoto T, Sakamoto M, Mitsumori M, Shibuya K, Araki N, et al. Clinical outcomes of a phase I/II study of 48 Gy of stereotactic body radiotherapy in 4 fractions for primary lung cancer using a stereotactic body frame. Int J Radiat Oncol Biol Phys. 2005;63(5):1427-31.
31. Baumann P, Nyman J, Hoyer M, Wennberg B, Gagliardi G, Lax I, Drugge N, Ekberg L, Friesland S, Johansson KA, et al. Outcome in a prospective phase II trial of medically inoperable stage I non-small-cell lung cancer patients treated with stereotactic body radiotherapy. J Clin Oncol. 2009;27(20):3290-6.
32. Fakiris AJ, McGarry RC, Yiannoutsos CT, Papiez L, Williams M, Henderson MA, Timmerman R. Stereotactic body radiation therapy for early-stage non-small-cell lung carcinoma: four-year results of a prospective phase II study. Int J Radiat Oncol Biol Phys. 2009;75(3):677-82.
33. Ricardi U, Filippi AR, Guarneri A, Giglioli FR, Ciammella P, Franco P, Mantovani C, Borasio P, Scagliotti GV, Ragona R. Stereotactic body radiation therapy for early stage non-small cell lung cancer: results of a prospective trial. Lung Cancer. 2010;68(1):72-7.
34. Timmerman R, Paulus R, Galvin J, Michalski J, Straube W, Bradley J, Fakiris A, Bezjak A, Videtic G, Johnstone D, et al. Stereotactic body radiation therapy for inoperable early stage lung cancer. JAMA. 2010;303(11):1070-6.
35. Bral S, Gevaert T, Linthout N, Versmessen H, Collen C, Engels B, Verdries D, Everaert H, Christian N, De Ridder M, et al. Prospective, risk-adapted strategy of stereotactic body radiotherapy for early-stage non-small-cell lung cancer: results of a Phase II trial. Int J Radiat Oncol Biol Phys. 2011;80(5):1343-9.
36. Grutters JP, Kessels AG, Pijls-Johannesma M, De Ruysscher D, Joore MA, Lambin P. Comparison of the effectiveness of radiotherapy with photons, protons and carbon-ions for non-small cell lung cancer: a meta-analysis. Radiother Oncol. 2010;95(1):32-40.
37. Kopek N, Paludan M, Petersen J, Hansen AT, Grau C, Hoyer M. Co-morbidity index predicts for mortality after stereotactic body radiotherapy for medically inoperable early-stage nonsmall cell lung cancer. Radiother Oncol. 2009;93(3):402-7.
38. Guckenberger M, Allgauer M, Appold S, Dieckmann K, Ernst I, Ganswindt U, Holy R, Nestle U, Nevinny-Stickel M, Semrau S, et al. Safety and efficacy of stereotactic body radiotherapy for stage i non-small-cell lung cancer in routine clinical practice: a patterns-of-care and outcome analysis. J Thorac Oncol. 2013;8(8):1050-8.
39. NCCN Clinical Practice Guidelines in Oncology: non-small cell lung cancer Version 1. 2013. http://www.nccn.org/.
40. Vansteenkiste J, De Ruysscher D, Eberhardt WEE, Lim E, Senan S, Felip E, Peters S. Early and locally advanced non-small-cell lung cancer (NSCLC): ESMO Clinical Practice Guidelines for diagnosis, treatment and follow-up. Ann Oncol. 2013;24 Suppl 6:vi89-98.
41. Renaud S, Falcoz PE, Olland A, Massard G. Is radiofrequency ablation or stereotactic abla-

tive radiotherapy the best treatment for radically treatable primary lung cancer unfi t for surgery? Interact Cardiovasc Thorac Surg. 2013;16(1):68-73.

42. Crabtree T, Puri V, Timmerman R, Fernando H, Bradley J, Decker PA, Paulus R, Putnum Jr JB, Dupuy DE, Meyers B. Treatment of stage I lung cancer in high-risk and inoperable patients: comparison of prospective clinical trials using stereotactic body radiotherapy (RTOG 0236), sublobar resection (ACOSOG Z4032), and radiofrequency ablation (ACOSOG Z4033). J Thorac Cardiovasc Surg. 2013;145(3):692-9.

43. Ginsberg RJ, Rubinstein LV. Randomized trial of lobectomy versus limited resection for T1 N0 non-small cell lung cancer. Lung Cancer Study Group. Ann Thorac Surg. 1995;60(3): 615-22; discussion 622-3.

44. Whitson BA, Groth SS, Andrade RS, Maddaus MA, Habermann EB, D'Cunha J. Survival after lobectomy versus segmentectomy for stage I non-small cell lung cancer: a population-based analysis. Ann Thorac Surg. 2011;92(6):1943-50.

45. Tsutani Y, Miyata Y, Nakayama H, Okumura S, Adachi S, Yoshimura M, Okada M. Oncologic outcomes of segmentectomy compared with lobectomy for clinical stage IA lung adenocarcinoma: propensity score-matched analysis in a multicenter study. J Thorac Cardiovasc Surg. 2013;146(2):358-64.

46. Grills IS, Mangona VS, Welsh R, Chmielewski G, McInerney E, Martin S, Wloch J, Ye H, Kestin LL. Outcomes after stereotactic lung radiotherapy or wedge resection for stage I nonsmall-cell lung cancer. J Clin Oncol. 2010;28(6):928-35.

47. Puri V, Crabtree TD, Kymes S, Gregory M, Bell J, Bradley JD, Robinson C, Patterson GA, Kreisel D, Krupnick AS, et al. A comparison of surgical intervention and stereotactic body radiation therapy for stage I lung cancer in high-risk patients: a decision analysis. J Thorac Cardiovasc Surg. 2012;143(2):428-36.

48. Verstegen NE, Oosterhuis JW, Palma DA, Rodrigues G, Lagerwaard FJ, van der Elst A, Mollema R, van Tets WF, Warner A, Joosten JJ, et al. Stage I-II non-small-cell lung cancer treated using either stereotactic ablative radiotherapy (SABR) or lobectomy by video-assisted thoracoscopic surgery (VATS): outcomes of a propensity score-matched analysis. Ann Oncol. 2013;24(6):1543-8.

49. Oshiro Y, Aruga T, Tsuboi K, Marino K, Hara R, Sanayama Y, Itami J. Stereotactic body radiotherapy for lung tumors at the pulmonary hilum. Strahlenther Onkol. 2010;186(5):274-9.

50. Lagerwaard FJ, Verstegen NE, Haasbeek CJ, Slotman BJ, Paul MA, Smit EF, Senan S. Outcomes of stereotactic ablative radiotherapy in patients with potentially operable stage I non-small cell lung cancer. Int J Radiat Oncol Biol Phys. 2012;83(1):348-53.

51. Guckenberger M, Baier K, Polat B, Richter A, Krieger T, Wilbert J, Mueller G, Flentje M. Dose-response relationship for radiation-induced pneumonitis after pulmonary stereotactic body radiotherapy. Radiother Oncol. 2010;97(1):65-70.

52. Ong CL, Palma D, Verbakel WF, Slotman BJ, Senan S. Treatment of large stage I-II lung tumors using stereotactic body radiotherapy (SBRT): planning considerations and early toxic-

ity. Radiother Oncol. 2010;97(3):431-6.
53. Haasbeek C, Palma D, Lagerwaard FJ, Slotman BJ, Senan S. Stereotactic Body Radiotherapy (SBRT) outcomes in stage I lung cancer patients with severe chronic obstructive pulmonary disease (GOLD III-IV). Int J Radiat Oncol Biol Phys. 2010;78(3):S183.
54. Dunlap NE, Cai J, Biedermann GB, Yang W, Benedict SH, Sheng K, Schefter TE, Kavanagh BD, Larner JM. Chest wall volume receiving>30 Gy predicts risk of severe pain and/or rib fracture after lung stereotactic body radiotherapy. Int J Radiat Oncol Biol Phys. 2010;76(3):796-801.
55. Stephans KL, Djemil T, Tendulkar RD, Robinson CG, Reddy CA, Videtic GM. Prediction of chest wall toxicity from lung stereotactic body radiotherapy (SBRT). Int J Radiat Oncol Biol Phys. 2012;82(2):974-80.
56. Woody NM, Videtic GM, Stephans KL, Djemil T, Kim Y, Xia P. Predicting chest wall pain from lung stereotactic body radiotherapy for different fractionation schemes. Int J Radiat Oncol Biol Phys. 2012;83(1):427-34.
57. Forquer JA, Fakiris AJ, Timmerman RD, Lo SS, Perkins SM, McGarry RC, Johnstone PA. Brachial plexopathy from stereotactic body radiotherapy in early-stage NSCLC:doselimiting toxicity in apical tumor sites. Radiother Oncol. 2009;93(3):408-13.
58. van derVoort van Zyp NC, Prevost JB, van der Holt B, Braat C, van Klaveren RJ, Pattynama PM, Levendag PC, Nuyttens JJ. Quality of life after stereotactic radiotherapy for stage I nonsmall- cell lung cancer. Int J Radiat Oncol Biol Phys. 2010;77(1):31-7.
59. Widder J, Postmus D, Ubbels JF, Wiegman EM, Langendijk JA. Survival and quality of life after stereotactic or 3D-conformal radiotherapy for inoperable early-stage lung cancer. Int J Radiat Oncol Biol Phys. 2011;81(4):e291-7.
60. Lagerwaard FJ, Aaronson NK, Gundy CM, Haasbeek CJ, Slotman BJ, Senan S. Patientreported quality of life after stereotactic ablative radiotherapy for early-stage lung cancer. J Thorac Oncol. 2012;7(7):1148-54.
61. Bolliger CT, Wyser C, Roser H, Soler M, Perruchoud AP. Lung scanning and exercise testing for the prediction of postoperative performance in lung resection candidates at increased risk for complications. Chest. 1995;108(2):341-8.
62. Swensen SJ, Silverstein MD, Ilstrup DM, Schleck CD, Edell ES. The probability of malignancy in solitary pulmonary nodules. Application to small radiologically indeterminate nodules. Arch Intern Med. 1997;157(8):849-55.
63. Patel VK, Naik SK, Naidich DP, Travis WD, Weingarten JA, Lazzaro R, Gutterman DD, Wentowski C, Grosu HB, Raoof S. A practical algorithmic approach to the diagnosis and management of solitary pulmonary nodules:part 2:pretest probability and algorithm. Chest. 2013;143(3):840-6.
64. Patel VK, Naik SK, Naidich DP, Travis WD, Weingarten JA, Lazzaro R, Gutterman DD, Wentowski C, Grosu HB, Raoof S. A practical algorithmic approach to the diagnosis and management of solitary pulmonary nodules:part 1:radiologic characteristics and imaging mo-

dalities. Chest. 2013;143(3):825-39.

65. Verstegen NE, Lagerwaard FJ, Haasbeek CJ, Slotman BJ, Senan S. Outcomes of stereotactic ablative radiotherapy following a clinical diagnosis of stage I NSCLC: comparison with a contemporaneous cohort with pathologically proven disease. Radiother Oncol. 2011;101(2): 250-4.

66. Sawada S, Yamashita MK, Eisaku N, Naoyuki O, Isao S, Yoshihiko ST. Evaluation of resected tumors that were not diagnosed histologically but were suspected of lung cancer preoperatively. J Thorac Oncol. 2007;2(8):S422.

67. Murai T, Shibamoto Y, Baba F, Hashizume C, Mori Y, Ayakawa S, Kawai T, Takemoto S, Sugie C, Ogino H. Progression of non-small-cell lung cancer during the interval before stereotactic body radiotherapy. Int J Radiat Oncol Biol Phys. 2012;82(1):463-7.

68. Stiles BM, Servais EL, Lee PC, Port JL, Paul S, Altorki NK. Point: clinical stage IA non-small cell lung cancer determined by computed tomography and positron emission tomography is frequently not pathologic IA non-small cell lung cancer: the problem of understaging. J Thorac Cardiovasc Surg. 2009;137(1):13-9.

69. Park HK, Jeon K, Koh WJ, Suh GY, Kim H, Kwon OJ, Chung MP, Lee KS, Shim YM, Han J, et al. Occult nodal metastasis in patients with non-small cell lung cancer at clinical stage IA by PET/CT. Respirology. 2010;15(8):1179-84.

70. Senthi S, Lagerwaard FJ, Haasbeek CJ, Slotman BJ, Senan S. Patterns of disease recurrence after stereotactic ablative radiotherapy for early stage non-small-cell lung cancer: a retrospective analysis. Lancet Oncol. 2012;13(8):802-9.

71. Seppenwoolde Y, Shirato H, Kitamura K, Shimizu S, van Herk M, Lebesque JV, Miyasaka K. Precise and real-time measurement of 3D tumor motion in lung due to breathing and heartbeat, measured during radiotherapy. Int J Radiat Oncol Biol Phys. 2002;53(4):822-34.

72. Ford EC, Mageras GS, Yorke E, Ling CC. Respiration-correlated spiral CT: a method of measuring respiratory-induced anatomic motion for radiation treatment planning. Med Phys. 2003;30(1):88-97.

73. Low DA, Nystrom M, Kalinin E, Parikh P, Dempsey JF, Bradley JD, Mutic S, Wahab SH, Islam T, Christensen G, et al. A method for the reconstruction of four-dimensional synchronized CT scans acquired during free breathing. Med Phys. 2003;30(6):1254-63.

74. Fredberg Persson G, Eklund Nygaard D, Munck Af Rosenschold P, Richter Vogelius I, Josipovic M, Specht L, Korreman SS. Artifacts in conventional computed tomography (CT) and free breathing four-dimensional CT induce uncertainty in gross tumor volume determination. Int J Radiat Oncol Biol Phys. 2011;80(5):1573-80.

75. Hurkmans CW, van Lieshout M, Schuring D, van Heumen MJ, Cuijpers JP, Lagerwaard FJ, Widder J, van der Heide UA, Senan S. Quality assurance of 4D-CT scan techniques in multicenter phase III trial of surgery versus stereotactic radiotherapy (radiosurgery or surgery for operable early stage (stage 1A) non-small-cell lung cancer [ROSEL] study). Int J Radiat Oncol Biol Phys. 2010;80(3):918-27.

76. Wolthaus JW, Sonke JJ, van Herk M, Belderbos JS, Rossi MM, Lebesque JV, Damen EM. Comparison of different strategies to use four-dimensional computed tomography in treatment planning for lung cancer patients. Int J Radiat Oncol Biol Phys. 2008;70(4):1229-38.
77. Guckenberger M, Krieger T, Richter A, Baier K, Wilbert J, Sweeney RA, Flentje M. Potential of image-guidance, gating and real-time tracking to improve accuracy in pulmonary stereotactic body radiotherapy. Radiother Oncol. 2009;91(3):288-95.
78. Ong CL, Verbakel WF, Cuijpers JP, Slotman BJ, Lagerwaard FJ, Senan S. Stereotactic radiotherapy for peripheral lung tumors: a comparison of volumetric modulated arc therapy with 3 other delivery techniques. Radiother Oncol. 2010;97(3):437-42.
79. Hurkmans CW, Cuijpers JP, Lagerwaard FJ, Widder J, van der Heide UA, Schuring D, Senan S. Recommendations for implementing stereotactic radiotherapy in peripheral stage IA nonsmall cell lung cancer: report from the Quality Assurance Working Party of the randomised phase Ⅲ ROSEL study. Radiat Oncol. 2009;4:1.
80. Guckenberger M, Baier K, Guenther I, Richter A, Wilbert J, Sauer O, Vordermark D, Flentje M. Reliability of the bony anatomy in image-guided stereotactic radiotherapy of brain metastases. Int J Radiat Oncol Biol Phys. 2007;69(1):294-301.
81. Purdie TG, Bissonnette JP, Franks K, Bezjak A, Payne D, Sie F, Sharpe MB, Jaffray DA. Conebeam computed tomography for on-line image guidance of lung stereotactic radiotherapy: localization, verification, and intrafraction tumor position. Int J Radiat Oncol Biol Phys. 2007;68(1):243-52.
82. Guckenberger M, Klement RJ, Allgauer M, Appold S, Dieckmann K, Ernst I, Ganswindt U, Holy R, Nestle U, Nevinny-Stickel M, et al. Applicability of the linear-quadratic formalism for modeling local tumor control probability in high dose per fraction stereotactic body radiotherapy for early stage non-small cell lung cancer. Radiother Oncol. 2013;109(1):13-20.
83. Onishi H, Araki T, Shirato H, Nagata Y, Hiraoka M, Gomi K, Yamashita T, Niibe Y, Karasawa K, Hayakawa K, et al. Stereotactic hypofractionated high-dose irradiation for stage I nonsmall cell lung carcinoma: clinical outcomes in 245 subjects in a Japanese multiinstitutional study. Cancer. 2004;101(7):1623-31.
84. Wulf J, Baier K, Mueller G, Flentje MP. Dose-response in stereotactic irradiation of lung tumors. Radiother Oncol. 2005;77(1):83-7.
85. Guckenberger M, Wulf J, Mueller G, Krieger T, Baier K, Gabor M, Richter A, Wilbert J, Flentje M. Dose-response relationship for image-guided stereotactic body radiotherapy of pulmonary tumors: relevance of 4D dose calculation. Int J Radiat Oncol Biol Phys. 2009;74(1):47-54.
86. Grills IS, Hope AJ, Guckenberger M, Kestin LL, Werner-Wasik M, Yan D, Sonke JJ, Bissonnette JP, Wilbert J, Xiao Y, et al. A collaborative analysis of stereotactic lung radiotherapy outcomes for early-stage non-small-cell lung cancer using daily online cone-beam computed tomography image-guided radiotherapy. J Thorac Oncol. 2012;7(9):1382-93.
87. Onimaru R, Fujino M, Yamazaki K, Onodera Y, Taguchi H, Katoh N, Hommura F, Oizu-

mi S, Nishimura M, Shirato H. Steep dose-response relationship for stage I non-small-cell lung cancer using hypofractionated high-dose irradiation by real-time tumor-tracking radiotherapy. Int J Radiat Oncol Biol Phys. 2008;70(2):374-81.

88. Zhang J, Yang F, Li B, Li H, Liu J, Huang W, Wang D, Yi Y, Wang J. Which is the optimal biologically effective dose of stereotactic body radiotherapy for Stage I non-small-cell lung cancer? A meta-analysis. Int J Radiat Oncol Biol Phys. 2011;81(4):e305-16.

89. McGarry RC, Papiez L, Williams M, Whitford T, Timmerman RD. Stereotactic body radiation therapy of early-stage non-small-cell lung carcinoma: phase I study. Int J Radiat Oncol Biol Phys. 2005;63(4):1010-5.

90. Timmerman R, McGarry R, Yiannoutsos C, Papiez L, Tudor K, DeLuca J, Ewing M, Abdulrahman R, DesRosiers C, Williams M, et al. Excessive toxicity when treating central tumors in a phase II study of stereotactic body radiation therapy for medically inoperable early-stage lung cancer. J Clin Oncol. 2006;24(30):4833-9.

91. Song SY, Choi W, Shin SS, Lee SW, Ahn SD, Kim JH, Je HU, Park CI, Lee JS, Choi EK. Fractionated stereotactic body radiation therapy for medically inoperable stage I lung cancer adjacent to central large bronchus. Lung Cancer. 2009;66(1):89-93.

92. Senthi S, Haasbeek CJ, Slotman BJ, Senan S. Outcomes of stereotactic ablative radiotherapy for central lung tumours: a systematic review. Radiother Oncol. 2013;106(3):276-82.

93. Haasbeek CJ, Lagerwaard FJ, Slotman BJ, Senan S. Outcomes of stereotactic ablative radiotherapy for centrally located early-stage lung cancer. J Thorac Oncol. 2011;6(12):2036-43.

94. Guckenberger M, Heilman K, Wulf J, Mueller G, Beckmann G, Flentje M. Pulmonary injury and tumor response after stereotactic body radiotherapy (SBRT): results of a serial follow-up CT study. Radiother Oncol. 2007;85(3):435-42.

95. Huang K, Dahele M, Senan S, Guckenberger M, Rodrigues GB, Ward A, Boldt RG, Palma DA. Radiographic changes after lung stereotactic ablative radiotherapy (SABR) - Can we distinguish recurrence from fibrosis? A systematic review of the literature. Radiother Oncol. 2012;102(3):335-42.

96. Chen F, Matsuo Y, Yoshizawa A, Sato T, Sakai H, Bando T, Okubo K, Shibuya K, Date H. Salvage lung resection for non-small cell lung cancer after stereotactic body radiotherapy in initially operable patients. J Thorac Oncol. 2010;5(12):1999-2002.

97. Neri S, Takahashi Y, Terashi T, Hamakawa H, Tomii K, Katakami N, Kokubo M. Surgical treatment of local recurrence after stereotactic body radiotherapy for primary and metastatic lung cancers. J Thorac Oncol. 2010;5(12):2003-7.

98. Peulen H, Karlsson K, Lindberg K, Tullgren O, Baumann P, Lax I, Lewensohn R, Wersall P. Toxicity after reirradiation of pulmonary tumours with stereotactic body radiotherapy. Radiother Oncol. 2011;101(2):260-6.

第5章
早期非小细胞肺癌围术期个体化化疗

作者:Simona Carnio,Paolo Bironzo,Silvia Novello,Giorgio Vittorio Scagliotti
译者:何哲浩

简介

外科手术是早期非小细胞肺癌(NSCLC)的重要治疗方式,术后 pIA 期患者 5 年生存率为 77%,pⅢA 期患者 5 年生存率为 23%[32]。仅靠外科手术无法达到肿瘤的最佳治疗效果,围术期全身性辅助化疗可以提高生存率。临床试验和荟萃分析已经证明:以顺铂为基础的辅助化疗可以提高早期非小细胞肺癌患者的总体生存期(OS)[2,3,23,103],5 年生存率平均提高 5%,但根据肿瘤分期不同存在一定差异($P=0.04$;ⅠA 期 HR 1.40,95%CI 0.95~2.06;ⅠB 期 HR 0.93,95%CI 0.78~1.10;Ⅱ期 HR 0.83,95%CI 0.73~0.95;Ⅲ期 HR 0.83,95%CI 0.72~0.94)[69]。因此,有学者建议对于Ⅱ~Ⅲ期非小细胞肺癌切除患者进行辅助性化疗[63,70,99,100]。

有研究显示,手术根治性切除的ⅠB 和Ⅱ期非小细胞肺癌复发率约为 50%,中位复发时间约为 1 年[48],复发与病理分期明显相关,ⅠA 期患者的复发率明显较少。根据以往的临床生存数据,我们需考虑两点:①20%~30%的Ⅰ期患者的预后较差,因此这部分患者可能从辅助性化疗中获益,而约 40%的Ⅱ期患者可通过单纯手术就可获得较好的预后,并不能从全身化疗中获益;② ⅢA 期肺癌行根治性手术或放疗的患者,尽管被归为同一分期,但存在明显的差异,如淋巴结转移数量等均存在差异。

20 世纪 90 年代两个随机试验表明诱导化疗可提高临床ⅢA 期(根据 1997 年之前的 TNM 分期)[79,80]的患者的生存率。而早期非小细胞肺癌患者是否需要行新辅助化疗目前仍在进行广泛的探讨和研究[20,26,30,71,82]。

多数关于新辅助化疗的临床Ⅲ期试验进行晚于术后辅助化疗的临床试验,当时已经确定术后辅助化疗可提高Ⅱ期和ⅢA 患者的预后,因此对于上述分期的根治性切除的患者不行术后辅助化疗,而行新辅助化疗,似乎不符合伦理。一项临床Ⅲ期试验认为新辅助化疗可以显著提高ⅡB~ⅢA 期肺癌患者的生存(3 年 PFS:36.1% vs 55.4%;$P=0.002$)[82],而另两个类似研究则认为新辅助化疗并不能使患者获益[26,71]。另有一项研究则发现相较于进展期肺癌，早期肺癌行新辅助化疗获益更大[20]。

2006年一项Meta分析评价了新辅助化疗在治疗早期肺癌的作用[9]，并在之后再次加入一项来自欧洲的临床试验进行汇总更新[30]。初期的Meta分析纳入了7项发表于1990~2005年间的随机试验，共包含988名患者，结果发现术前化疗提高了患者的生存率，HR为0.82(95%CI 0.69~0.97)，5年生存率提高了6%。纳入新的研究后，该Meta分析的结果发生了改变，HR为0.87(95% CI 0.76~1.01)，不存在显著性生存差异。之后Meta分析纳入另两项临床试验（NATCH和CHEST）的结果出来之后，该研究共纳入10项临床试验，共2200例患者，结果显示术前新辅助化疗可提高患者生存，HR为0.89(95% CI 0.81~0.98, $P=0.02$)。该Meta分析结果提示术前化疗获益量与术后辅助化疗相似。

关于术前新辅助化疗与术后辅助化疗孰优孰劣，有meta分析纳入32项临床试验，纳入患者均为手术可切除患者，结果显示，两种化疗方式治疗肺癌的总体生存，无疾病生存均无显著性差异[55]。近期法国的研究确认对于Ⅰ~Ⅱ期患者，术前化疗和术后辅助化疗患者的生存并不存在显著性差异[102]。

制定早期肺癌患者的个体化围术期全身治疗方案的目的是优化收益毒性比(toxicity ratio optimization)，通俗地讲，即使低复发风险患者避免行全身性治疗，而使高复发风险患者（包括Ⅰ期高复发风险患者）接受全身性治疗。

非小细胞肺癌主要预后因素为分期、性别、年龄以及体力状态评分[34,51,94]，而个体化的治疗则需要准确了解肺癌的分子基因特征。有研究评估了一系列分子标记物对于肺癌患者预后的预测机制，结果显示部分分子标记物对于患者生存预后或复发转移有一定的预测价值。其中一项最大的回顾性研究纳入了515例行手术切除的Ⅰ期非小细胞肺癌患者，结果表明多种生物分子标记物，包括表皮生长因子受体(EGFR)、HER2/neu、bcl-2、p53以及血管生成标记物等与患者生存间无显著相关性[68]。

最近，人类基因组项目批准了基因组测序的临床应用及开发，包括全面分析基因表达、拷贝数变异、DNA甲基化、microRNA、基因签名等变异情况，评估上述分子指标在早期肺癌的预后预测价值。上述生物标记物不久就可以用于指导个体化治疗。本章将回顾目前的临床研究结果，评述生物标记物在肺癌个体化治疗中的价值。

基因组特性：基因签名的作用

肿瘤生长包含正常创伤修复的众多方面。一个创伤反应(WR)包含512个基因，在多种肿瘤中（例如乳腺癌和肺癌），上述基因重新启动表达[14]。在早期乳腺癌和肺腺癌中，WR特征可预测肿瘤预后及转移。侵袭性基因签名(IGS)包括186个基因，是乳腺癌和其他肿瘤（包括肺癌）的预后预测因子。IGS包括NF-κB通路、

RAS-MAPK通路以及基因表达表观控制所涉及的基因，IGS仅有6个与WR签名重叠[56]。

肺癌基因表达谱与腺癌的复发密切相关，而与鳞状细胞癌复发的相关性稍弱[112]。这些结果由构成多种不同平台的微阵技术获得。对来源于7个微阵研究的数据组进行meta分析，进而识别一个由64个基因构成的表达签名，该签名可以预测患者生存，准确度高达85%[60]。

虽然在一个或者多个独立患者群体中，这些签名大多数已经得以验证，但是基因组间微阵数据集重叠几率极小，分析其原因可能为样本收集方法、处理方案、单中心研究对象、小样本量以及不同微阵平台的特性。为了弥补上述不足，进行了大样本的多中心联合研究，纳入肺腺癌患者以评估部分基因联合或不联合相关临床指标（分期、性别和年龄）是否能够用于预测肺腺癌患者的生存状况，结果发现相关风险评分与患者生存密切相关，特别是临床和分子基因指标能更好地评估早期肺癌患者预后[87]。

最近研究人员开发了一项经验模型以评估肺癌特异性生物标记物的预测价值，但并不是用于预测患者的生存时间，有假说认为决定肿瘤细胞命运的是两组功能失衡的基因（阴和阳），而非单个基因，阴和阳基因最终决定患者的生存时间。对比正常肺组织样本和肺癌组织样本，进而挑选出可能的阴和阳基因，该模型在四个独立肺癌数据集中测试，结果显示该模型可以对患者进行准确分层，分为高风险和低风险生存组，并且预测Ⅱ期和Ⅲ期的化疗效果[105]。

10年前加拿大有学者通过对181例行辅助化疗患者肿瘤标本的mRNA测定，筛选出15种基因用于区分非小细胞肺癌，将肺癌患者区分成高风险组与低风险组，研究者将该15种基因于另181例早期肺癌患者进行验证，该181例患者包含不同类型的非小细胞肺癌病理学类型，结果发现，高风险组与低风险组总体生存期（OS）存在显著差别（$HR=1.92, P=0.012$）。亚组分析显示，该模型成功预测了127名Ⅰ期患者及其亚组，48例ⅠA期患者的生存率（$HR=5.61, P=0.014$）。该基因签名对恶性腺瘤和鳞状细胞癌均适用（$HR=1.76, P=0.058$；$HR=4.19$，$P=0.045$）[21]。

在另外一个研究中，使用挑选出的两个基因（TTF1和NKX2-8）对患者进行分层，进而对比患者相关的预后信息，结果发现与TTF1和NKX2-8的超表达与顺铂、紫杉烷、吉西他滨及长春瑞滨的耐药相关，但是同培美曲塞的治疗反应呈正相关[39]。

miRNAs可调控转基因转录后的过程，因此可作为肿瘤转移过程的上游调控因子。在非小细胞肺癌中，miRNAs的组织表达与预后具有相关性[107]。研究显示miR-486、miR30d、miR-1和miR-499的表达量可作为Ⅰ～ⅢA期非小细胞肺癌的独立预测因子，与生存率相关[40]。已有研究评估在早期非小细胞肺癌患者血清中

miRNA 的预后重要性：miR-660、miR-140-5p、miR-451、miR-28-3p、miR-30c 和 mi-92a 是常见的常见的 miRNA。有研究构建了一组 miRNA 以探讨 miRNA 表达的作用并且明确对预后的影响，同时用于诊断非小细胞肺癌时的价值[8]。最近还有研究按照特定 miRNAs 的表达谱，将早期非小细胞肺癌患者进行分组，并检测其与预后的相关性[15,37,91]。在另一项研究中，以完全切除的合并 EGFR 突变非小细胞肺癌患者为对象，评估 miRNAs 表达谱与生存期、疾病进展及对吉非替尼治疗反应之间的关联，结果发现 miR-21 和 mi10b 与疾病进展、生存期及对吉非替尼的辅助治疗的反应有关[88]。

免疫靶点

近年来，临床试验表明免疫治疗对于包括肺癌在内的部分实体瘤有一定效果[38,46]。START 为一项纳入 1500 例 III 期非小细胞肺癌患者随机安慰剂对照 III 期试验，放化初始治疗部分缓解或稳定的患者随机接受 tecemotide（免疫药物）或者安慰剂，主要研究终点为总体生存期，结果发现 tecemotide 免疫治疗并不能提高患者总体生存，但亚组分析显示，806 名接受 tecemotide 联合放化治疗 III 期患者中位生存时间增加 10.2 个月（$HR=0.78; 95\%CI: 0.64\sim0.95; P=0.016$）[10]。

MAGE-A3 为肿瘤特异性抗原，因其在多种实体肿瘤中表达，而正常组织中无表达，因此是免疫治疗的理想靶点。MAGE-A3 在 35% 可切除非小细胞肺癌患者中表达。一项临床 II 期试验纳入 182 例完全切除 MAGE-A3 阳性 I B-II 期非小细胞肺癌，以无疾病生存期（DFI）为主要研究终点，结果显示，MAG3-A3 免疫治疗组患者术后 44 月的复发率为 35%，而安慰剂组则为 43%，两组患者在多项研究指标间均无明显区别，无疾病生存期（$HR=0.75, 95\%CI: 0.46\sim1.23; P=0.254$），无病生存率（DFS）（$HR=0.76; 95\%CI: 0.48\sim1.21; P=0.248$）或者总体生存期（$HR=0.81; 95\%CI: 0.47\sim1.40; P=0.454$），术后 70 个月的随访数据也并未发现明显的差异。MAGE-A3 治疗患者未出现显著毒副反应[99,100]。

通过微阵检测使用 MAGE-A3 抗原特异性免疫治疗的黑色素瘤标本，并经 qRT-PCR 验证，发现一种基因签名与临床预后相关，可预测患者总体生存期。该基因签名也被用于检测经 MAGE-A3 抗原特异性免疫治疗 I B~II 期肺癌切除标本中，结果发现该基因签名与无疾病生存期（DFI）相关（$HR=0.42; 95\%CI: 0.17\sim1.03; P=0.06$）。尽管所有患者，包含合并或不合并该基因签名的患者，MAGE-A3 免疫治疗并不能提高总生存期，但存在阳性基因签名的患者，MAGE-A3 免疫治疗可能使患者获益（$HR=0.63; 95\%CI: 0.22\sim1.78; P=0.38$）[97]。

另有一项临床 III 期随机双盲对照试验（MAGRIT），将 MAG3-A3 免疫用于非小细胞肺癌的辅助治疗（图 5.1），该研究共计划纳入超过 9300 例 I~IIIA 期肺癌手术切除患者，筛选出 MAGE-A3 表达阳性患者，再根据患者术后是否接受辅助性

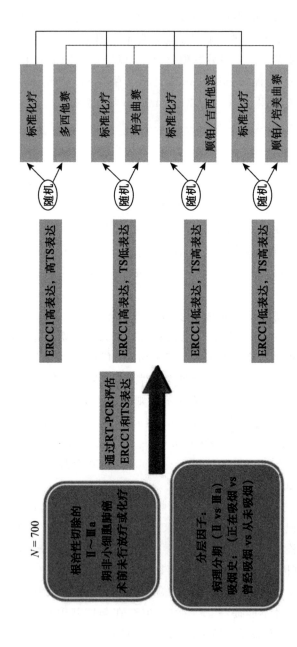

图5.1 ITACA（国际个体化辅助化疗试验），Ⅲ期多中心临床随机对照研究，根治性切除Ⅱ–Ⅲa期非小细胞肺癌术后基于基因表达的个体化方案辅助化疗与标准辅助化疗的对照研究

化疗进行分层后随机分配到 MAGE-A3 治疗组或安慰剂对照组,该研究目前已招募 2270 例患者,结果待近期公布。

EGFR 靶向药物在早期非小细胞肺癌围术期的应用

目前,Ⅳ期 EFFR 突变患者的标准治疗是 EGFR 酪氨酸激酶抑制剂(TKI),其在早期肺癌围术期应用也引起了极大的关注,但目前尚未形成定论。纪念斯隆凯特林癌症中心(MSKCC)开展了一项回顾性研究,纳入 167 例Ⅰ～Ⅲ期 EGFR 突变患者,56 例术前或术后使用 EGFR-TKI 治疗,另 111 例则未使用 EGFR-TKI 治疗,结果发现 EGFR-TKI 可使早期肺癌患者获益,虽然两组患者总体生存率相似(≥90),但治疗组患者 2 年无疾病生存率为 89%,而对照组患者则为 72%,差异具有显著性($P=0.06$)[42]。纪念斯隆凯特林癌症中心的另一个回顾性研究发现,辅助 EGFR-TKI 治疗不能增加治愈率,但可推迟复发时间[67]。

由于吉非替尼辅助治疗肺癌的研究多为回顾性研究或前瞻性研究中的亚组分析,因此将吉非替尼作为辅助性治疗肺癌方法目前尚未形成定论[33,47]。来自中国的一项小样本临床试验,纳入 60 例ⅢA-N2 期合并敏感型 EGFR 突变的手术切除治疗患者,术后接受 4 个疗程的辅助性卡铂和培美曲塞联合化疗,之后一组患者接受 6 个月的吉非替尼治疗(PC-G 组),另一组则未接受其他治疗(PC 组),结果发现同 PC 组相比,其中位无疾病生存期明显提高(39.8vs 27.0月,$P=0.014$,HR=0.37),但是 OS 并没有明显差异(41.6月 vs 32.6月,$P=0.066$)。PC-G 组中,两年 PFS 和 OS 比率分别为 78.9%和 92.4%,PC 组则分别为 54.2%和 77.4%[101]。RADIANT 试验旨在研究厄洛替尼辅助治疗肺癌的临床效果(图 5.2),目前已完成患者招募工作[64]。该Ⅲ期临床试验纳入 945 例Ⅰ～ⅢA 期肺癌,经免疫组化确认肿瘤组织存在 EGFR 表达或经荧光原位免疫杂交技术确认存在 EGFR 基因拷贝数增加,经手术切除和术后辅助化疗,以 2∶1 的比例将患者分配到厄洛替尼治疗组或安慰剂对照组,治疗时间共 2 年,初步结果即将公布。另有一项相关研究也正在进行中,即 SELECTⅡ期试验[64],纳入了 36 例ⅠA～ⅢA 期合并 EGFR 突变的手术切除患者,在术后辅助标准放疗或化疗结束后使用 150mg/d 的厄洛替尼治疗 2 年,结果 10 例患者因药物副反应需减少厄洛替尼剂量,随访后发现,2 年无疾病生存率为 94%(95% CI80%,99%),10 例患者出现肿瘤复发,但大部分患者对后续的 EGFR-TKI 治疗仍有一定效果[65]。随后该试验扩大了样本量,共纳入 100 例患者,预计结果将在近内公布(图 5.3)。另有一些关于使用新一代或老一代 EGFR-TKI 药物术前或术后辅助治疗早期 EGFR 突变肺癌的研究,如 ALCHEMIST 试验拟研究厄洛替尼和 EML4-ALK 融合靶向药物克唑替尼治疗合并相关突变肺癌的临床效果,该试验今后也将纳入一些新的分子靶点相关药物。

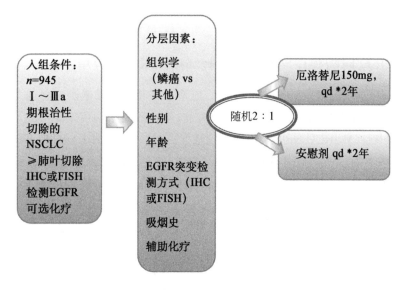

图5.2 RADIANT 研究[RADIANT(Randomized Double-Blind Trial in Adjuvant NSCLC with Tarceva) 特罗凯辅助治疗非小细胞肺癌的随机对照双盲研究]

[EGFR(epidermal growth factor receptor) 表皮生长因子受体，FISH (fluorescence in situ hybridization) 荧光原位杂交技术，IHC(immunohisto-chemistry) 免疫组化]

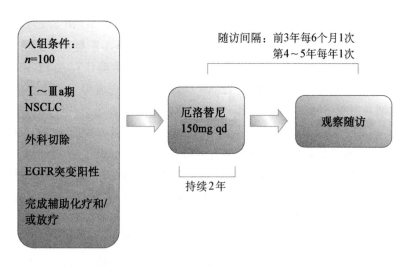

图5.3 SELECT 研究

化疗相关基因

核苷酸切除修复途径相关蛋白可修复铂类药物造成的细胞 DNA 损伤,其中最重要的是切除修复交叉互补基因(ERCC)家族,可通过核苷酸切除修复机制减少 DNA 损伤[98]。目前可使用免疫组化、qRT-PCR、AQUA 等多种方法检测 ERCC1 基因活性,由于缺乏对比数据,因此截至目前尚未明确上述哪一种检测方法更好[17,22]。ERCC1 的预后价值最先在行铂类药物化疗的晚期肺癌患者评估[13,58]。而后,有研究检测了行手术切除的 I A～Ⅲ B 期肺癌标本中的 ERCC1 信使 RNA(mRNA)表达量,结果发现 mRNA 高表达患者中位总生存期为 94.6 个月(>50 无单位比率),而低表达的患者中位生存期明显偏低,仅为 35.5 个月($P=0.01$),因此该 mRNA 可以作为独立危险因素预测患者预后[92]。另有一项关于肺癌辅助化疗的研究,使用免疫组化检测了 761 例肺癌 ERCC1 表达,结果发现,ERCC1 不表达或低表达的患者行铂类药物为基础的化疗效果明显较好($P=0.009$),患者的无疾病生存期(DFS)和总生存期(OS)明显高于 ERCC1 表达阳性的患者(死亡相关 HR,0.65;95% CI,0.50～0.86;$P=0.002$)。在对照组中,患者未行铂类药物化疗,发现 ERCC1 表达阳性患者预后明显较好,5 年总生存率明显高于 ERCC1 表达阴性患者(HR,0.66;95% CI,0.49～0.90;$P=0.009$)[1,2]。也有研究使用 AQUA 检测 ERCC1 水平,结果同上类似,发现 ERCC1 高分值患者预后好于低评分患者,但由于样本量等原因,差异尚缺乏显著性(HR=0.77,$P=0.10$)[6]。

Muts 同源蛋白 2(MSH2)是错配修复通路的一个主要修复成分,ERCC1 和 MSH2 均阴性检测可增加预后评估的价值,有研究发现,ERCC1、MSH2 双阴性肿瘤接受铂类药物化疗获益更加明显[44]。但该研究结果在近期的一项大样本研究中并未得到相似结果,这可能是由于 ERCC1 存在四种亚型,而仅其中一种亚型参与 DNA 切除修复和铂类药物耐药机制,但目前使用的单克隆抗体无法区分上述四种亚型[28],目前 ERCC1 不作为辅助化疗的常规检测项目。

ERCC1 的研究目前多限于术后辅助化疗,而在术前新辅助化疗中,研究甚少。有一项研究认为 ERCC1 可预测以铂类药物为基础的术前新辅助化疗肺癌患者的预后($P \leqslant 0.05$)[45]。另有一项研究发现,ERCC1 mRNA 表达量与肿瘤行铂类药物化疗的客观缓解率(OR)相关,但与局部或远处转移无关[61]。还有一项相关研究发现 ERCC1 表达量与新辅助化疗患者的预后明显相关,该研究共纳入 113 例老年非小细胞肺癌患者,ERCC1 表达阴性的患者中位生存期为 53 个月,明显高于 ERCC1 表达阳性患者 37 个月的中位生存期,因此 ERCC1 可作为患者预后的独立预测因子($P<0.05$),该研究同时发现新辅助化疗可诱导肿瘤 ERCC1 表达,而 ERCC1 高表达患者行铂类药物化疗客观缓解率明显偏低[53]。

乳腺癌易感基因 1(BRCA1)同核苷酸切除修复(NER)参与基因转录,可调控紫杉醇和长春花碱等抗微管化疗药物诱导的凋亡，介导对铂类等 DNA 损伤药物的耐药[19]。有研究检测了行初始化疗的早期非小细胞肺癌患者的 BRCA1 mRNA 表达量，发现该 mRNA 高表达患者生存明显较差，mRNA 表达量可以作为预测患者生存的独立危险因子[76]。

最近，有 Meta 分析研究了 BRCA1 的预后预测价值，结果发现，对于铂类药物化疗的患者，BRCA1 高表达患者客观缓解率（HR=1.70）、总生存期（HR 1.58）、无事件生存（HR 2.39）均明显劣于 BRCA1 低表达或不表达的患者，而对于紫杉醇化疗的患者，BRCA1 高表达患者则客观缓解率明显更高（HR 0.41），但由于纳入的研究缺乏总生存期、无事件生存期等相关数据，该 Meta 分析未进一步评估这两项指标。有研究使用 BRCA1 表达量来指导化疗方案的选择，如来自西班牙的一项的临床 Ⅱ 期试验，纳入了行术后辅助化疗的完全切除 Ⅱ～ⅢA 期肺癌患者，BRCA1 mRNA 高表达量接受多西他赛治疗，而低表达患者则接受铂类药物化疗，结果发现两组患者总生存期无明显差异[16]。

PAP80 也是一种 DNA 修复蛋白，与 BRCA1 表达量同患者无进展生存期，总体生存期等明显相关，可作为预测总生存期的独立预测因子[75]。PAP80 在早期肺癌患者中的预后预测、治疗选择中的价值仍需要评估，西班牙的临床 Ⅲ 期相关研究已开始开展，该研究拟比较术后辅助标准化疗方案与 RAP80，BRCA1 指导选择化疗方案的生存差别，将于不久公布。

核糖核苷酸还原酶 M1(RRM1) 可作为核糖核苷酸还原酶的关键组分催化还原核糖核苷二磷酸为相应的脱氧核糖核苷酸[77]。目前有研究发现 RRM1 可以预测肿瘤对吉西他滨和铂类药物等的治疗效果[25]。曾有数项研究评估了 RRM 对于早期肺癌患者的预后预测价值[111]，以及肺癌对吉西他滨联合顺铂化疗治疗效果的预测价值[5,7]，有研究发现 RRM1 表达同肿瘤治疗缓解呈逆相关，但未发现与生存之间的相关性[74]。近期回顾性研究发现 ERCC1 和 RRM1 表达量与术后行辅助化疗或未行辅助化疗的完全切除肺癌患者的肿瘤复发率和总体生存期之间无显著相关性[95]。

ERCC1 表达与 RRM1 和 BRCA1 水平密切相关[77,78,109]，研究发现 70%～80% 的患者上述三种蛋白表达存在异质性[29]。

胸苷酸合成酶（TS）将四氢叶酸氧化为二氢叶酸，可以加速脱氧尿苷酸（dUMP）脱氧胸苷一磷酸（TMP），研究发现，TS 高表达肿瘤对 5-FU 耐药性先关[43,52,90]，通过对晚期肺癌患者的研究发现，TS 蛋白和 mRNA 低表达的非鳞癌患者对培美曲塞的治疗反应较好，预后也较好，在鳞癌或小细胞肺癌患者中，TS 蛋白和 mRNA 高表达的缓和治疗反应较差[12,13,62,81]。

TS 对于早期手术切除的肺癌患者拟行初始化疗，也有一定的指导价值，有研究发现该 mRNA 高表达，则患者的无疾病生存期较短，但该蛋白表达量则未发现明确意义,而另一项研究结果则发现 TS 蛋白也有预测价值,通过 AQUA 检测 TS 蛋白表达,发现 TS 蛋白高表达的患者预后相对较好[89,110]。

目前仅有少量前瞻性临床研究正在开展,拟确定上述相关基因在指导化疗方案选择中的价值。国际定向辅助化疗(ITACA)研究是其中一个主要代表性研究(图 5.3),该研究拟比较完整切除 Ⅱ～ⅢA 期非小细胞肺癌患者行标准化疗和 ERCC1 和 TS 检测评估指导化疗的优劣,该研究已基本完成 700 多例患者的招募和随机分配工作[66]。

其他生物标记物

关于 K-ras 突变对于早期肺癌的预后预测价值目前尚有争论,仅少数研究认为早期非小细胞肺癌患者的 K-ras 突变可能同不良预后有关[50],但多数其他研究并未发现类似结果,甚至是相反的结果[11,96]。来自意大利的一项研究,共有 227 例非鳞癌患者,单因素分析发现 K-ras 突变患者生存期明显较短,但多因素分析则无统计学差异[83]。

TP53 基因突变在肺癌发生发展中发挥着重要作用,但其蛋白 P53 检测的敏感性,以及通过免疫组化检测 P53 表达量对于肺癌预后的评估价值目前尚未完全明确,仅有少数研究发现 P53 蛋白表达可作为辅助化疗的效果独立预测因子,但 TP53 基因则缺乏相关意义[84]。

βTubⅢ 表达可预测晚期非小细胞肺癌患者对于抗微管化疗药物的治疗反应[24,85]。βTubⅢ 高表达提示患者是无复发生存期较短[86]。回顾性研究也证明了该蛋白对于辅助或新辅助化疗的预后预测价值[72,108]。

P27^{kip1} 是细胞周期依赖性激酶抑制剂,其上调可接到肿瘤对于铂类药物治疗耐药,P27^{kip1} 蛋白低表达患者预后较好[27,73]。通过对 Ⅲ 期手术切除肺癌患者研究发现,细胞周期蛋白 D2 同患者无复发生存相关[49]。而早期非小细胞肺癌中,通过 FISH 或免疫组化技术检测胰岛素的生长因子受体(IGR1R)与 EGFR 阳性的患者其无疾病生存期明显较短($P=0.05$)[59]。而对于手术切除 Ⅰ～Ⅲ 期初始化疗的非小细胞肺癌患者,肝细胞生长因子受体(c-MET)主可作为鳞癌患者的独立预后不良预测因子[31]。HER2 在 ⅠB～ⅡA 期肺癌中的表达提示预后较差[104]。CXCR7 在 Ⅰ 期肺癌中的表达提示肿瘤转移可能性大,预后较差[41],而 CXCR4 也对患者预后评估有一定价值[93]。在 Ⅰ 期肺癌中发现了一组甲基化状态可变基因与患者预后相关[15,87]。BRCA1 甲基化也可能作为根治性切除 Ⅰ 期非小细胞肺癌术后的预后预测因子[36]。而血管内皮生长因子过表达提示早期肺癌患者进展,预后较差[4,54]。

结论

早期肺癌围术期个体化治疗是临床研究热点,目前研究尚不充分,已有的研究结果存在争议,多为回顾性研究,且分子检测方法存在差异,导致研究之间的异质性明显。目前只能基于患者的临床特征、组织病理学特征和肿瘤分期来实现围术期全身治疗的个体化,正在进行的随机临床试验的结果可以在今后为实现更精确的个体化治疗提供指导性建议。

参考文献

1. Arriagada R, Dunant A, Pignon JP, et al. Long term results of the international adjuvant lung cancer trial evaluating adjuvant cisplatin-based chemotherapy in resected lung cancer. J Clin Oncol. 2010;28:35-42.

2. Arriagada R, Auperin A, Burdett S, et al.; NSCLC Meta-analyses Collaborative Group. Adjuvant chemotherapy, with or without postoperative radiotherapy, in operable non- small cell lung cancer: two meta-analyses of individual patient data. Lancet. 2010;375(9722):1267-77.

3. Arriagada R, Bergman B, Dunant A, et al.; International Adjuvant Lung Cancer Trial Collaborative Group. Cisplatin-based adjuvant chemotherapy in patients with completely resected non-small-cell lung cancer. N Engl J Med. 2004;350(4):351-60.

4. Baillie R, Carlile J, Pendleton N, et al. Prognostic value of vascularity and vascular endothelial growth factor expression in non small cell lung cancer. J Clin Pathol. 2001;54:116-20.

5. Bepler G, Kusmartseva I, Sharma S, et al. RRM1 modulated in vitro and in vivo efficacy of gemcitabine and platinum in non-small-cell lung cancer. J Clin Oncol. 2006;24:4731-7.

6. Bepler G, Olaussen KA, Vataire AL, et al. ERCC1 and RRM1 in the international adjuvant lung trial by automated quantitative in situ analysis. Am J Pathol. 2011;178:69-78.

7. Bepler G, Sommers KE, Cantor A, et al. Clinical efficacy and predictive molecular markers of neoadjuvant gemcitabine and pemetrexed in resectable non-small cell lung cancer. J Thorac Oncol. 2008;3:1112-8.

8. Boeri M, Verri C, Conte D, et al. MicroRNA signatures in tissues and plasma predict development and prognosis of computed tomography detected lung cancer. Proc Natl Acad Sci U S A. 2011;108:3713-8.

9. Burdett S, Stewart L, Rydzewska L. A systematic review and meta-analysis of the literature: chemotherapy and surgery versus surgery alone in non-small cell lung cancer. J Thorac Oncol. 2006;1:611-21.

10. Butts CA, Socinski M, Mitchell P, et al. START: A phase Ⅲ study of L-BLP25 cancer immu-notherapy for unresectable stage Ⅲ non-small cell lung cancer. J Clin Oncol. 2013;31(No 15s): abstr 7500, 458s.

11. Capelletti M, Wang XF, Gu L, et al. Impact of KRAS mutations on adjuvant carboplatin/paclitaxel in surgically resected stage IB NSCLC: CALGB 9633. J Clin Oncol. 2010;28(No 15s): abstr 7008, 516s.

12. Ceppi P, Volante M, Saviozzi S, et al. Squamous cell carcinoma of the lung compared with other histotypes shows higher messenger RNA and protein levels for thymidylate synthase.

Cancer. 2006;107:1589-96.
13. Ceppi P, Volante M, Novello S, et al. ERCC1 and RRM1 gene expressions but not EGFR are predictive of shorter survival in advanced non-small cell lung cancer treated with cisplatin and gemcitabine. Ann Oncol. 2006;17(12):1818-25.
14. Chen Q, Si Q, Xiao S, et al. Prognostic significance of serum miR-17-5p in lung cancer.Med Oncol. 2013;30:353.
15. Cobo M, Massuti B, Moran T, et al. Spanish customized adjuvant trial (SCAT) based on BRCA1 mRNA levels. J Clin Oncol. 2008;26(No 15 Suppl): abstract 7533, 405s.
16. De Castro Jr G, Pasini FS, Siqueira SA, et al. ERCC1 protein, mRNA expression and T19007C polymorphism as prognostic markers in head and neck squamous cell carcinoma patients treated with surgery and adjuvant cisplatin-based chemoradiation. Oncol Rep. 2011;25: 693-9.
17. De Fraipont F, Levallet G, Creveuil C, et al. An apoptosis methylation prognostic signature for early lung cancer in the IFCT-0002 trial. Clin Cancer Res. 2012;18(10):2976-86.
18. Deng CX. BRCA1: cell cycle checkpoint, genetic instability, DNA damage response and cancer evolution. Nucleic Acids Res. 2006;34:1416-26.
19. Depierre A, Milleron B, Moro-Sibilot D, et al. Preoperative chemotherapy followed by surgery compared with primary surgery in resectable stage I (except T1N0), II, and Ⅲa non-small-cell lung cancer. J Clin Oncol. 2002;20:247-53.
20. Der SD, Sykes J, Pintilie M, et al. Validation of a histology-independent prognostic gene signature for early-stage, non-small-cell lung cancer including stage IA patients. J Thorac Oncol. 2014;9(1):59-64.
21. Doll CM, Prystajecky M, Eliasziw M, et al. Low ERCC1 mRNA and protein expression are associated with worse survival in cervical cancer patients treated with radiation alone. Radiother Oncol. 2010;97:352-9.
22. Douillard JY, Rosell R, De Lena M, et al. Adjuvant vinorelbine plus cisplatin versus observation in patients with completely resected stage IB-ⅢA non-small-cell lung cancer (Adjuvant Navelbine International Trialist Association [ANITA]): a randomized controlled trial. Lancet Oncol. 2006;7(9):719-27.
23. Dumontet C, Isaac S, Souquet PJ, et al. Expression of class Ⅲ beta tubulin in non-small cell lung cancer is correlated with resistance to taxane chemotherapy. Bull Cancer. 2005;92:E25-30.
24. Fairman JW, Wijerathna SR, Ahmad MF, et al. Structural basis for allosteric regulation of human ribonucleotide reductase by nucleotide-induced oligomerization. Nat Struct Mol Biol. 2011;18:316-22.
25. Felip E, Rosell R, Maestre JA, et al. Preoperative chemotherapy plus surgery versus surgery plus adjuvant chemotherapy versus surgery alone in early-stage non-small-cell lung cancer. J Clin Oncol. 2010;28:3138-45.
26. Filipits M, Pirker R, Dunant A, et al. Cell cycle regulators and outcome of adjuvant cispla-

tin- based chemotherapy in completely resected non-small-cell lung cancer: the International Adjuvant Lung Cancer Trial Biologic Program. J Clin Oncol. 2007;25:2735-40.
27. Friboulet L, Olaussen KA, et al. ERCC1 isoform expression and DNA repair in non-small-cell lung cancer. N Engl J Med. 2013;368:1101-10.
28. Gandara DR, Grimminger PP, Mack PC, et al. Histology- and gender-related associations of ERCC1, RRM1, and TS biomarkers in 1,802 patients with NSCLC: implications for therapy. J Clin Oncol. 2010;28(No 15s): abstr 7513, 541s.
29. Gilligan D, Nicolson M, Smith I, et al. Preoperative chemotherapy in patients with resectable non-small cell lung cancer: results of the MRC LU22/NVALT 2/EORTC 08012 multicentre randomized trial and update of systematic review. Lancet. 2007;369:1929-37.
30. Go H, Jeon YK, Park HJ,et al. High MET gene copy number leads to shorter survival in patients with non-small cell lung cancer. J Thorac Oncol. 2010;5:305-13.
31. Goldstraw P, Crowley J, Chansky K, et al. The IASLC Lung Cancer Staging Project: proposals for the revision of the TNM stage groupings in the forthcoming (seventh) edition of the TNM Classification of malignant tumours. J Thorac Oncol. 2007;2(8):706-14.
32. Goss GD, O'Callaghan C, Lorimer I, et al. Gefitinib versus placebo in completely resected non- small-cell lung cancer: results of the NCIC CTG BR19 Study. J Clin Oncol. 2013;31:3320-6.
33. Graziano SL. Non-small cell lung cancer: clinical value of new biological predictors. Lung Cancer. 1997;17:S37-58.
34. Greenblatt MS, Bennett WP, Hollstein M, et al. Mutations in the P53 tumor suppressor gene: clues to cancer etiology and molecular pathogenesis. Cancer Res. 1994;54(4855):4878.
35. Harada H, Miyamoto K, Yamashita Y, et al. Methylation of breast cancer susceptibility gene 1 (BRCA1) predicts recurrence in patients with curatively resected stage I non-small cell lung cancer. Cancer. 2013;119(4):792-8.
36. Heegaard NH,Schetter AJ, Welsh JA, et al. Circulating micro-RNA expression profiles in early stage non small cell lung cancer. Int J Cancer. 2012;130:1378-86.
37. Hodi FS, O'Day SJ, McDermott DF, et al. Improved survival with ipilimumab in patients with metastatic melanoma. N Engl J Med. 2010;363:711-23.
38. Hsu DS, Acharya CR,Balakumaran BS, et al. Characterizing the developmental pathways TTF-1, NKX2-8, and PAX9 in lung cancer. Proc Natl Acad Sci U S A. 2009;106:5312-7.
39. Hu Z, Chen X, Zhao Y, et al. SerummicroRNA signatures identified in a genome-wide serum microRNA expression profiling predict survival of non-small-cell lung cancer. J Clin Oncol. 2010;28:1721-6.
40. Iwakiri S, Mino N, Takahashi T, et al. Higher expression of chemokine receptor CXCR7 is linked to early and metastatic recurrence in pathological stage I non small cell lung cancer. Cancer. 2009;115(11):2580-93.
41. Janjigian YY, Park BJ, Zakowski MF, et al. Impact on disease-free survival of adjuvant erlotinib or gefitinib in patients with resected lung adenocarcinomas that harbor EGFR muta-

tions. J Thorac Oncol. 2011;6:569-75.

42. Johnston PG, Lenz HJ, Leichman CG, et al. Thymidylate synthase gene and protein expression correlate and are associated with response to 5-fluorouracil in human colorectal and gastric tumors. Cancer Res. 1995;55:1407-12.

43. Kamal NS, Soria JC, Mendiboure J, et al. MutS homologue 2 and the long-term benefit of adjuvant chemotherapy in lung cancer. Clin Cancer Res. 2010;16:1206-15.

44. Kang CH, Jang BG, Kim DW, et al. The prognostic significance of ERCC1, BRCA1, XRCC1, and betaⅢ-tubulin expression in patients with non-small cell lung cancer treated by plati- num- and taxane-based neoadjuvant chemotherapy and surgical resection. Lung Cancer. 2010;68(3):478-83.

45. Kantoff PW, Higano CS, Shore ND, et al. Sipuleucel-T immunotherapy for castration- resistant prostate cancer. N Engl J Med. 2010;363:411-22.

46. Kelly K, Chansky K, Gaspar LE, et al. Phase Ⅲ trial of maintenance gefitinib or placebo after concurrent chemoradiotherapy and docetaxel consolidation in inoperable stage Ⅲ non-small- cell lung cancer: SWOG S0023. J Clin Oncol. 2008;26:2450-6.

47. Kelsey CR, Marks LB, Hollis D, et al. Local recurrence after surgery for early stage lung cancer: an 11-year experience with 975 patients. Cancer. 2009;115:5218-27.

48. Ko E, Kim Y, Park SE, et al. Reduced expression of cyclin D2 is associated with poor recurrence-free survival independent of cyclin D1 in stageⅢ non-small cell lung cancer. Lung Cancer. 2012;77(2):401-6.

49. Kosaka T, Yatabe Y, Onozato R, et al. Prognostic implication of EGFR, KRAS, and TP53 gene mutations in a large cohort of Japanese patients with surgically treated lung adenocarcinoma. J Thorac Oncol. 2009;4(1):22-9.

50. Lau CL, D'Amico DA, Harpole DH, et al. Clinical and molecular prognostic factors and models for non-small cell lung cancer. In: Lung cancer principles and practice. 2nd ed. Philadelphia: Lippincott Williams & Wilkins; 2000. p. 602-11.

51. Leichman CG, Lenz HJ, Leichman L, et al. Quantification of intratumoral thymidylate synthase expression predicts for disseminated colorectal cancer response and resis- tance to protracted-infusion fluorouracil and weekly leucovorin. J Clin Oncol. 1997;15:3223-9.

52. Li GF, Deng SJ, Weng WW, et al. ERCC1 expression and outcomes of neo-adjuvant chemotherapy in elderly patients with non-small cell lung cancer. Nan Fang Yi Ke Da Xue Xue Bao. 2010;30(9):2131-3.

53. Liao M, Wang H, Lin Z, et al. Vascular endothelial growth factor and other biological predictors related to the postoperative survival rate on non-small cell lung cancer. Lung Cancer. 2001;33:125-32.

54. Lim E, Harris G, Patel A, et al. Preoperative versus postoperative chemotherapy inpatients with resectable non-small cell lung cancer: systematic review and indirect comparison meta-analysis of randomized trials. J Thorac Oncol. 2009;4(11):1380-8.

55. Liu R, Wang X, Chen GY, et al. The prognostic role of a gene signature from tumorigenic

breast-cancer cells. N Engl J Med. 2007;356:217-26.
56. Lokk K, Vooder T, Kolde R, et al. Methylation markers of early stage non-small cell lung cancer. PLoS One. 2012;7(6):e39813.
57. Lord RV, Brabender J, Gandara D, et al. Low ERCC1 expression correlates with prolonged survival after cisplatin plus gemcitabine chemotherapy in non-small cell lung cancer. Clin Cancer Res. 2002;8(7):2286-91.
58. Ludovini V, Flacco A, Bianconi F, et al. Concomitant high gene copy number and protein over- expression of IGF1R and EGFR negatively affect disease-free survival of surgically resected non-small-cell-lung cancer patients. Cancer Chemother Pharmacol. 2013;71(3):671-80.
59. Lu Y, Lemon W, Liu PY, et al. A gene expression signature predicts survival of patients with stage I nonsmall cell lung cancer. PLoS Med. 2006;3:e467.
60. Marra A, Kemming D, Krueer T, et al. ERCC1 as a predictor of response to induction therapy for stage III non-small cell lung cancer. J Clin Oncol. 2013;31(15s): abstr 18511.
61. Maus MK, Mack PC, Astrow SH, et al. Histology-related associations of ERCC1, RRM1, and TS biomarkers in patients with non-small-cell lung cancer: implications for therapy. J Thorac Oncol. 2013;8(5):582-6.
62. NCCN Clinical practice guidelines in oncology. Non small cell lung cancer. V. 1. 2011. Accessed at http://www. nccn. org/professionals/physiciangls/PDF. nscl. pdf.
63. NCT00373425 - Study of tarceva after surgery with or without adjuvant chemotherapy in Non-Small Cell Lung Carcinoma (NSCLC) patients who have Epidermal Growth Factor Receptor (EGFR) positive tumors (RADIANT) at www. clinicaltrials. gov.
64. Neal JW, Pennell NA, Govindan R, et al. The SELECT study: a multicenter phase II trial of adjuvant erlotinib in resected epidermal growth factor receptor (EGFR) mutation-positive non-small cell lung cancer (NSCLC). J Clin Oncol. 2012;30: abstr 7010.
65. Novello S, Manegold C, Grohe C, et al. International tailored chemotherapy adjuvant trial: Itaca trial. J Clin Oncol. 2012;30(No 15s): abstr TPS7109.
66. Oxnard GR, Janjigian YY, Arcila ME, et al. Maintained sensitivity to EGFR tyrosine kinase inhibitors in EGFR-mutant lung cancer recurring after adjuvant erlotinib or gefitinib. Clin Cancer Res. 2011;17:6322-8.
67. Pastorino U, Andreola S, Tagliabue E, et al. Immunocytochemical markers in stage I lung cancer: relevance to prognosis. J Clin Oncol. 1997;15:2858-65.
68. Pignon JP, Tribodet H, Scagliotti GV, et al. Lung adjuvant cisplatin evaluation: a pooled analysis by the LACE Collaborative Group. J Clin Oncol. 2008;26(21):3552-9.
69. Pisters KM, Evans WK, Azzoli CG et al. ; American Society of Clinical Oncology. Cancer Care Ontario and American Society of Clinical Oncology adjuvant chemotherapy and adjuvant radiation therapy for stages I-IIIA resectable non small-cell lung cancer guideline. J Clin Oncol. 2007;25(34):5506-18.
70. Pisters KMW, Vallieres E, Crowley JJ, et al. Surgery with or without preoperative paclitaxel and carboplatin in early-stage non small- cell lung cancer: Southwest Oncology Group Trial

S9900, an intergroup, randomized, phase Ⅲ trial. J Clin Oncol. 2010;28:1843-9.
71. Reiman T, Sève P, Vataire A, et al. Prognostic value of class Ⅲ B-tubulin (Tubb3) in operable non-small cell lung cancer (NSCLC) and predictive value for adjuvant cisplatin-based che- motherapy (CT): a validation study on three randomized trials. J Clin Oncol. 2008;26 (15 Suppl): abstr 7506, 398s.
72. Rekhtman N, Azzoli CG, Kris MG, et al. Patterns of co-expression of ERCC1 and P27 in resected non-small cell lung cancer by immunohistochemistry. J Clin Oncol. 2008;26(15 Suppl): abstr 7595, 420s.
73. Reynolds C, Obasaju C, Schell MJ, et al. Randomized phase Ⅲ trial of gemcitabine-based chemotherapy with in situ RRM1 and ERCC1 protein levels for response prediction in non-small-cell lung cancer. J Clin Oncol. 2009;27:5808-15.
74. Rosell R, Perez-Roca L, Sanchez JJ, et al. Customized treatment in non-small-cell lung cancer based on EGFR mutations and BRCA1 mRNA expression. PLoS One. 2009;4:e5133.
75. Rosell R, Skrzypski M, Jassem E, et al. BRCA1: a novel prognostic factor in resected non-small-cell lung cancer. PLoS One. 2007;2:e1129.
76. Rosell R, Danenberg KD, Alberola V, et al. Ribonucleotide reductase messenger RNA expression and survival in gemcitabine/cisplatin-treated advanced non-small cell lung cancer patients. Clin Cancer Res. 2004;10(4):1318-25.
77. Rosell R, Felip E, Taron M, et al. Gene expression as a predictive marker of outcome in stage ⅡB-ⅢA-ⅢB non-small cell lung cancer after induction gemcitabine-based chemotherapy followed by resectional surgery. Clin Cancer Res. 2004;10:4215s-9.
78. Rosell R, Camps C, Maestre J, et al. A randomized trial comparing preoperative plus surgery with surgery alone in patients with non-small-cell lung cancer. N Engl J Med. 1994;330:153-8.
79. Roth JA, Fossella F, Komaki R, et al. A randomized trial comparing perioperative chemotherapy and surgery with surgery alone in resectable stage ⅢA non-small-cell lung cancer. J Natl Cancer Inst. 1994;86:673-80.
80. Scagliotti G, Hanna N, Fossella F, et al. The differential efficacy of pemetrexed according to NSCLC histology: a review of two phase Ⅲ studies. Oncologist. 2009;14:253-63.
81. Scagliotti GV, Pastorino U, Vansteenkiste JF, et al. Randomized phase Ⅲ study of surgery alone or surgery plus preoperative cisplatin and gemcitabine in stages IB to ⅢA non-small-cell lung cancer. J Clin Oncol. 2012;30:172-8.
82. Scagliotti GV, Fossati R, Torri V, et al. Randomized study of adjuvant chemotherapy for completely resected stage I, II or ⅢA non-small cell lung cancer. J Natl Cancer Inst. 2003; 95(19):1453-61.
83. Schiller JH, Adak S, Feins RH, et al. Lack of prognostic significance of P53 and K-RAS mutations in primary resected non-small-cell lung cancer on E4592: a laboratory ancillary study on an Eastern Cooperative Oncology Group prospective randomized trial of postopera- tive adjuvant therapy. J Clin Oncol. 2001;19:448-57.
84. Sève P, Mackey J, Isaac S, et al. ClassⅢ beta-tubulin expression in tumor cells predicts re-

sponse and outcome in patients with non-small cell lung cancer receiving paclitaxel. Mol Cancer Ther. 2005;4:2001-7.
85. Sève P, Lai R, Ding K, et al. Class Ⅲ beta-tubulin expression and benefit from adjuvant cisplatin/vinorelbine chemotherapy in operable non-small cell lung cancer: analysis of NCIC JBR. 10. Clin Cancer Res. 2007;13:994-9.
86. Shedden K, Taylor JM, Enkemann SA, et al. Gene expression-based survival prediction in lung adenocarcinoma: a multi-site, blinded validation study: Director's Challenge Consortium for the molecular classification of lung adenocarcinoma. Nat Med. 2008;14(8):822-7.
87. Shen Y, Tang D, Yao R, et al. microRNA expression profiles associated with survival, disease progression, and response to gefitinib in completely resected non-small-cell lung cancer with EGFR mutation. Med Oncol. 2013;30(4):750.
88. Shintani Y, Ohta M, Hirabayashi H, et al. New prognostic indicator for non-small-cell lung cancer, quantitation of thymidylate synthase by real-time reverse transcription polymerase chain reaction. Int J Cancer. 2003;104:790-5.
89. Shirota Y, Stoehlmacher J, Brabender J, et al. ERCC1 and thymidylate synthase mRNA levels predict survival for colorectal cancer patients receiving combination oxaliplatin and fluorouracil chemotherapy. J Clin Oncol. 2001;19:4298-304.
90. Silva J, Garcia V, Zaballos A, et al. Vesicle-related microRNAs in plasma of nonsmall cell lung cancer patients and correlation with survival. Eur Respir J. 2011;37:617-23.
91. Simon GR, Sharma S, Cantor A, et al. ERCC1 expression is a predictor of survival in resected patients with non-small cell lung cancer. Chest. 2005;127:978-83.
92. Spano JP, Andre F, Morat L, et al. Chemokine receptor CXCR4 and early-stage non small cell lung cancer: pattern of expression and correlation with outcome. Ann Oncol. 2004; 15(4):613-7.
93. Takise A, Kodama T, Shimosato Y, et al. Histopathologic prognostic factors in adenocarcino-mas of the peripheral lung less than 2 cm in diameter. Cancer. 1988;2083-2088.
94. Tantraworasin A, Saeteng S, Lertprasertsuke N, et al. The prognostic value of ERCC1 and RRM1 gene expression in completely resected non-small cell lung cancer: tumor recurrence and overall survival. Cancer Manag Res. 2013;3(5):327-36.
95. Tsao MS, Aviel-Ronen S, Ding K, et al. Prognostic and predictive importance of P53 and RAS for adjuvant chemotherapy in non small-cell lung cancer. J Clin Oncol. 2007;25: 5240-7.
96. Ulloa-Montoya F, Louahed J, Dizier B, et al. Predictive gene signature in MAGE-A3 antigen- specific cancer immunotherapy. J Clin Oncol. 2013;31:2388-95.
97. van Duin M, de Wit J, Odijk H, et al. Molecular characterization of the human excision repair gene ERCC-1: cDNA cloning and amino acid homology with the yeast DNA repair gene RAD10. Cell. 1986;44:913-23.
98. Vansteenkiste J, De Ruysscher D, Eberhardt WEE, et al. ; ESMO Guidelines Working Group. Early and locally advanced non-small-cell lung cancer (NSCLC): ESMO Clinical Practice Guidelines for diagnosis, treatment and follow-up. Ann Oncol. 2013;24(6):vi89-

vi98.
99. Vansteenkiste J, Zielinski M, Linder A, et al. Adjuvant MAGE-A3 immunotherapy in resected non-small-cell lung cancer: phase II randomized study results. J Clin Oncol. 2013;31: 2396-403.
100. Wang SY, Ou W, Li N, et al. Pemetrexed-carboplatin adjuvant chemotherapy with or withoutgefitinib in resected stage ⅢA-N2 non-small cell lung cancer harboring EGFR mutations: a randomized phase II study. J Clin Oncol. 2013;31(15 Suppl): abstr 7519, 462s.
101. Westeel V, Quoix E, Puyraveau M. et al.; Intergroupe Francophone de Cancérologie Thoracique. A randomised trial comparing preoperative to perioperative chemotherapy in early stage non-small-cell lung cancer (IFCT 0002 trial). Eur J Cancer. 2013;49(12): 2654-64.
102. Winton T, Livingston R, Johnson D, et al. Vinorelbine plus cisplatin vs observation in resected non-small-cell lung cancer. N Engl J Med. 2005;352(25):2589-97.
103. Xia Q, Zhu Z, Wang J, et al. Expression and association of HER2 with prognosis in early-stage (T1-T2N0M0) non small cell lung cancer. Tumour Biol. 2012;33(5):1719-25.
104. Xu W, Banerji S, Davie JR, et al. Yin Yang gene expression ratio signature for lung cancer prognosis. PLoS One. 2013;8(7):e68742.
105. Yang Y, Xie Y, Xian L. Breast cancer susceptibility gene 1 (BRCA1) predict clinical outcome in platinum- andtaxol-based chemotherapy in non-small-cell lung cancer (NSCLC) patients: a system review and meta-analysis. J Exp Clin Cancer Res. 2013;32:15-24.
106. Yu SL, Chen HY, Chang GC, et al. MicroRNA signature predicts survival and relapse in lung cancer. Cancer Cell. 2008;13:48-57.
107. Zalcman G, Levallet G, Bergot E, et al. Evaluation of class Ⅲ beta-tubulin (bTubⅢ) expres- sion as a prognostic marker in patients with resectable non-small cell lung cancer (NSCLC) treated by perioperative chemotherapy (CT) in the phase Ⅲ trial IFCT-0002. J Clin Oncol. 2009;27(No 15s): abstr 7526, 388s.
108. Zhang GB, Chen J, Wang LR, et al. RRM1 and ERCC1 expression in peripheral blood versus tumor tissue in gemcitabine/carboplatin-treated advanced non-small cell lung cancer. Cancer Chemother Pharmacol. 2012;69:1277-87.
109. Zheng Z, Li X, Schell MJ, et al. Thymidylate synthase in situ protein expression andsurvival in stage I non-small-cell lung cancer. Cancer. 2008;112:2765-73.
110. Zheng Z, Chen T, Li X, et al. DNA synthesis and repair genes RRM1 and ERCC1 in lung cancer. N Engl J Med. 2007;356:800-8.
111. Zhu CQ, Pintilie M, John T, et al. Understanding prognostic gene expression signatures in lung cancer. Clin Lung Cancer. 2009;10:331-40.

第三部分
局部晚期非小细胞肺癌治疗新进展

第6章
局部晚期 NSCLC 的放射治疗进展

作者：Juliette Thariat，Ariane Lapierre，Martin Früh，
　　　Francoise Mornex
译者：许亚萍　林　钢　闫茂慧

前言

手术是治疗非小细胞肺癌(non-small cell lung cancer, NSCLC)的最有效治疗方法,但仅有30%的患者可行根治性手术[1]。术后是否行辅助放疗和(或)辅助化疗取决于术后病理分期及手术切除情况。约50%的肺癌患者只能接受姑息性治疗,其中大部分患者为晚期肺癌伴远处转移。姑息性治疗包括局部减瘤放射治疗、全身化疗、对症支持治疗以及上述方法的综合。剩余的20%为局部晚期 NSCLC 患者,肿块局限在胸廓内,没有远处转移,但已侵犯胸廓内结构,或已经侵及同侧或对侧纵隔,无法行根治性手术切除。伴一站以上纵隔淋巴结转移的ⅢA期及ⅢB期局部晚期 NSCLC 患者多接受非手术治疗。由于局部复发率(80%)和远处转移率(60%)均较高,局部晚期 NSCLC 患者需要局部联合全身的多学科综合治疗[2],通常需接受胸部放疗(radiotherapy, RT)和(或)化疗[3]。

20世纪60年代,早期的放疗多使用200～260 kV级的X射线或钴60,但这些方式往往无法给予肿瘤足够的照射剂量,其放疗疗效存在争议。随后尝试了增加放疗剂量的研究,退伍军人医院肺癌研究协会(VALG)纳入800例不可手术的、卡氏评分(Karnofsky performance status, KPS)大于50%的 NSCLC 患者(多数因为肿块较大),随机分为放疗组、安慰剂组及化疗组,放疗计划剂量为40～50 Gy

(33%的患者实际放疗剂量<40 Gy,1年生存率从14%提高到18%[4]。1990年范德比尔特试验[5]纳入319例不可手术的局部晚期NSCLC患者,随机分为单纯化疗组(长春地辛每周方案)、放疗组(60 Gy/2 Gy/fx)及放化疗组。结果显示三组的中位生存时间(8.6个月 vs 9.4个月 vs 10.1个月)和5年生存率(3% vs 3% vs 1%)均相似,但放疗可提高疾病的局部控制率(放疗组30%,放化疗组34%,化疗组10%)。RTOG关于放疗剂量的相关研究结果显示肿瘤局部控制率与放疗的生物等效剂量(Biologically equivalent dose, BED)相关($P<0.0001$),从而影响生存期[6]。近年来,立体定向放疗(stereotacticradiotherapy)使用BED>100 Gy治疗早期NSCLC取得较好的疗效,说明BED与局部控制率的相关性。由于肿瘤体积和危及器官(organs at risk, OAR)的原因,Ⅲ期患者的高剂量大分割放疗并不安全。提高局部晚期NSCLC局部控制率的方法包括:改变分割方式缩短总的治疗时间(加速放疗)、应用现代放疗技术如调强放射治疗技术(Intensity modulated radiation therapy, IMRT)根据正常器官的耐受剂量行个体化放射治疗剂量递增。其他的方法包括目前在临床实践中联合化疗以及在临床试验中联合靶向治疗等。

本章主要介绍局部晚期NSCLC多学科综合治疗中放化疗联合治疗的作用以及放疗在肿瘤局部控制及延长生存方面的研究进展。

放化疗联合治疗

化疗与放疗的联合以放疗为基础

20世纪70~80年代,虽然放疗疗效不理想,但放射治疗是治疗局部晚期NSCLC的标准治疗方式。80年代铂类广泛应用为肺癌治疗带来新的曙光,CALGB8433试验第一次验证了化疗所带来的益处,该试验自1984年到1987年,纳入体力状态评分较好的患者接受顺铂+长春碱化疗后行放疗,中位无进展生存时间和总生存时间均有所提高,总生存时间提高了4个月[7],虽然不能改善局控率,但显著提高了患者生存率和无远处转移生存时间。Kubota等的一项研究显示,胸部放疗联合以铂类为基础的化疗与单纯化疗相比,尽管总生存期无显著提高,但放疗组长期生存患者数显著增加[8]。1992年EORTC试验显示以顺铂为主的3周方案化疗联合同步放疗并不能改善生存(2年生存率26% vs 13%)[9]。最近的研究比较了诱导化疗联合放疗与同步放化疗的结果,提示同步放化疗在生存方面更有优势。1995年,非小细胞肺癌协作小组发表了第一个Meta分析结果,从52项非小细胞肺癌协作小组的随机对照临床试验中提取数据,其中22项研究为局部晚期NSCLC。结果显示化疗联合放疗改善患者生存(HR=0.90),2年和5年生存率分别提高3%和2%[10]。应用铂类化疗可获得更好疗效[10-12],但化疗方案是否需双药联合仍有争议。Delbaldo等2004年发表的一篇Meta分析提示,在化疗联合放疗中,双药联合化疗较单药化疗可显著提高治疗疗效和生存期。加入第三种化疗药物后在增加毒副反应的同时,虽然提高了肿瘤的控制率,但对生存时间并无显著影响[13]。因此,标准的治疗方案为以铂类为基础的双药联合方案。是否卡铂或顺铂为基础无明显差异[11],可根据患者情况个体化选择。

肺癌患者诊断中位年龄是 71 岁(其中 35% 的患者≥75 岁),但很少有随机对照临床试验纳入大于 70 岁、体力状态差的患者,而且有伴发疾病的患者大部分不能耐受同步放化疗,所以,尽管有高级别证据支持放化疗联合治疗,合适的老年患者,同步放化疗可行的结果也可见报道[14],但老年患者行同步放化疗仍需严格筛选和仔细观察。日本的Ⅲ期临床试验结果显示,大于 70 岁且 PS 评分在 0～2 分的患者予以含低剂量卡铂方案的同步放化疗较单纯放疗可提高生存期,为老年患者选择合适的治疗方案提供了依据(中位总生存时间:22.4 个月 vs 16.9 个月,HR=0.68,$P=0.0179$)[15]。

化疗的最佳时机

20 世纪 80 年代到本世纪初,随着放疗地位的不断提高,提出了化疗与放疗的时序问题。不到 10 年时间,有 12 个随机对照试验结果公布,其结果基本一致:同步放化疗可提高患者总生存期和无进展生存期(progression free survival,PFS)。2010 年,Aupérin 等发表了一篇 Meta 分析,汇总 6 项试验(纳入 1205 例患者)[16],同步化放疗较序贯化放疗有显著的生存获益:3 年生存率提高了 5.7%(HR=0.84;95% CI:0.74～0.95)。同步放化疗组有提高无疾病进展生存时间的趋势(HR=0.90;95% CI:0.79～1.01)。3 年局部进展率在同步放化疗组降低了 6.0%(HR=0.77;95% CI:0.62～0.95),但远处转移并无差异。局部控制和生存优势明显,但远处转移无明显优势,说明局部控制对生存的重要影响。最新的一项 Meta 分析证实非手术的 NSCLC 患者行化疗联合放疗 2 年和 5 年生存率可提高 4% 和 2.2% (HR=0.89;95% CI:0.81～0.98)[11]。同步放化疗可带来更多的生存获益,尤其是同步含铂类化疗方案。ASCO 指南推荐对Ⅲ期 NSCLC 予以含铂类药物为基础的方案化疗[17]。

综上所述,局部晚期 NSCLC 同步放化疗是标准治疗模式。同步放化疗毒副反应相对较多,3～4 级食管毒副反应发生率为 18%(相对风险度为 4.9),但肺部毒副反应增加不明显[16]。

放化疗疗效优于单纯放疗已基本明确,但治疗时间选择仍不明确。一些临床试验研究诱导化疗或巩固化疗的疗效[18,19,102,103],结果显示诱导化疗或巩固化疗并无生存获益,但毒副反应明显增多。CALGB 39801 试验提示 PS 评分较差或体重下降明显的患者可从诱导化疗中获益,但此项研究的患者总体生存率较低[18]。PulmonArt 试验提示以顺铂为基础的巩固化疗可以提高患者 PFS[19]。一项回顾性研究评估了诱导化疗和巩固化疗的疗效,提示足量放射治疗疗程的完成情况是影响预后的一个重要因素,与化放疗顺序无关[20]。在2013年的国际肺癌世界大会上,Van Houtte报告了对6个随机对照试验进行Meta分析评估诱导化疗与巩固化疗的疗效(规范放疗)(Abstract P2.24-021),结果显示在生存期和无病生存期方面两者均无明显差异。诱导化疗可以在放疗前缩小肿瘤体积,增加行放射治疗的机会。但应用诱导化疗会延长放疗前的等待时间。此外,诱导化疗有助于评估肿瘤对放疗的敏感性。

放射治疗进展

肿瘤靶区(gross tumor volume,GTV)可因摆位误差而发生改变。肿瘤在治疗过程中因呼吸运动可出现缩小、增大、移位等变化。应用影像引导可以确保放疗靶区的准确性[21]。图像引导放射治疗(image-guided radiation therapy,IGRT)可以解决上述问题。

影像引导放射治疗(IGRT)

器官运动可引起剂量沿着运动路径分布改变。适当控制治疗过程中肿瘤运动可以减少正常组织受照射体积,目前使用的主要方法包括腹部加压技术、主动呼吸运动控制技术、呼吸门控技术及实时跟踪放射治疗技术(AAPM工作组76)。

肿瘤运动的评估

慢速CT、呼气相CT、吸气相CT、4D或呼吸相关CT可以显示出肿瘤在呼吸运动时的边界。快速CT会增加系统误差,因为扫描时肿瘤的位置可能不是其平均位置,因此需用呼气和吸气控制技术、呼吸门控技术、呼吸相关及4D CT技术来解决呼吸运动导致的肿瘤位置改变。4D-CT应用外部红外线标记测量气流,获取多个呼吸时相的图像,图像采集与呼吸信号采集同步,呼吸周期某一时段的一系列图像整合成一个完整的3D-CT图像,而不同呼吸周期时相图像叠加在一起形成4D-CT图像。4D-CT图像可帮助确定肿瘤平均位置及具体运动范围。最大密度投影(maximum intensity projections,MIPs),指呼吸周期中所有时相的每个像素的最大值,利用每个扫描时相上人工像素显示的最大投影,勾画每个扫描时相上的肿瘤影像,从而形成一个融合的肿瘤靶区,即内靶区(internal target volume,ITV)。

肿瘤运动控制技术

浅呼吸或主动呼吸运动控制技术

体部立体框架不能完全消除呼吸引起的移位,在前后左右5mm、头尾10mm处约会有15%的靶体积会丢失,主动呼吸控制技术在为患者提供准确治疗技术的同时增加治疗时间。

呼吸同步技术

外部呼吸运动信号与内在靶区运动需建立准确关联。内部肿瘤运动可以应用"慢速"CT 成像技术评估，因为它采集数据时间较长，使得肿瘤位置的信息可以获取。缺点是运动伪影和模糊的肿瘤边界。快速薄层螺旋 CT 可以采集到肿瘤在呼吸周期的某一时刻的位置，这些图像可以行呼吸周期重建。呼吸运动是不规则的，并且个体化的呼吸模式不可能完全在治疗前评估出来。

呼吸运动可以通过外在实时监测信号观察，如患者体表的红外线反射标记。将标记放置于肿瘤位置或其附近，或某指定器官处（如膈肌），肿瘤运动也可以被测量到。呼吸门控还包括放疗实施过程中呼吸周期中的特殊的间隔范围，一般被称为射线区或"门控窗"（gating window）[22]。在应用呼吸门控技术时，被选中的某一时段的肿瘤位置用于描绘肿瘤的体积，而患者在 CT 扫描时的呼吸运动并不能准确地代表在整个治疗过程中的呼吸运动，外部信号与体内肿瘤也不能保证完全一致（不规则的呼吸、肿瘤的变化和基线位移引起）。门控宽度应考虑选择运动最小幅度和照射时间。其他控制呼吸运动的方法还有肿瘤跟踪，即在治疗过程中随着肿瘤的运动动态改变射线束的位置。该技术可以通过直线加速器的准直系统与靶目标运动同步来完成。多叶准直系统，准直装置实现叶片的运动与肿瘤运动的长轴一致，然而这种方法仅能实现在单方向修正肿瘤运动。全面 3D 修正的实现还依赖于加速器在行全身立体定向放射治疗时安装一个"机械臂"来跟踪呼吸运动。跟踪方法需依赖呼吸运动的精确预测模型以确定肿瘤的位置。

通常应用 X 线透视检测在治疗期间验证肿瘤位置，或者正侧位 X 线图像与相应的数字重建影像（DRR）对比。

调强放疗（IMRT）

调强放疗的优势和原理

局部晚期肺癌放射治疗主要受限于邻近肿瘤的重要脏器（如心脏、脊髓、食管及骨质结构等）、受照靶区大小以及正常肺组织的耐受量，另外还有剂量传递至靶区运动相关的物理不确定性。IMRT 通过调整剂量分布，使 PTV 的剂量适形度更好，同时避免正常结构受到高剂量照射。Liu 等进行了一项关于剂量学的回顾性研究，显示对于绝大多数局部晚期肺癌患者，IMRT 计划可以降低心脏、脊髓及食管的剂量，进而降低肺的 V20，如图 6.1 所示[23]。

虽然没有 3DCRT 与 IMRT 在肺癌中应用的前瞻性随机对照研究结果发表，但是回顾性研究显示，与 3DCRT 相比，IMRT 在总生存期（IMRT 组中位生存时间 1.4 年 vs 3DCRT 组 0.85 年）、无远处转移生存时间及毒副反应（HR=0.33）等相似[24]。

IMRT 的基本原理是通过调整来自多个方向不同强度的射线束使肿瘤内剂量

均匀,与常规放疗相比,适形度更好,尤其在凹形或者形状复杂的靶区中,从而和附近正常组织分开。IMRT 通过改变每一个入射射线束的强度来实现最佳吸收剂量分布,通常是将每一个射线束分割成更小的射线,并且分别将它们调整成所需的强度。此外通过 IMRT 治疗计划,可以获得个体化的吸收剂量分布,通过一系列参数设置优化剂量分布[26](附录彩图 6.1)。

IMRT 不确定性的处理

剂量梯度陡变存在一定的缺点,包括传递剂量至运动靶区和沿着射线路径剂量异质性模式变化两方面的不确定性。第一个原因是呼吸运动,动态 IMRT(相对于静态 IMRT)在剂量递送过程中使用移动光栅,当肿瘤与多叶光栅同时运动时,不能确定肿瘤是精确地接受了计划剂量还是在整个治疗过程中被光栅所遮挡。多次分割治疗后,这种所谓的相互影响效应能够引起剂量分布模糊,外周光束半影增加,从而导致适形剂量分布减少[26]。摆位误差及放疗分次间和分次内位移增加了模糊效应,而在实际治疗计划实施过程中,对剂量分布的影响则有限[26]。模糊效应可能对大器官运动的影响会较明显,因此有必要应用肿瘤门控或实时跟踪影像。

最新一代直线加速器尤其在行立体定向放疗时通常使用无均准滤过器技术(flattening filter free,FFF),使得上述情况加剧。FFF 的作用是在允许变更的范围内,使参考深度的光子束剂量分布一致,且显著降低光子束剂量率。FFF 光束允许较高的剂量率,在单次分割中有助于缩短治疗时间,减少器官移动[27],然而 FFF 光束进行大照射野治疗时可能导致靶区剂量分布不均匀。当运用动态 IMRT 时,FFF 光束会更容易引起这种相互影响效应,可通过增加照射野数目和分割次数能弥补此不足[28]。

呼吸门控技术或肿瘤跟踪技术可以部分弥补肿瘤和器官运动对剂量分布的影响,在整个治疗过程中还会有其他的变化,如解剖结构上的变化(患者靶区几何形状改变、肿瘤退缩、肺组织密度改变等)。在剂量学研究中,解剖结构改变对实际剂量传递的影响比放疗分次间基线移位对其影响大,CTVT 的平均剂量绝对差异大于 1%[29]。导致以上差异的原因可能是 PTV 考虑了呼吸运动,最好通过定期 4D-CT 扫描评估解剖结构改变和基线位移。由于这种评估技术实施起来较麻烦,而且消耗时间,因此推荐对需要进行剂量调整的患者在治疗期间行 4D-CT 扫描。

IMRT 的另一个问题是剂量的不均匀性。通过增加照射野的数量,虽然可以使 PTV 的剂量适形度更高,但是剂量分布却更不均匀。增加对均质性剂量的限制(如在 3DCRT 中见到的剂量分布标准偏差小于 3%)可在保证满足危及器官限量的同时增加 PTV 剂量[30]。

IMRT 中的低剂量

由于 IMRT 增加了照射野数目,Liao 等回顾性研究显示肺 V20 显著降低(3DCRT 37% vs IMRT 34%)[24]。另有研究得到了相似的结果,运用 IMRT 治

第6章 ■ 局部晚期NSCLC的放射治疗进展

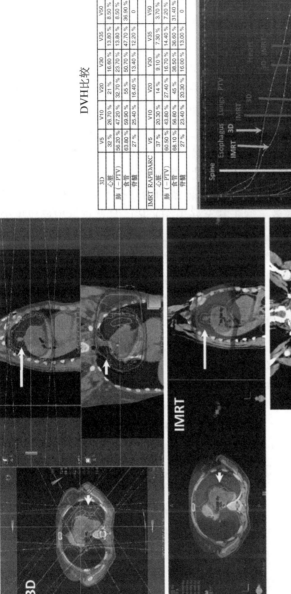

DVH比较

3D	V5	V10	V20	V30	V35	V50	V66
心脏	32 %	26.70 %	21 %	16.60 %	13.80 %	8.50 %	0.90 %
肺（-PTV）	56.20 %	47.20 %	32.70 %	23.70 %	13.80 %	8.50 %	4.40 %
食管	63.80 %	59.90 %	55 %	50.70 %	47.70 %	36.90 %	3 %
脊髓	27 %	25.40 %	16.40 %	13.40 %	12.20 %	0	0

IMRT RAPIDARC	V5	V10	V20	V30	V35	V50	V66
心脏	37 %	20.30 %	14 %	9.10 %	7.30 %	3.70 %	1.10 %
肺（-PTV）	60.50 %	43.80 %	27.40 %	16.70 %	14.40 %	7.20 %	0
食管	68.10 %	56.80 %	45 %	38.50 %	36.60 %	31.40 %	5 %
脊髓	27 %	23.40 %	20.30 %	16.00 %	13.00 %	0	0

图6.1　局部晚期不可手术非小细胞肺癌IMRT计划的剂量分布

疗,肺和其他关键结构受量减低,但因为 IMRT 照射野数目增加,肺 V5 则较高(57% vs 65%)[24-31]。IMRT 毒副反应多发生于肺组织接受较大范围的低剂量照射,可出现肺纤维化等晚期副反应,美国安德森肿瘤中心的回顾性研究显示,仅 5% 的患者在治疗 18 个月后发生 2 级(有症状)及以上肺纤维化[32]。其他毒副反应也是可控的,美国安德森肿瘤中心患者中 3 级及以上食管毒副反应发生率低于 20%,3 级及以上皮肤毒副反应低于 10%,并且 60% 以上的患者治疗过程中 KPS 评分保持稳定[32]。在头颈部肿瘤等其他类型肿瘤 IMRT 的类似研究中,由于增加了照射入射点,沿着射束路径的预期外毒副反应可能会增加。当剂量限制过于苛刻时,高剂量点可能会落在正常组织上,如椎体、肋骨或正常肺组织等。Uyterlinde 等最近报道应用 IMRT 同步化疗治疗 NSCLC,大量患者发生了椎体骨折,占 8%[33],虽然该研究样本量较小,但提醒我们在应用任何新技术时应意识到非预期毒副反应的发生。综上,尽管 IMRT 应用于肺癌的研究多为回顾性或纯理论研究,尚缺乏临床前瞻性研究,但仍应将其视为前景的治疗技术,初步研究显示 IMRT 治疗局部晚期肺癌显示其疗效等同于甚至好于 3DCRT,且严重毒副反应更少。

IMRT 的治疗模式

SEER 数据库分析[34]显示,IMRT 治疗 III 期肺癌患者的数量从 2001 年的 0.5% 增加到 2007 年的 14.7%。这种增长与临床患者分期改变没有明显关系,主要是由于很多治疗中心(非大学附属医院)在尝试应用高科技的放疗技术(享有医疗保险报销)治疗局部晚期肺癌,该研究还显示 IMRT 并没有增加放射性肺炎和食管炎的发生。

除了肺上沟、椎旁和心脏旁肿瘤,IMRT 在肺癌中的应用并未得到完全肯定,但是部分医学中心 100% 的局部晚期肺癌患者尝试使用 IMRT。

治疗模式在迅速的发生变化,IMRT 应用的证据级别在提高。为了限制肿瘤运动幅度≤1cm、减小 CTV/PTV 范围,4D 计划是必需的。靠近危及器官(如脊髓、臂丛神经、食管、纵隔)的大肿瘤应用 IMRT 治疗比适形放疗更为有效。要关注靶区的冷热点,努力降低肺组织的低剂量,也要仔细了解组织异质性,剂量计算算法和受影响的光束。从制定计划到剂量给予的每一步都要进行重复性验证,有必要严格保证各个步骤的质量。到目前为止,一些新技术的优势尚不明确,如 4DCT 与 3DCT 哪个更适合行 IMRT,目前正在进行相关方面的随机对照研究(临床试验注册号:NCT00520702),另外相同环境下图像引导自适应光子治疗和质子治疗的优劣对比(临床试验注册号:NCT00495170)。仍需要更多的前瞻性随机临床试验的研究结果来支持这些新技术的使用,已经有一些前瞻性研究在 NCI 临床试验网站上注册,如 NCT00921739,NCT01836692,NCT01166204,NCT00497250,NCT01617980,NCT01577212,NCT00938418,NCT00690963,NCT01411098747,NCT01429766,NCT01822496,NCT01912625,NCT01024829,NCT01059188,

NCT01391260，NCT01494415，NCT01580579。

剂量

剂量递增

RTOG 7301研究确立了NSCLC行2D放疗的标准剂量模式为60 Gy，2 Gy/次[35]，但患者中位生存时间仅10个月，3年生存率低于10%。20世纪80年代一些研究试图提高总剂量以提高肿瘤局部控制率，结果显示，局部晚期NSCLC放疗总剂量与局部控制及总生存期显著相关[36]。RTOG 8311 Ⅰ/Ⅱ期随机试验纳入了848例患者，行1.2 Gy/次，2次/天超分割放疗，探索放疗剂量递增(60，64.8，69.6，74.5，及79.2 Gy)的疗效，发现69.6 Gy组较低剂量组效果更好，而高于70 Gy的较高剂量组并没有提高患者生存期，反而由于正常肺组织受照体积较大发生放射性肺损伤增加[37]。随后有研究应用适形放疗将放疗剂量从65 Gy提高到102 Gy[2]，3~4级急性肺损伤和食管毒性毒副反应的发生率较少(4%~12%)，但远期放疗毒副反应结果未见报道[38,39]。剂量递增较常规剂量放疗提高了局部控制率(50%~60%)，2年生存率约40%，高剂量引起的食管毒副反应并没有使放疗延迟或终止。50例患者应用高达74 Gy的放疗剂量放疗发生急性心脏毒性的概率为8%[38,39]。2007年Memorial Slogan Kettering癌症中心的一项回顾性研究分析了82例不可手术Ⅰ~ⅢB期NSCLC应用适形放疗序贯化疗，放疗剂量≥80 Gy治疗的疗效[40]，结果显示增加放疗剂量使Ⅲ期患者的5年局部控制率(39%)和生存率(31%)均增加，与其他研究结果相似。Kong等的研究[41]也认为增加放疗总剂量对患者5年生存和局部控制均增加。Rosenzweig等发表了一项Ⅰ期临床研究，104例患者(65%为Ⅲ期患者，6%为复发患者)接受总剂量≥80.0 Gy的适形放疗，其中16%的患者接受诱导化疗，未行同步放化疗[42]，结果显示7%的患者发生晚期放射性肺损伤，25% NTCP的最大限量为84.0 Gy。RTOG 84-07(1984~1989年)Ⅰ/Ⅱ期临床试验给予原发肿瘤灶及淋巴结区域45 Gy放疗，再给予肿瘤局部及受累淋巴结加量18~63 Gy，总剂量由63 Gy递增到70.2 Gy/5.5周或5周[43]，结果显示早期和晚期放疗毒副反应均在可接受范围内，生存期并无显著不同。CALGB 8433临床试验纳入Ⅲ期、KPS>70、无体重减轻的患者，结果显示2年总生存率约20%。

随后的一些研究，如CALGB 30105 Ⅱ期临床试验，研究对象为Ⅲ期NSCLC，放疗剂量74 Gy、1次/天、2 Gy/次，同步放化疗后继续巩固化疗[44]，随机分组接受卡铂联合吉西他滨联合化疗或卡铂联合紫杉醇化疗，结果显示由于吉西他滨的放疗增敏作用，发生4~5级放射性肺损伤概率很高，超出了可接受范围，而卡铂联合紫杉醇组的患者中位生存时间为24个月，3级及以上放射性肺损伤的发生率为12%[44]，该临床试验结果为开展RTOG 0617 Ⅲ期试验奠定了基础。

RTOG 0617 Ⅲ期随机对照试验，对ⅢA/ⅢB期NSCLC患者进行2×2析因试验设计,比较标准剂量(60 Gy)与高剂量(74 Gy)适形放疗的疗效,同步行每周方案卡铂联合紫杉醇化疗,然后行2周期卡铂加紫杉醇巩固化疗,同时加或不加西妥昔单抗治疗,结果高剂量组因患者生活质量严重影响而提前结束[104],高剂量组显著增加了死亡风险(60 Gy组和74 Gy组中位生存时间分别为28.7个月和19.5个月,$P=0.0007$),高剂量组局部失败率37%,高剂量组有增加治疗相关性死亡的趋势(10 vs 2)[105]。RTOG 0617 III期试验结果与之前的 II 期试验结果不一致的原因有待进一步分析。虽然影响结果的确切原因还未明确,但这些结果与患者生活质量一致(ASTRO 2013),分析其原因可能包括:放疗周期的延长加剧了肿瘤细胞再增殖,在高剂量组肺和心脏接受了较高剂量的照射引发肺、心脏治疗相关死亡事件增加,以及高剂量放疗与西妥昔单抗可能存在的负性相互作用。

改变分割模式

局部晚期肺癌放疗常用的改变分隔模式有同步局部加量、超分割、加速放疗、加速超分割等。CHART试验显示加速超分割放疗(54 Gy,3次/每天*12天)较常规放疗有显著的生存获益[45]。然而3次/天*12天的加速超分割放疗模式在实际临床应用中受到限制。RTOG 9204 II期临床试验应用2次/天的放疗模式(同步化疗)提高了局部控制率,但食管放射性损伤发生率较高[46]。最近一项纳入了10项随机试验(2000例患者)的Meta分析比较了超分割联合或不联合加速放疗与常规分割放疗的结果,结果显示非常规分割模式5年生存率提高了3%。欧盟框架计划7(FP7)核心资助项目PET提升计划(NCT0102482)使用功能性显像进行剂量递增和重新分配。通过小剂量增加单次放疗剂量至规定的正常组织限量,患者随机分组接受标准方案放疗(66 Gy/24F,2.75Gy/次),原发肿瘤灶整体加量或根据治疗前FDG-PET/CT显示的SUVmax区域的50%面积予以加量。

放疗区域的确定

研究结果显示增加放疗剂量可以提高肿瘤局部控制率,放疗毒副反应(放射性食管及肺部损伤)与放疗体积相关。局部晚期NSCLC不行淋巴结区域预防照射可以最大限度地提高肿瘤放疗剂量和减少正常组织损伤。应用正电子发射断层扫描评估肿瘤体积有利于获得更准确的肿瘤分期。部分回顾性研究、III期随机试验及一项纳入了4项RTOG试验(7811,7917,8311,8407)共1705例患者的Meta分析显示放疗区域内的区域淋巴结复发率低于10%[47-49]。因此推荐治疗前行PET/CT检查以明确区域淋巴结的诊断,为淋巴结区域放疗靶区确定提供准确依据[50]。

放疗的多种成像技术

计划和剂量曲线

PET/CT在放疗计划中的应用

PET/CT已成为局部晚期肺癌放射治疗方案设计的重要参考,见图6.2[50,51]

附录彩图 6.2，PET/CT 有助于区分肿瘤和肺不张，较 CT 可获得更准确的分期[52,53]。PET/CT 扫描可使患者在不增加放疗剂量的前提下获得更大的收益，也明确了 1/3 拟行根治性放疗的患者实际无法行根治性放疗[54]，但也有研究认为 PET/CT 评估肿瘤分期存在移行性，如有研究评估了 120 天内重复行 PET/CT 检

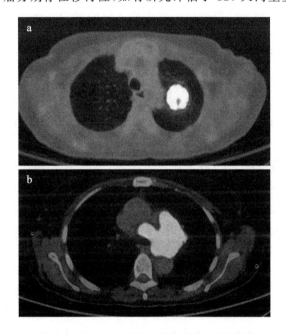

图 6.2　PET/CT 应用于放射治疗方案设计

查的结果差异，结果显示过一半的患者行第二次 PET/CT 检查显示肿瘤分期明显上调，SUV 值可预测肿瘤分期上调，但上调组和未上调组患者 SUV 值不存在明显统计学差异[55]。

放疗中缺氧的评估

缺氧与肿瘤放疗抵抗和血管生成相关。可通过血管灌注来评估血流量，用以间接测量肿瘤的血管生成。有研究使用动态增强 CT(dynamic contrast enhanced CT,DCE-CT)评估肿瘤血管浸润情况，PET/CT 评估肿瘤代谢活性，可以发现肿瘤内在的异质性，但与肿瘤血流灌注量无显著相关性[54]。

动态 PET/CT 应用 18F-FMISO（半衰期 110 分钟）作为肿瘤缺氧示踪剂。评估含氧量测量值与 18F-FMISO 摄取量之间的相关性。初步研究表明 FMISO 高摄取率提示肿瘤复发风险较高，重复行 PET/CT 测得 FMISO 摄取量减少可预测疗效。HIL 试验（海德堡团队，NCT01617980）纳入Ⅲ期 NSCLC 患者行 4D-CT 的调强放疗，探讨应用 18F-FMISO PET/CT 和功能性 MRI 进行肿瘤乏氧显像的相关性。另外，有研究将[(18)F]HX4 作为 PET 的缺氧示踪剂[56]，15 例 NSCLC 患

者出现[(18)F]HX4的大量摄取,这种特异性的摄取模式在PET显像2~4小时比较稳定,4小时左右出现摄取高峰。

缺氧区域立体定向放疗加量

立体定向放疗目前主要用于不适合手术的局限期患者。对于可手术的早期肺癌患者,对比立体定向放疗与外科手术治疗疗效的Ⅲ期临床试验正在进行中。立体定向放疗是应用立体定向设备行大分割模式放疗。局部晚期NSCLC因肿瘤体积较大等原因,使得其行立体定向放射治疗(stereotactic ablative radiation therapy,SABR)受到限制。SABR被越来越多地应用于局部加量(+/−剂量递增)[57]或残留病灶、复发部位的放疗。Ⅲ期患者(包括N2)的回顾性资料表明,可以使用SABR(50 Gy适形放疗+25 Gy/5F的立体定向放疗)提高总治疗剂量[57]。这种剂量追加模式可以特别针对缺氧区域。大分割调强放疗是SABR的最佳选择模式,但约有25%的患者出现中、重度急性毒副反应。另一项前瞻性研究应用SABR行残留病灶加量[58],对无远处转移患者,放化疗至60 Gy后,原发肿瘤灶或淋巴结转移区域仍有的残留灶(≤5cm)行SABR加量。依据RTOG 0813研究,残余肿瘤病灶总的生物等效剂量需>100Gy,可行10 Gy*2F或6.5 Gy*3F加量。研究中位随访13个月,在33例患者中有4例患者发生3级急性放射性肺炎,1例发生3级慢性放射性肺损伤,原发肿瘤部位的局部控制率为83%。NSCLC行根治性同步放化疗后仍有残留者,应用直线加速器行SBRT予以残留灶加量是可行的,与标准放射治疗相比并没有增加毒副反应。需应用IGRT采取合适的分割模式;采用肿瘤跟踪技术监控其内部运动也十分重要[59],特别是当采用大分割放疗时。

一些探讨立体定向放疗在局部晚期NSCLC中的应用的Ⅰ/Ⅱ期临床试验目前正在进行中(NCI clinicaltrials.gov:NCT01657617,NCT01656460,NCT01746810,NCT01300299,NCT01463423,NCT01051037,NCT01899989,NCT01781741,NCT01345851,NCT00945451,NCT01711697,NCT01543672)。

未来新药

培美曲塞

培美曲塞作为一种叶酸代谢拮抗剂,竞争性抑制酶与核苷酸的结合。相比吉西他滨,培美曲塞联合顺铂可提高转移性非鳞状细胞NSCLC的总生存期[60]。初期临床研究提示培美曲塞具有放射增敏作用,增敏作用取决于药物浓度和肿瘤类型,在LXI肺肿瘤细胞系中其增强比为1.6[61]。相关的Ⅰ期和Ⅱ期临床研究显示,联合培美曲塞同步放疗发生的毒副反应均为中度[62-64],是局部晚期(Ⅲ期)NSCLC安全有效的治疗方法[65,66]。CALGB 30407试验提示鳞状细胞NSCLC应用培美曲塞不能从中获益[66],随后只纳入非鳞状细胞NSCLC作为研究对象。2008年启动的PROCLAIM临床Ⅲ期试验,比较顺铂联合培美曲塞与顺铂联合依托泊苷,同步66 Gy放疗,联合巩固化疗[67],该研究纳入了近600例患者,拟明确同步培美曲塞联合顺铂是否有生存获益。放疗剂量强度两组相似,初步结果显示培美曲塞联合顺铂组总体不良事件显著减少,毒副反应包括中性粒细胞减少和感染[106]。有待包括潜在的晚期毒性反应的所有研究结果的公布。2010年法国胸部肿瘤学组(IFCT)启动IFCT 0803临床Ⅲ期试验,比较顺铂联合培美曲塞,同步66 Gy放疗,联合或不联合西妥昔单抗[68]。即"最佳"方案整合了目前最新的肿瘤治疗方案,包括放化疗、诱导化疗、高剂量(66 Gy)放疗、培美曲塞、西妥昔单抗和以铂类为基础的化疗。但IFCT 0803试验招募106例患者后终止。Garrido等最近公布了非鳞状NSCLC行培美曲塞联合顺铂(培美曲塞$500mg/m^2$+顺铂$75mg/m^2$,d1 q21d)诱导化疗后同步化放疗的Ⅱ期临床试验数据,1年无进展生存期为51%,与其他铂类药物为基础的诱导化疗后同步放化疗结果相似,总体缓解率为59%,有3%的患者疾病进展。71%的患者行高剂量强度放疗。局部晚期NSCLC接受根治性放化疗后,10%的患者发生3~4级毒副反应(食管炎,中性粒细胞减少症)。

西妥昔单抗

西妥昔单抗是表皮生长因子受体(EGFR)单克隆抗体靶向药物,FLEX临床Ⅲ期试验表明该药物治疗EGFR高表达患者(免疫组化检查)效果优于低表达患者[69]。相关临床前研究[67]和RTOG 0324研究为放化疗期间加西妥昔单抗治疗提供了有利的证据。而在第十五届世界肺癌大会上公布的RTOG 0617试验的初步结果(摘要PL03 2013)提示,不能手术切除的Ⅲ期NSCLC患者放化疗联合西妥昔单抗并不能使患者获益更多。

联合西妥昔单抗可增加治疗相关毒副反应,有研究纳入465例肺癌患者,行每周卡铂和紫杉醇方案化疗加西妥昔单抗治疗,同期放疗,中位随访19个月,结果显示中位总生存期23个月,18个月时生存率为60%,中位无进展生存期为10个月。总的不良事件发生率行西妥昔单抗组为85%,未行西妥昔单抗组为70%,非血液学不良事件发生率2组分别为71%和51%($P<0.0001$)。

新的靶向治疗和其他治疗

EGFR突变局部晚期NSCLC患者放疗和(或)化疗后局部复发率较低,因此有假设提出EGFR抑制剂对EGFR突变患者可能有放疗增敏作用[70,71]。研究显示,放化疗期间予以标准剂量的EGFR抑制剂如厄洛替尼和吉非替尼等,并不明显增加毒副反应[72,73]。然而,到目前为止,多数放化疗联合EGFR-TKI的研究结论都不尽如人意,生存率低于或接近单纯放化疗[73-77]。特别是SWOG S0023研究,Ⅲ期NSCLC行顺铂联合依托泊苷化疗同步63 Gy放疗+多西他赛巩固治疗后,继续吉非替尼治疗,对比安慰剂组,结果显示平均生存时间安慰剂组较试验组高(35个月 vs 23个月),导致试验提前关闭[74]。另一项研究也得出相似的结果,Ⅲ期NSCLC患者术后行吉非替尼辅助治疗未延长患者生存[78]。这些研究结果提示,未经 EGFR 突变选择的Ⅲ期 NSCLC 患者使用 EGFR-TKI 治疗疗效不确定,今后研究应更关注 EGFR 突变患者行 EGFR-TKI 治疗联合化疗的疗效。

现有的证据提示,NSCLC 发生 EGFR 突变[79-86]和间变性淋巴瘤激酶(ALK)基因重排[87,88],可行个性化靶向药物治疗。

ALK 基因重排的患者口服 ALK 抑制剂如克唑替尼靶向治疗,是非小细胞肺癌治疗中的一个突破性进展。晚期非小细胞肺癌患者发生 ALK 重排,无论之前是否接受过治疗,行克唑替尼治疗疗效均优于标准化疗[107]。此外,初步的回顾性资料表明,克唑替尼不仅可与放疗联合应用,而且与放化疗联合应用也可提高寡进展晚期肺癌的局部控制率[89,90]。一项Ⅲ期临床试验结果提示,仅有 4% 的 NSCLC 患者表现为 ALK 阳性。目前一项Ⅱ期随机临床试验正在Ⅲ期 NSCLC 患者中进行(RTOG1306)。

抗血管生成药物如贝伐单抗在其他许多肿瘤中已成为一线治疗方案,贝伐单抗联合化疗治疗转移性 NSCLC 患者的结果令人鼓舞[91,92]。然而,贝伐单抗与放疗同时使用会增加气管食管瘘、肺出血的发生,尤其是在鳞状细胞癌患者中,使用贝伐单抗未见生存获益[93,94]。肺癌患者放疗联合贝伐单抗,由于严重并发症的发生,目前没有相关临床试验在开展,建议放射治疗期间应避免使用贝伐单抗。其他抗血管生成药物联合放化疗或放疗应用于治疗 NSCLC 的疗效也有被评估。如 AE-941 或沙利度胺,相关研究结论显示增加了血栓栓塞的发生率,未提高患者生存期[95,96]。

另外还有其他靶向药物也在进行临床试验中,如乙丙昔罗可克服肿瘤缺氧,降低血红蛋白的氧亲和力,增加组织氧分压。一项研究在诱导化疗后予乙丙昔罗联合放疗,结果显示生存期为 20.6 个月,毒副反应发生率较低[97]。一项Ⅱ期临床试验,将一种新疫苗 MUC-1,L-BP25 应用于ⅢB、Ⅳ期 NSCLC,结果显示提高了ⅢB 期患者的中位生存时间(30.6 个月 vs 13.3 个月)[98]。基于这些结果,START Ⅲ期试验,研究纳入 1320 例不能手术切除的Ⅲ期 NSCLC 患者,患者行一线放化疗后随机分为 L-BP25(Stimuvax)组和安慰剂组,联合环磷酰胺 300mg/m² 治疗[108],主要研究终点总生存期无显著差异(25.6 个月 vs 22.3 个月,HR 0.88,$P=0.12$)。亚组分析($n=806$)比较了接受标准同步放化疗的患者与序贯放化疗患者的疗效,结果同步放化疗组总生存期提高约 10 个月(30.8 个月 vs 20.6 个月,HR 0.78,$P=0.016$)。一项Ⅲ期临床试验(START 2)已启动,入组患者为完成标准同步放化疗的患者。

一项Ⅱ期临床研究提示应用免疫治疗显著提高治疗有效患者的总生存期(19 个月 vs 3.5 个月)[99],目前 GV 1001(端粒酶肽疫苗)用于肺癌放化疗后的Ⅲ期临床研究正在开展中。

质子治疗

质子的物理特性使其可以使肿瘤剂量更精确化(有利于保护正常组织。但目前质子治疗的明确适应证有限,主要包括眼部肿瘤、颅底脊索瘤/软骨肉瘤、一些儿童的肿瘤和肉瘤等,质子治疗应用于肺部肿瘤的治疗,肿瘤运动控制、组织成分和密度的不同以及图像引导等是目前研究的重点。Lopez Guerra 等分析了 250 例 NSCLC 患者行 66 Gy 光子治疗或 74 Gy 等效(Gy Equivalent, GyE)质子治疗的疗效[100]。比较他们 1 年后一氧化碳肺弥散能力(DLCO),结果显示适形放疗组 DLCO 较质子治疗组显著下降。Sejpal 等研究了 202 例局部晚期 NSCLC 行放射治疗的疗效,分别行 74 GyE 质子治疗和 63 Gy 的 IMRT 或适形放化疗放疗,中位随访时间 1.5 年[101]。结果显示质子治疗组、IMRT 和适形放化疗组的中位生存期分别为 24 个月、18 个月和 18 个月。据 NCI 临床试验数据库资料报道,关于局部晚期 NSCLC 质子治疗的 8 项 I/II 期临床试验和 1 项 III 期随机临床试验目前正在进行中(NCI clinicaltrials.gov NCT00881712,NCT01770418,NCT00915005,NCT01629498,NCT01993810,NCT01386697,NCT01076231,NCT01108666,NCT01565772)。到目前为止,质子治疗还仅局限于临床试验阶段。

结论和展望

目前,局部晚期非小细胞肺癌的标准治疗模式依然是放疗(60~66 Gy)联合以顺铂为基础的化疗。可以选择性使用诱导或巩固化疗。今后的研究将致力于确定在最佳的多模态影像(如 PET-CT、自适应图像及运动控制等)引导下行各种放疗新技术如 IMRT、立体定向放疗、质子治疗等的临床疗效,优化放疗联合化疗和靶向药物的治疗模式,以进一步提高肿瘤局部控制率和患者生存率。在目前局部晚期非小细胞肺癌的治疗中需综合考虑患者生活质量、治疗疗效、成本效益比及患者的个体情况等。

参考文献

1. Little AG, et al. Patterns of surgical care of lung cancer patients. AnnThorac Surg. 2005;80:2051-6; discussion 2056.
2. Girard N, Mornex F. Radiotherapy for locally advanced non-small cell lung cancer. Eur J Cancer (Oxf Engl). 2009;199045 Suppl 1:113-25.
3. Mauguen A, et al. Surrogate endpoints for overall survival in chemotherapy and radiotherapy trials in operable and locally advanced lung cancer: a re-analysis of meta-analyses of individual patients' data. Lancet Oncol. 2013;14:619-26.
4. Roswit B, et al. The survival of patients with inoperable lung cancer: a large-scale randomized study of radiation therapy versus placebo. Radiology. 1968;90:688-97.

5. Johnson DH, et al. Thoracic radiotherapy does not prolong survival in patients with locally advanced, unresectable non-small cell lung cancer. Ann Intern Med. 1990;113:33-8.
6. Machtay M, et al. Defining local-regional control and its importance in locally advanced nonsmall cell lung carcinoma. J Thorac Oncol. 2012;7:716-22.
7. Dillman RO, et al. A randomized trial of induction chemotherapy plus high-dose radiation versus radiation alone in stage Ⅲ non-small-cell lung cancer. N Engl J Med. 1990;323:940-5.
8. Kubota K, et al. Role of radiotherapy in combined modality treatment of locally advanced non-small-cell lung cancer. J Clin Oncol. 1994;12:1547-52.
9. Schaake-Koning C, et al. Effects of concomitant cisplatin and radiotherapy on inoperable non-small-cell lung cancer. N Engl J Med. 1992;326:524-30.
10. Chemotherapy in non-small cell lung cancer:a meta-analysis using updated data on individual patients from 52 randomised clinical trials. Non-small Cell Lung Cancer Collaborative Group. BMJ. 1995;311:899-909.
11. Aupérin A, et al. Concomitant radio-chemotherapy based on platin compounds in patients with locally advanced non-small cell lung cancer (NSCLC):a meta-analysis of individual data from 1764 patients. Ann Oncol. 2006;17:473-83.
12. Okawara G, Mackay JA, Evans WK, Ung YC, Lung Cancer Disease Site Group of Cancer Care Ontario's Program in Evidence-based Care. Management of unresected stage Ⅲ nonsmall cell lung cancer:a systematic review. J Thorac Oncol. 2006;1:377-93.
13. Delbaldo C, et al. Benefits of adding a drug to a single-agent or a 2-agent chemotherapy regimen in advanced non-small-cell lung cancer:a meta-analysis. JAMA. 2004;292:470-84.
14. Topkan E, Parlak C, Topuk S, Guler OC, Selek U. Outcomes of aggressive concurrent radiochemotherapy in highly selected septuagenarians with stage ⅢB non-small cell lung carcinoma:retrospective analysis of 89 patients. Lung Cancer. 2013;81:226-30.
15. Atagi S, et al. Thoracic radiotherapy with or without daily low-dose carboplatin in elderly patients with non-small-cell lung cancer:a randomised, controlled, phase 3 trial by the Japan Clinical Oncology Group (JCOG0301). Lancet Oncol. 2012;13:671-8.
16. Aupérin A, et al. Meta-analysis of concomitant versus sequential radiochemotherapy in locally advanced non-small-cell lung cancer. J Thorac Oncol. 2010;28:2181-90.
17. Pisters KMW, et al. Cancer Care Ontario and American Society of Clinical Oncology adjuvant chemotherapy and adjuvant radiation therapy for stages I-ⅢA resectablenon small-cell lung cancer guideline. J Thorac Oncol. 2007;25:5506-18.
18. Belani CP, et al. Combined chemoradiotherapy regimens of paclitaxel and carboplatin for locally advanced non-small-cell lung cancer:a randomized phase Ⅱ locally advanced multi- modality protocol. J Thorac Oncol. 2005;23:5883-91.
19. Van Meerbeeck JP, et al. Mature results of PulmonArt:involved-field 3D radiotherapy (RT) and docetaxel/cisplatin chemotherapy (CT) in a randomised phase 2 study comparing concurrent CT-RT followed by consolidation CT, with induction CT followed by concurrent CT-RT in patients (pts) with stage Ⅲ non-small cell lung cancer (NSCLC):B5-06. J Thorac Oncol.

2007;2(8):S349-50.
20. Garrido P, et al. Predictors of long-term survival in patients with lung cancer included in the randomized Spanish Lung Cancer Group 0008 phase II trial using concomitant chemoradiation with docetaxel and carboplatin plus induction or consolidation chemotherapy. Clin Lung Cancer. 2009;10:180-6.
21. Guckenberger M, Wilbert J, Richter A, Baier K, Flentje M. Potential of adaptive radiotherapy to escalate the radiation dose in combined radiochemotherapy for locally advanced non-small cell lung cancer. Int J Radiat Oncol Biol Phys. 2011;79:901-8.
22. Giraud P, et al. Respiratory gating techniques for optimization of lung cancer radiotherapy. J Thorac Oncol. 2011;6:2058-68.
23. Liu HH, et al. Feasibility of sparing lung and other thoracic structures with intensitymodulated radiotherapy for non-small-cell lung cancer. Int J Radiat Oncol Biol Phys. 2004;58(4): 1268-79.
24. Liao ZX, et al. Influence of technologic advances on outcomes in patients with unresectable, locally advanced non-small-cell lung cancer receiving concomitant chemoradiotherapy. Int J Radiat Oncol Biol Phys. 2010;76(3):775-81.
25. Prescribing, recording, and reporting photon-beam intensity-modulated radiation therapy (IMRT):contents. J ICRU. 2010;10:NP-NP.
26. Bortfeld T, Jiang SB, Rietzel E. Effects of motion on the total dose distribution. Semin Radiat Oncol. 2004;14(1):41-51.
27. Thomas EM, et al. Effects of flattening filter-free and volumetric-modulated arc therapy delivery on treatment efficiency. J Appl Clin Med Phys. 2013;14:4328.
28. Ong CL, Dahele M, Slotman BJ, Verbakel WFAR. Dosimetric impact of the interplay effect during stereotactic lung radiation therapy delivery using flattening filter-free beams and volumetric modulated arc therapy. Int J Radiat Oncol Biol Phys. 2013;86:743-8.
29. SchmidtML, Hoffmann L, Kandi M, Møller DS, Poulsen PR. Dosimetric impact of respiratory motion, interfraction baseline shifts, and anatomical changes in radiotherapy of nonsmall cell lung cancer. Acta Oncol. 2013;52:1490-6.
30. Schwarz M, et al. Impact of geometrical uncertainties on 3D CRT and IMRT dose distributions for lung cancer treatment. Int J Radiat Oncol Biol Phys. 2006;65(4):1260-9.
31. Chapet O, et al. Potential benefits of using non coplanar field and intensity modulated radiation therapy to preserve the heart in irradiation of lung tumors in the middle and lower lobes. Radiother Oncol. 2006;80:333-40.
32. Jiang Z-Q, et al. Long-term clinical outcome of intensity-modulated radiotherapy for inoperable non-small cell lung cancer: the MD Anderson experience. Int J Radiat Oncol Biol Phys. 2012;83(1):332-9.
33. Uyterlinde W, Chen C, Sonke JJ, De Bois J, Belderbos J, Van Den Heuvel M. Vertebral fractures in NSCLC patients treated with IMRT and concurrent chemotherapy. World lung cancer 2013;O14.02.

34. Shirvani SM, et al. Intensity modulated radiotherapy for stage Ⅲ non-small cell lung cancer in the United States:predictors of use and association with toxicities. Lung Cancer. 2013;82: 252-9.
35. Perez CA, Bauer M,Edelstein S, Gillespie BW, Birch R. Impact of tumor control on survival in carcinoma of the lung treated with irradiation. Int J Radiat Oncol Biol Phys. 1986; 12:539-47.
36. Bayman N,Blackhall F, McCloskey P, Taylor P, Faivre-Finn C. How can we optimise concurrent chemoradiotherapy for inoperable stage Ⅲ non-small cell lung cancer? Lung Cancer. 2014;83:117-25.
37. Cox JD, et al. A randomized phase I/II trial of hyperfractionated radiation therapy with total doses of 60. 0 Gy to 79. 2 Gy:possible survival benefit with greater than or equal to 69. 6 Gy in favorable patients with Radiation Therapy Oncology Group stage Ⅲ non-small-cell lung carcinoma:report of Radiation Therapy Oncology Group 83-11. J Clin Oncol. 1990;8;1543-55.
38. Kong F-M, Zhao L, Hayman JA. The role of radiation therapy in thoracic tumors. Hematol Oncol Clin North Am. 2006;20:363-400.
39. Bellière A, et al. Feasibility of high-dose three-dimensional radiation therapy in the treatment of localised non-small-cell lung cancer. Cancer Radiother. 2009;13:298-304.
40. Sura S, Yorke E, Jackson A, Rosenzweig KE. High-dose radiotherapy for the treatment of inoperable non-small cell lung cancer. Cancer J. 2007;13:238-42.
41. Kong F-M, et al. High-dose radiation improved local tumor control and overall survival in patients with inoperable/unresectable non-small-cell lung cancer:long-term results of a radiation dose escalation study. Int J Radiat Oncol Biol Phys. 2005;63:324-33.
42. Rosenzweig KE, et al. Results of a phase I dose-escalation study using three-dimensional conformal radiotherapy in the treatment of inoperable nonsmall cell lung carcinoma. Cancer. 2005;103:2118-27.
43. Byhardt RW, et al. A phase I/II study to evaluate accelerated fractionation via concomitant boost for squamous, adeno, and large cell carcinoma of the lung:report of Radiation Therapy Oncology Group 84-07. Int J Radiat Oncol Biol Phys. 1993;26:459-68.
44. Salama JK, et al. Pulmonary toxicity in Stage Ⅲ non-small cell lung cancer patients treated with high-dose (74 Gy) 3-dimensional conformal thoracic radiotherapy and concurrent chemotherapy following induction chemotherapy: a secondary analysis of Cancer and Leukemia Group B (CALGB) trial 30105. Int J Radiat Oncol Biol Phys. 2011;81:e269-74.
45. Hatton M, et al. Induction chemotherapy and continuous hyperfractionated accelerated radiotherapy (chart) for patients with locally advanced inoperable non-small-cell lung cancer:the MRC INCH randomized trial. Int J Radiat Oncol Biol Phys. 2011;81:712-8.
46. Komaki R, et al. Randomized phase II chemotherapy and radiotherapy trial for patients with locally advanced inoperable non-small-cell lung cancer:long-term follow-up of RTOG 92-04. Int J Radiat Oncol Biol Phys. 2002;53:548-57.
47. Rosenzweig KE, Sura S, Jackson A, Yorke E. Involved-field radiation therapy for inoperable

non small-cell lung cancer. J Clin Oncol. 2007;25:5557-61.

48. Yuan S, et al. A randomized study of involved-field irradiation versus elective nodal irradiation in combination with concurrent chemotherapy for inoperable stage Ⅲ nonsmall cell lung cancer. Am J Clin Oncol. 2007;30:239-44.

49. Emami B, et al. The impact of regional nodal radiotherapy (dose/volume) on regional progression and survival in unresectable non-small cell lung cancer:an analysis of RTOG data. Lung Cancer. 2003;41:207-14.

50. De Ruysscher D, Nestle U, Jeraj R, Macmanus M. PET scans in radiotherapy planning of lung cancer. Lung Cancer. 2012;75:141-5.

51. De Ruysscher D, et al. Effects of radiotherapy planning with a dedicated combined PET-CTsimulator of patients with non-small cell lung cancer on dose limiting normal tissues and radiation dose-escalation:a planning study. Radiother Oncol. 2005;77:5-10.

52. MacManus M, et al. Use of PET and PET/CT for radiation therapy planning:IAEA expert report 2006－2007. Radiother Oncol. 2009;91:85-94.

53. Mac Manus MP, et al. The use of fused PET/CT images for patient selection and radical radiotherapy target volume definition in patients with non-small cell lung cancer:results of a prospective study with mature survival data. Radiother Oncol. 2013;106:292-8.

54. Van Elmpt W, et al. Characterization of tumor heterogeneity using dynamic contrast enhanced CT and FDG-PET in non-small cell lung cancer. Radiother Oncol. 2013;109:65-70.

55. Geiger GA, et al. Stage migration in planning PET/CT scans in patients due to receive radiotherapy for non-small-cell lung cancer. Clin Lung Cancer. 2013. doi:10.1016/j.cllc.2013.08.004.

56. Zegers CML, et al. Hypoxia imaging with [18F]HX4 PET in NSCLC patients:defining optimal imaging parameters. Radiother Oncol. 2013;109:58-64.

57. Karam SD, et al. Dose escalation with stereotactic body radiation therapy boost for locally advanced non small cell lung cancer. Radiat Oncol. 2013;8:179.

58. Feddock J, et al. Stereotactic body radiation therapy can be used safely to boost residual disease in locally advanced non-small cell lung cancer:a prospective study. Int J Radiat Oncol Biol Phys. 2013;85:1325-31.

59. Udrescu C, Mornex F, Tanguy R, Chapet O. ExacTrac Snap Verification:a new tool for ensuring quality control for lung stereotactic body radiation therapy. Int J Radiat Oncol Biol Phys. 2013;85:e89-94.

60. Scagliotti GV, et al. Phase Ⅲ study comparing cisplatin plus gemcitabine with cisplatin plus pemetrexed in chemotherapy-naive patients with advanced-stage non-small-cell lung cancer. J Clin Oncol. 2008;26(21):3543-51.

61. Bischof M, Weber K-J, Blatter J, Wannenmacher M, Latz D. Interaction of pemetrexed disodium (ALIMTA, multitargetedantifolate) and irradiation in vitro. Int J Radiat Oncol Biol Phys. 2002;52:1381-8.

62. Cardenal F, et al. Phase I study of concurrent chemoradiation with pemetrexed and cisplatin followed by consolidation pemetrexed for patients with unresectable stage Ⅲ non-small cell

lung cancer. Lung Cancer. 2011;74:69-74.
63. Mornex F. Pemetrexed (PEM) and Cisplatin (CIS) in concurrent combination with high dose of thoracic Radiation (RT), after induction Chemotherapy (CT), in patients (PTS) with locally advanced Non-Small Cell Lung Cancer (NSCLC):a phase I study. Int J Radiat Oncol Biol Phys. 2010;78(3):S501-2.
64. Seiwert TY, et al. A phase I study of pemetrexed, carboplatin, and concurrent radiotherapy in patients with locally advanced or metastatic non-small cell lung or esophageal cancer. Clin Cancer Res. 2007;13:515-22.
65. Choy H, et al. Phase 2 study of pemetrexed plus carboplatin, or pemetrexed plus cisplatin with concurrent radiation therapy followed by pemetrexed consolidation in patients with favorableprognosis inoperable stage ⅢA/B non-small-cell lung cancer. J Thorac Oncol. 2013;8:1308-16.
66. Govindan R, et al. Randomized phase II study of pemetrexed, carboplatin, and thoracic radiation with or without cetuximab in patients with locally advanced unresectable non-small-cell lung cancer:Cancer and Leukemia Group B trial 30407. J Clin Oncol. 2011;29:3120-5.
67. Vokes EE, Senan S, Treat JA, Iscoe NA. PROCLAIM:a phase Ⅲ study of pemetrexed, cisplatin, and radiation therapy followed by consolidation pemetrexed versus etoposide, cisplatin, and radiation therapy followed by consolidation cytotoxic chemotherapy of choice in locally advanced stage Ⅲ non-small-cell lung cancer of other than predominantly squamous cell histology. Clin Lung Cancer. 2009;10:193-8.
68. Tredaniel J, et al. A phase II study of cetuximab, pemetrexed, cisplatin, and concurrent radiotherapy in patients with locally advanced, unresectable, stage Ⅲ, non squamous, non-small cell lung cancer (NSCLC). Rev Mal Respir. 2011;28:51-7.
69. Pirker R, et al. Cetuximab plus chemotherapy in patients with advanced non-small-cell lung cancer (FLEX):an open-label randomised phase Ⅲ trial. Lancet. 2009;373:1525-31.
70. Mak RH, et al. Outcomes after combined modality therapy for EGFR-mutant and wild-type locally advanced NSCLC. Oncologist. 2011;16:886-95.
71. Chinnaiyan P, et al. Mechanisms of enhanced radiation response following epidermal growth factor receptor signaling inhibition by erlotinib (Tarceva). Cancer Res. 2005;65:3328-35.
72. Choong NW, et al. Phase I trial of erlotinib-based multimodality therapy for inoperable stage Ⅲ non-small cell lung cancer. J Thorac Oncol. 2008;3:1003-11.
73. Rothschild S, et al. Gefitinib in combination with irradiation with or without cisplatin in patients with inoperable stage Ⅲ non-small cell lung cancer:a phase I trial. Int J Radiat Oncol Biol Phys. 2011;80:126-32.
74. Kelly K, et al. PhaseⅢ trial of maintenance gefitinib or placebo after concurrent chemoradiotherapy and docetaxel consolidation in inoperable stage Ⅲ non-small-cell lung cancer:SWOG S0023. J Clin Oncol. 2008;26:2450-6.
75. Komaki R, et al. Phase II trial of erlotinib and radiotherapy following chemoradiotherapy for patients with stage Ⅲ non-small cell lung cancer. ASCO Meet abstract. 2011. 29:7020.

76. Ready N, et al. Chemoradiotherapy and gefitinib in stage Ⅲ non-small cell lung cancer with epidermal growth factor receptor and KRAS mutation analysis: cancer and leukemia group B (CALEB) 30106, a CALGB-stratified phase II trial. J Thorac Oncol. 2010;5:1382-90.
77. Stinchcombe TE, et al. Induction chemotherapy with carboplatin, irinotecan, and paclitaxel followed by high dose three-dimension conformal thoracic radiotherapy (74 Gy) with concurrent carboplatin, paclitaxel, and gefitinib in unresectable stage ⅢA and stage ⅢB nonsmall cell lung cancer. J Thorac Oncol. 2008;3:250-7.
78. Goss GD, et al. Gefitinib versus placebo in completely resected non-small-cell lung cancer: results of the NCIC CTG BR19 study. J Clin Oncol. 2013;31:3320-6.
79. Lynch TJ, et al. Activating mutations in the epidermal growth factor receptor underlying responsiveness of non-small-cell lung cancer to gefitinib. N Engl J Med. 2004;350:2129-39.
80. Maemondo M, et al. Gefitinib or chemotherapy for non-small-cell lung cancer with mutated EGFR. N Engl J Med. 2010;362:2380-8.
81. Mitsudomi T, et al. Gefitinib versus cisplatin plus docetaxel in patients with non-small-cell lung cancer harbouring mutations of the epidermal growth factor receptor (WJTOG3405): an open label, randomised phase 3 trial. Lancet Oncol. 2010;11:121-8.
82. Zhou C, et al. Erlotinib versus chemotherapy as first-line treatment for patients with advanced EGFR mutation-positive non-small-cell lung cancer (OPTIMAL, CTONG-0802): a multicentre, open-label, randomised, phase 3 study. Lancet Oncol. 2011;12:735-42.
83. Rosell R, et al. Erlotinib versus standard chemotherapy as first-line treatment for European patients with advanced EGFR mutation-positive non-small-cell lung cancer (EURTAC): a multicentre, open-label, randomised phase 3 trial. Lancet Oncol. 2012;13:239-46.
84. Yang JC-H, et al. Afatinib for patients with lung adenocarcinoma and epidermal growth factor receptor mutations (LUX-Lung 2): a phase 2 trial. Lancet Oncol. 2012;13:539-48.
85. Sequist LV, et al. Phase Ⅲ study of afatinib or cisplatin plus pemetrexed in patients with metastatic lung adenocarcinoma with EGFR mutations. J Clin Oncol. 2013;31:3327-34.
86. Wu Y-L, et al. Afatinib versus cisplatin plus gemcitabine for first-line treatment of Asian patients with advanced non-small-cell lung cancer harbouring EGFR mutations (LUX-Lung 6): an open-label, randomised phase 3 trial. Lancet Oncol. 2014;15:213-22.
87. Shaw AT, et al. Crizotinib versus chemotherapy in advanced ALK-positive lung cancer. N Engl J Med. 2013;368:2385-94.
88. Kwak EL, et al. Anaplastic lymphoma kinase inhibition in non-small-cell lung cancer. N Engl J Med. 2010;363:1693-703.
89. Gan GN, et al. Stereotactic radiation therapy can safely and durably control sites of extracentral nervous system oligoprogressive disease in anaplastic lymphoma kinase-positive lung cancer patients receiving crizotinib. Int J Radiat Oncol Biol Phys. 2014. doi:10.1016/j.ijrobp.2013.11.010.
90. Weickhardt AJ, et al. Local ablative therapy of oligoprogressive disease prolongs disease control by tyrosine kinase inhibitors in oncogene-addicted non-small-cell lung cancer. J Thorac

Oncol. 2012;7:1807-14.
91. Sandler A, et al. Paclitaxel-carboplatin alone or with bevacizumab for non-small-cell lung cancer. N Engl J Med. 2006;355:2542-50.
92. Reck M, et al. PhaseⅢ trial of cisplatin plus gemcitabine with either placebo or bevacizumab as first-line therapy for nonsquamous non-small-cell lung cancer:AVAil. J Clin Oncol. 2009; 27:1227-34.
93. Spigel DR, et al. Tracheoesophageal fistula formation in patients with lung cancer treated with chemoradiation and bevacizumab. J Clin Oncol. 2010;28:43-8.
94. Stinchcombe T, et al. Phase I/II trial of bevacizumab (B) and erlotinib (E) with induction (IND) and concurrent (CON) carboplatin (Cb)/paclitaxel (P) and 74 Gy of thoracic conformal radiotherapy (TCRT) in stage Ⅲ non-small cell lung cancer (NSCLC). ASCO Meet Abstr. 2011;29:7016.
95. Hoang T, et al. Randomized phase Ⅲ study of thoracic radiation in combination with paclitaxel and carboplatin with or without thalidomide in patients with stage Ⅲ non-small-cell lung cancer:the ECOG 3598 study. J Clin Oncol. 2012;30:616-22.
96. Lu C, et al. Chemoradiotherapy with or without AE-941 in stage Ⅲ non-small cell lung cancer:a randomized phase Ⅲ trial. J Natl Cancer Inst. 2010;102:859-65.
97. Choy H, et al. Phase II multicenter study of induction chemotherapy followed by concurrent efaproxiral (RSR13) and thoracic radiotherapy for patients with locally advanced non-small-cell lung cancer. J Clin Oncol. 2005;23:5918-28.
98. Butts C, et al. A multi-centre phase IIB randomized controlled study of BLP25 liposome vaccine (L-BLP25 or Stimuvax) for active specific immunotherapy of non-small cell lung cancer (NSCLC):updated survival analysis:B1-01. J Thorac Oncol. 2007;2:S332-3.
99. Brunsvig PF, et al. Telomerase peptide vaccination in NSCLC:a phase II trial in stage Ⅲ patients vaccinated after chemoradiotherapy and an 8-year update on a phase I/II trial. Clin Cancer Res. 2011;17:6847-57.
100. Lopez Guerra JL, et al. Changes in pulmonary function after three-dimensional conformal radiotherapy, intensity-modulated radiotherapy, or proton beam therapy for non-small-cell lung cancer. Int J Radiat Oncol Biol Phys. 2012;83:e537-43.
101. Sejpal S, et al. Early findings on toxicity of proton beam therapy with concurrent chemotherapy for nonsmall cell lung cancer. Cancer. 2011;117:3004-13.
102. Park K, Ahn YC, Ahn JS, et al. A multinational phase Ⅲ randomized trial with or without consolidation chemotherapy using docetaxel and cisplatin after concurrent chemoradiation in inoperable stage Ⅲ non-small cell lung cancer. J Clin Oncol 32:5s, 2014 (suppl; abstr 7500).
103. Huber RM, Engel-Riedel W, Kollmeier J, et al. GILT study:Oral vinorelbine (NVBo) and cisplatin (P) with concomitant radiotherapy (RT) followed by either consolidation (C) with NVBo plus P plus best supportive care (BSC) or BSC alone in stage (st) Ⅲ non-small cell lung cancer (NSCLC):Final results of a phase (ph) Ⅲ study. J Clin Oncol 30, 2012 (suppl;

abstr 7001).

104. Bradley JD, Paulus R, Komaki R, et al. Randomized phase Ⅲ comparison of standard-dose (60 Gy) versus high-dose (74 Gy) conformal chemoradiotherapy ± cetuximab for stage ⅢA/ⅢB non-small cell lung cancer: Preliminary findings on radiation dose in RTOG 0617. Abstract LBA2. 53rd ASTRO Annual Meeting, 2011.

105. Bradley JD, Paulus R, Komaki R, et al. A randomized phase Ⅲ comparison of standard-dose (60 Gy) versus high-dose (74 Gy) conformal chemoradiotherapy with or without cetuximab for stage Ⅲ non-small cell lung cancer: Results on radiation dose in RTOG 0617. J Clin Oncol 31, 2013 (suppl; abstr 7501).

106. Vokes E, Wang L, Vansteenkiste J, et al. Preliminary Safety and Treatment Delivery Data During Concurrent Phase of Chemoradiation Therapy of the PROCLAIM Trial: A Phase 3 Trial of Pemetrexed, Cisplatin, and Radiotherapy Followed by Consolidation Pemetrexed Versus Etoposide, Cisplatin, and Radiotherapy Followed by Consolidation Cytotoxic Chemotherapy of Choice in Patients With Stage Ⅲ Nonsquamous Cell Lung Cancer. J Thor Oncol 8, 2013 (suppl 2; abstr P1. 09-009).

107. Mok T, Kim DW, Wu YL, et al. First-line crizotinib versus pemetrexed-cisplatin or pemetrexed-carboplatin in patients (pts) with advanced ALK-positive non-squamous non-small cell lung cancer (NSCLC): results of a phase Ⅲ study (PROFILE 1014). J Clin Oncol 32: 5s, 2014 (suppl; abstr 8002).

108. Butts CA, Socinski MA, Mitchell P, et al. START: A phase Ⅲ study of L-BLP25 cancer immunotherapy for unresectable stage Ⅲ non-small cell lung cancer. J Clin Oncol 31, 2013 (suppl; abstr 7500).

第7章
局部晚期非小细胞肺癌外科治疗

作者:Philippe G. Dartevelle,Sacha Mussot
译者:汪路明

肺癌侵犯胸壁

胸壁侵犯在肺癌中并不罕见,据统计,5%~8%的非小细胞肺癌患者术中会发现合并胸壁侵犯[1]。由于CT或骨骼ECT往往无法准确判定是否存在肋骨侵犯,因此往往需要依靠患者临床表现来判断评估。有研究证实CT扫描在评估壁层胸膜侵犯时会产生误判[2]。Rendina等[3]研究显示CT扫描胸膜增厚对判断胸膜侵犯并无裨益,但胸膜外脂肪垫消失可作为特异性指征。另外,直接侵犯导致肋骨破坏是胸壁侵犯的特异性指征。尽管MRI不作为常规检查手段,但理论上MRI对判断有无肌层侵犯存在优势。PET用于筛查有无远处转移,但由于分辨率原因,对于局部侵犯并不敏感。McCaughan等[4]报道在34%局部晚期患者中存在血清碱性磷酸酶的升高,但并非特异性指标。肺功能检查及肺灌注扫描可以帮助判断患者能否耐受手术及是否需重建反常运动的胸壁。

手术的目标是完整切除原发肿瘤及周围软组织,保证手术切缘阴性,并重建胸壁维持正常的呼吸功能。术前充分评估肿瘤侵犯胸壁的范围和部位,不仅可以避免在病灶附近开胸,导致肿瘤破溃,也可以帮助判断肿瘤侵犯范围和选择合适重建胸壁的材料。一般来说,侵犯胸壁肿瘤(除外侵犯胸廓入口及前胸壁的肿瘤)多采用标准后外侧切口。手术切除范围包括肿瘤侵犯的肋骨(连同相关肋间肌)及上下各一正常肋骨部分切除,切缘距肿瘤3~5cm。为避免肿瘤播散,肿瘤需行整块切除。一般来说,小范围侵犯胸壁切除后行肺切除相对容易。对于大范围侵犯来说,先用切割闭合器楔形切除肿瘤,连同胸壁组织完整切除肿瘤后,切除残余肺叶相对容易操作,术中冰冻切片检查可保证肿瘤完整切除。

大部分的胸壁切除患者不需要假体重建。肩胛骨的支撑能减少胸壁切除对功能及外观的影响,因此,不超过3根后肋的切除范围很少需要假体材料替代。大范围缺失,特别是位于前外侧的低位肋骨缺失,往往需要假体重建。但是,需权衡假体替代感染风险与功能外观受益之间的利弊。

胸壁重建可应用像聚四氟乙烯补片等软性材料来完成。对于较大和无支撑的缺损,可使用钛合金肋骨桥加强胸壁硬度[5]。目前,肌皮瓣重建胸壁已经很少应用[6]。重建材料的选择主要基于两点:绝对的无菌和最少的漏气。

所有 T3 期的肿瘤都是可切除的,但是预后取决于侵犯部位,在完整切除的所有 T3 肿瘤中,胸壁侵犯是预后最好的。R0 切除的 T3(胸壁侵犯)N0 期肺癌 5 年生存率超过 50%(表 7.1)。根据现有的文献报道,合并胸壁侵犯的肺癌患者 5 年生存率的决定因素为 R0 切除,胸壁浸润深度及淋巴结转移情况。非 R0 切除生存时间多低于 2.5 年[4,7-19],胸壁侵犯深度影响预后,仅有壁层胸膜侵犯患者 5 年生存率是深层侵犯患者的近 2 倍(62% vs 35%)[4]。局限于壁层胸膜侵犯的患者是否可行胸膜外切除(不切除相关软组织及骨组织,但切缘阴性)仍存在争议,McCaughan 等[4]研究证实对仅有壁层胸膜侵犯患者行胸膜外切除疗效确切,而 Piehler 等[8]报道该类患者行胸膜外切除局部复发率较高。Chapelier 等[16]也发现肿瘤累及壁层胸膜患者 5 年生存率显著优于胸壁深层侵犯患者。N2 阳性患者则多无法获得 5 年生存,而 N0 患者 5 年生存率可超过 50%,因此,PET 及纵隔镜可用于有胸壁侵犯且淋巴结肿大患者,如术前证实 N2 阳性,建议接受术前化疗或放化疗,根据是否降期来决定下一步治疗。

表 7.1 NSCLC 侵犯胸壁根治切除结果

作者	年	患者数量	手术死亡率(%)	5 年生存率(%)			
				所有患者	N0	N1	N2
Piehler [8]	1982	66	15.2	32.9	54.0	7.4[a]	7.4[a]
Patterson [9]	1982	35	8.5	38.0	NS	NS	0.0
McCaughan [4]	1985	125	4.0	40.0	56.0	21.0[a]	21.0[a]
Ratto [93]	1991	112	1.7	NS	50.0	25.0	0.0
Allen [10]	1991	52	3.8	26.3	29.0	11.0	NS
Shah and Goldstraw [11]	1995	58	3.4	37.2	45.0	38.0	0.0
Downey [12]	1999	175	6.0	36.0	56.0	13.0	29.0
Facciolo [13]	2001	104	0.0	61.4	67.0	100.0	17.0
Magdeleinat [14]	2001	201	7.0	21.0	25.0	21.0	20.0
Burkhart [8]	2002	94	6.3	38.7	44.0	26[a]	26.0[a]
Chapelier [16]	2000	100	1.8	18	22	9	0
Riquet [17]	2002	125	7	22.5	30.7	0	11.5
Roviaro [18]	2003	146	0.7	NS	78.5	7.2[a]	7.2[a]
Matsuoka [19]	2004	97	NS	34.2[b]	44.2	40.0	6.2

NS:原文未列出;[a]:N1 与 N2 未区分;[b]:完整切除

侵犯胸壁的肺癌患者是否需行术前及术后放疗目前存在广泛争议。术前放疗的潜在优势包括：使不可手术切除的肿瘤降期后存在切除可能，降低肿瘤切缘阳性率，降低手术时肿瘤种植风险[20]。然而，有研究认为术前放射治疗可降低该类患者的存活率[10,14]。目前，放疗主要非 R0 切除及肺门或纵隔淋巴结阳性患者的补救治疗，以降低肿瘤局部复发率。目前的研究认为辅助化疗对生存没有明显的影响，但可能是由于样本量偏少，尚不能获得统计学意义。

上沟瘤

上沟瘤指累及胸廓入口的良性及恶性肿瘤，常引起持续剧烈的肩臂痛，疼痛部位根据第八颈神经和第一、第二胸神经分布，也可导致 Horner 综合征和上肢肌无力及萎缩，临床又称为 Pancoast-Tobias 综合征。支气管肺癌为最常见的上沟瘤，其中非小细胞肺癌所占比例不到 5%，肿瘤起源于两肺上叶，外侵累及壁层胸膜、胸内筋膜、锁骨下血管、臂丛神经、椎体和第一肋骨。上沟瘤的临床表现取决于肿瘤部位，位于前斜角肌前的肿瘤常累及颈阔肌和胸锁乳突肌、颈内和颈前静脉、肩胛舌骨肌下部、锁骨下静脉和颈内静脉及其主要分支、前斜角肌脂肪垫。侵犯第一肋间神经及第一肋骨较侵犯膈神经及上腔静脉更常见，病人往往存在前上胸壁疼痛。

位于前斜角肌和中斜角肌之间的肿瘤可侵犯前斜角肌前方的膈神经，锁骨下动脉及后肩胛动脉的主要分支，臂丛神经干和中斜角肌（附录彩图 7.1）。肿瘤侵犯臂丛神经，可出现 T1（手臂尺侧和肘部）和 C8 神经根（前臂尺骨表面、小指和无名指）压迫相关的临床症状。

中斜角肌和后斜角肌之间的肿瘤常位于肋椎沟，可能侵犯 T1 神经根，锁骨下动脉和椎动脉后方，椎旁的交感神经链，颈下（星状）神经节和椎骨前肌肉。此类肿瘤可侵犯横突和椎体，如紧邻肋脊角或延伸至椎间孔但并未累及椎管内，则仍可手术切除。因上沟瘤多位于肺外周，肺部症状，如咳嗽、咯血和呼吸困难在初期并不常见。T2 肋间臂神经压迫导致腋窝及上臂中部感觉异常及疼痛也较为常见。随着肿瘤增大进展，患者可出现典型的 Pancoast 综合征。

上沟瘤在初期阶段诊断比较困难，Pancoast-Tobias 综合征出现到诊断平均周期约 6 个月。患者在 X 线胸片上表现为隐藏在锁骨和第一肋骨后面的肺尖部小肿瘤。确诊需结合病史、体格检查、生化检测、X 线胸片、气管镜、痰细胞学检查、经胸或经皮细针穿刺活检及胸部 CT。如 X 线胸片有证据显示纵隔淋巴结肿大，建议行胸部 CT 或 PET-CT 扫描、组织病理学确诊。对 N2 期患者应放弃手术治疗。神经系统检查，MRI 和 PET 检查可明确肿瘤有无累及臂丛神经、膈神经和硬膜外腔。血管造影、锁骨下动脉造影、多普勒超声检查（脑血管异常可能影响椎血管判断）和 MRI 常用于评估有无血管侵犯。当肿瘤长入椎间孔时需常规行 MRI 检查

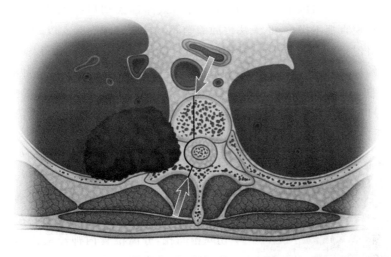

图 7.1　左上沟支气管肺癌侵犯胸廓入口，包括锁骨下动脉。箭头示达到 R0 切除的切除范围

以排除硬膜外腔侵犯。

任何肺切除术前初步评估还包括常规心肺功能评估和有无远处转移相关检查。

外科手术是根治上沟瘤的唯一方法，但上沟瘤的治疗仍需进一步优化，目前上沟瘤的传统治疗模式是 45 年前确定的术前辅助放疗联合手术治疗，该治疗模式的临床证据是基于与历史对照获得相对较好的短期生存[21]。有研究尝试使用大剂量初始放疗[22]，三明治治疗模式，即术前及术后放疗[23]，术后单用放疗[24]，术中短距离放疗联合术前放疗和手术治疗[25]等方式治疗上沟瘤。2001 年，SWOG 9416（Intergroup 0160）[26]开始开展多中心的研究，以评估诱导放化疗和手术治疗上沟瘤的临床效果，并于 2003 年发表研究结果[27]。随后多个中心开始尝试使用术前同期放化疗[28,29]，结果发现 92% 患者获得完整切除，明显优于传统治疗模式平均 66% 的切除率[26,30]。尽管没有随机对照研究比较两种方法的优劣[31]，目前的研究结果认为术前放化疗优于单纯放疗，可作为 Pancoast 肿瘤新的标准治疗模式。我们认为可对新诊断上沟瘤患者先手术切除，因为术前放化疗无疑会增加手术难度及术后并发症发生率，放疗可用于术后辅助治疗。

上沟瘤手术绝对禁忌证：①胸腔外转移；②N2 淋巴结转移；③广泛的 T1 神经根以上的颈段气管、食管和臂丛神经浸润。上述情况表明难以达到局部完全 R0 切除或提示需行截肢手术。目前，锁骨下血管侵犯不再作为手术禁忌证考虑。术前诊断的广泛椎体侵犯提示无法完全切除。椎间孔累及但未侵犯椎管的上沟瘤可行手术切除。

未累及胸廓入口的上沟瘤一般均可经后入路邵氏切口手术切除[21]。因后路切口无法实现直视下操作,也无法按肿瘤学间隙结构解剖胸廓入口,上沟瘤一旦出现胸廓入口侵犯建议行前路经颈入路切口[24,32]。该手术入路目前已作为所有良恶性上沟瘤的标准入路,包括非气管肿瘤(如第一肋骨肉瘤和臂丛神经肿瘤)。该入路也可以良好显露上胸椎前外侧面。该手术入路的禁忌证为:①胸腔外转移;②T1神经根以上的臂丛神经侵犯;③广泛的斜角肌和胸外肌侵犯;④纵隔淋巴结转移;⑤严重的心肺疾病。

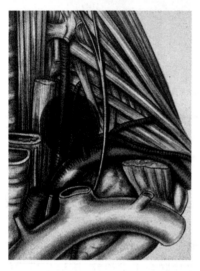

图7.2 右胸顶肿瘤侵犯肋横突间隙、椎间孔和部分同侧椎体;先行前路切口分离肿瘤,然后经后中线切口行半椎体切除

我们曾报道适用于位于后侧的侵犯椎间孔但未累及椎管的上沟瘤切除技术[33],该技术术中需与脊柱外科医生合作。该手术通过前经颈入路和后中线入路联合完成,关键在于能通过切除椎间孔,分离椎管内神经根达到肿瘤的完整切除(附录彩图7.2)。该术式手术并发症发生率为7%~38%,手术死亡率为5%~10%[34-48]。

隆突切除

外科手术器械的改进及支气管袖式肺叶切除的开展为隆突切除及重建奠定了基础。但由于手术并发症多,技术操作要求高,且临床证据支持少,目前仅有少数中心拥有安全开展该术式的经验。但是,近期的一系列研究证实隆突切除在经验丰富的中心能安全开展,围术期死亡率低于10%,部分患者可获得良好的长期生存。目前研究结果大大优于早期系列报道,可能与手术及麻醉技术的提高相关。

合适手术患者选择和对病灶的详细评估是隆突切除患者获得良好生存的关键。所有患者均需评估以确保能耐受手术及肺实质切除。术前评估包括:X线胸片、胸部CT扫描、肺功能检查、动脉血气分析、通气/灌注扫描、心电图和超声心动图,必要时可行最大耗氧量及运动耐量试验。

隆突切除手术为择期手术,术前准备包括:胸部理疗、深呼吸训练和停止吸烟;气道阻塞、支气管痉挛及并发肺部感染的治疗;术前停止应用激素。术前需行软质或硬质气管镜检查以评估肿瘤大小,残留气道长度是否足够行无张力吻合。对支气管肺癌患者除完善常规检查以排除胸外转移外,术中我们常规行纵隔镜检查以明确有无N2或N3转移。

表 7.2 上沟瘤患者手术切除结果

作者及发表时间	患者数量(例)	5 年生存率(%)	死亡率(%)
Paulson,1985 [35]	79	35	3
Anderson,1986 [36]	28	34	7
Devine,1986 [37]	40	10	8
Miller,1987 [38]	36	31	NS
Wright,1987 [39]	21	27	—
Shahian,1987 [23]	18	56	—
McKneally,1987 [40]	25	51	NS
Komaki,1990 [22]	25	40	NS
Sartori,1992 [41]	42	25	2.3
Maggi,1994 [42]	60	17.4	5
Ginsberg,1994 [43]	100	26	4
Okubo 1995 [44]	18	38.5	5.6
Dartevelle,1997 [45]	70	34	—
Martinod,2002 [46]	139	35	7.2
Alifano,2003 [47]	67	36.2	8.9
Goldberg,2005 [48]	39	47.9	5%
总计	807	34.5±11.7[a]	5.6±2.2[a]

NS:原文未说明

[a] 平均数±标准差

另外右上肺前段来源的隆突肿瘤需行肺血管成像,因为肿瘤侵犯右上肺动脉往往提示侵犯上腔静脉后方。上腔静脉可能受侵患者需行上腔静脉造影以明确诊断。经食管超声检查有时可用于评估有无后纵隔侵犯,特别是食管或左心房。

适应证及禁忌证

下段气管和对侧主支气管之间的安全切除长度一般是 4cm。这对右全肺及隆突切除,气管远端与左主支气管端端吻合尤为重要。主动脉弓干扰易造成吻合口张力过高,因此,左主支气管上移距离有限。

隆突切除适用于肿瘤侵犯主支气管距离隆突小于 1cm、下段气管侧壁、隆突或对侧主支气管的患者。该术式多用于右侧支气管肿瘤,因为左侧支气管较长且主动脉弓下空间较小,肿瘤常见大范围周围组织侵犯,而仅有隆突累及少见。由于 N2 或 N3 期支气管肺癌患者隆突切除长期生存较差,因此,一旦术前纵隔镜确诊纵隔淋巴结转移常作为手术禁忌证。诱导治疗可使部分患者获益,但我们的经验证实诱导治疗可以增加手术的技术难度并增加围术期死亡率,尤其是涉及隆突重建的全肺切除。

外科技术

关于隆突切除手术技术我们已在相关文献中详细叙述[49,50],在此仅强调部分关键点,术中通气是隆突切除手术的技术关键,我们的技术和 Grillo 等[51]的报道类似。首先,利用一根增长的经口气管插管进入对侧支气管以实现单肺通气。隆突切除后,台上将无菌气管插管插到对侧主支气管并连接无菌通气系统。该插管可以安全移动以腾出缝合气管空间。

入路

手术入路因隆突切除方式而改变。

如 Pearson 等的报道[51-53],隆突切除无需切肺,而且一般经正中胸骨切口入路。我们发现,该入路也适合所有肺切除手术,包括左全肺切除。

隆突切除同时行肺切除术式的手术入路取决于肺切除术式。右侧经第五肋间后外侧切口可以很好的暴露主气管下段及两侧主支气管起始段。对左侧而言,暴露主气管下段及右侧主支气管受主动脉弓影响,这就是选择正中胸骨切开入路行左侧隆突重建的全肺切除的原因。

隆突重建类型

1. 单纯隆突切除不合并肺切除　隆突切除不合并肺切除仅限于肿瘤位于隆突或左右主支气管起始段。根据侵犯范围不同可采用不同的重建方式。对位于隆突的小肿瘤,可将左右主支气管内侧壁重建隆突后与主气管吻合(附录彩图 7.3)。如果侵犯范围更大,需要切除更长段气管,端端吻合或端侧吻合是较合理的选择。

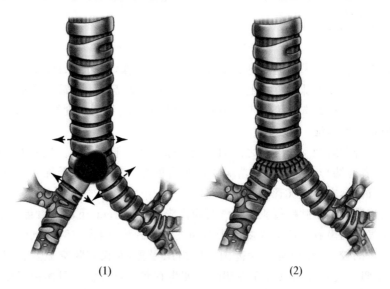

图 7.3　隆突切除后"新隆突"重建(1),隆突病灶小范围侵犯主气管(1)。虚线为拟切割线(1)。左右主支气管内侧壁用 4-0 PDS 缝线行间断缝合成"新隆突"(2)

2. 右全肺切除隆突重建　右全肺切除隆突重建是支气管肺癌隆突切除最常见的术式。

3. 隆突切除合并肺叶切除　右上肺肿瘤侵犯隆突及下段主气管时需行该术式。

4. 左全肺切除隆突重建　左全肺切除隆突重建受主动脉弓影响解剖相对困难。对于术前预计行该术式的患者我们的经验是行正中胸骨切开入路[54]，而不是早期的左侧开胸入路。

支气管肺癌切除隆突重建的手术治疗效果有所改善。近期报道显示对有经验的中心经选择病人隆突切除相对安全且可获得满意的长期生存。本中心中位死亡率小于7%，中位5年生存率可达到43.3%（表7.3）。

表7.3　全肺切除隆突重建患者的死亡率及5年生存率

作者及发表时间	患者数量(例)	手术死亡率(%)	5年生存率(%)
Jensik,1982 [55]	34	29	15
Deslauriers,1989 [56]	38	29	13
Tsuchiya,1990 [57]	20	40	59（2年生存率）
Mathisen,1991 [58]	37	18.9	19
Roviaro,1994 [59]	28	4	20
Dartevelle,1995 [60]	60	6.6	43.3
Mitchell,1999 [61]	143	12.7	42
Roviaro,2001 [62]	49	8.2	24.5
Porhanov,2002 [63]	231	16	24.7
Regnard,2005 [64]	65	7.7	26.5
de Perrot,2006 [54]	119	7.6	44
Macchiarini,2006 [65]	50	4	51
总计	874	10.4±11.6	25.6±15.2

合并纵隔淋巴结转移患者的预后较差，因此，该类患者被认为是隆突切除相对禁忌证。需进一步研究以确定诱导治疗对合并N2转移支气管肺癌患者的作用，目前认为若可使纵隔淋巴结阳性转阴，术前诱导治疗可改善预后，但另一方面，诱导治疗可增加右全肺切除隆突重建患者的手术并发症发生率及死亡率。近期我们的研究发现诱导治疗使右全肺切除隆突重建患者手术相关死亡率从6.7%增加到13%[54]。Martin等[66]则报道诱导治疗后的右全肺切除死亡率高达24%。

上腔静脉侵犯

上腔静脉综合征是良性或恶性疾病阻塞上腔静脉回流所引起的临床症状。右侧支气管肺癌侵犯上腔静脉占肺癌手术患者的1%[67]。由于手术预后较差、缺乏合适的重建材料、上腔静脉阻断技术顾虑、移植物血栓以及感染问题的存在,上腔静脉综合征一直被认为是手术的绝对禁忌证。但近期实验及临床进步使上腔静脉重建技术得以普及,胸腔恶性肿瘤患者的手术适应证得以扩大[66-78]。尽管上腔静脉切除重建对技术要求较高,但经选择的局部晚期肺癌患者手术预后良好。

上腔静脉综合征患者的临床症状及体征相对典型,不易混淆。最常见症状依次为:呼吸困难、充血、咳嗽、上肢及颜面部水肿。不常见症状包括:胸痛、吞咽困难、晕厥、咯血和头痛。最常见体征为颜面部及上肢水肿、颈部及胸壁静脉曲张、发绀和多血症。在多数患者,上腔静脉综合征隐匿并缓慢进展。短期内出现的上腔静脉综合征一般病因为恶性肿瘤或导管相关血栓栓塞所致。而慢性症状往往与导管血栓以外的非恶性疾病相关。对于恶性疾病患者从上腔静脉综合征初发症状到症状明显时间为 3.2~6.5 周。

纵隔肿瘤患者往往表现为 X 线胸片检查发现上纵隔增宽。胸部 CT 能显示上腔静脉及其分支等相关解剖结构。横断面、冠状面及矢状面磁共振成像能清晰呈现肿瘤与周围血管的关系。上腔静脉造影(两上肢同时注射造影剂)应作为外科手术前常规检查。超声心动图检查可以排除延伸至右心房、颈静脉或腋静脉的血栓。脑 CT 扫描可以排除夹闭上腔静脉时可能引起脑水肿的脑部疾病。痰细胞学检查、气管镜、锁骨上淋巴结活检、胸腔穿刺活检、纵隔镜检查、骨髓穿刺活检和开胸活检等可以明确组织学诊断。

术前评估重点为充分评估肿瘤及血管侵及范围,注意静脉钳闭后的血流动力学变化并选择合适的上腔静脉重建材料,可以提高上腔静脉切除重建手术的安全有效性。

血管适应证

术后可能形成移植物血栓,造成肺栓塞风险并产生严重后果。上腔静脉重建只有在颅内静脉床开放良好的情况下进行。

上腔静脉阻断后的血流动力学影响

上腔静脉阻断对血流动力学影响因上腔静脉阻塞程度不同而不同,Dartevelle 等[69]证实减少静脉阻断时间并给予抗凝治疗可逆转上腔静脉阻断导致的血流动力学影响。

Spaggiari 等[79]回顾 109 例行上腔静脉切除肺癌患者文献资料,分析其预后相关因素,发现围术期并发症发生率为 30%,死亡率为 12%,5 年生存率 21%,中位生存期为 11 个月,术前诱导治疗患者主要并发症发生率增加。肺切除术式(如全肺切除)和上腔静脉切除术式(如全部切除假体置换)[80]是影响患者术后生存的预后因素。

最近,Suzuki 等[77]和 Shargall 等[78]报道了 55 例肺癌合并上腔静脉综合征患者行手术切除的死亡率为 12%,并发症发生率和死亡率与是否行全肺切除隆突重建等相关,而与是否行上腔静脉切除无明显相关性。

侵犯左心房、主动脉及肺动脉主干

肿瘤侵犯左心房、主动脉和肺动脉主干的患者,完整切除肿瘤比较困难,且围术期死亡率较高。对于这类 T4 期肺癌患者手术价值尚缺乏统一定论。大动脉侵犯的 T4 期肺癌长期生存极差。完全切除的心包内肺动脉主干或左心房局部侵犯患者 5 年生存率为 20%～30%[81]。一般来说,心包内侵犯距离小于 1～1.5cm 都能保证 R0 切除及血管断端安全闭合。多数专家认为需要体外循环(CPB)辅助的胸部肿瘤切除应列为相对禁忌证,但近期也有研究表明体外循环支持下行扩大肺切除,可获得更高的完整切除率[70,82-90]。据统计目前仅有不到 0.1% 的胸部肿瘤切除手术使用体外循环。

外科根治手术应基于患者体质和多学科评估讨论后制定,胸腔外转移为手术禁忌。治疗方案的选择应以有效为目的,部分患者可选用姑息性治疗。

大部分局部晚期肺癌的切除并不需要体外循环。体外循环主要适用于癌瘤侵犯主动脉弓、降主动脉、肺动脉分叉、左心房及隆突。体外循环对肺功能及其他脏器功能的副作用在文献中已详细阐述,但是否会引起肿瘤播散目前知之甚少。部分恶性肿瘤画着经体外循环辅助肿瘤切除后可获得长期无疾病生存,表明使用体外循环并不增加肿瘤播散风险,但也有少量个案报道认为体外循环可使肿瘤发生播散[82]。如何选择合适适应证患者是局部晚期肿瘤行体外循环支持下切除的关键。

术前评估

胸部 CT 是术前评估最基本的检查手段。术前完整的生化及影像学检查可以排除颅脑、腹部和骨骼转移。主动脉弓和弓上分支血管造影和经食管超声检查可以明确有无左锁骨下动脉和食管壁侵犯。颈动脉和椎动脉的多普勒检查可以确保四支血管的畅通。磁共振成像可以排除椎间孔侵犯。

非小细胞肺癌侵犯左心房在根治性开胸手术患者中所占比例不到 4%。肿瘤直接侵犯左心房较癌栓从肺静脉延伸至左心房更常见。对大部分患者,可在血管钳钳夹左心房后切除肿瘤及肺静脉,而后一般可以直接缝合左心房缺损。如左心房侵犯范围较大,肿瘤往往沿心肌肌层浸润而无法根治切除。因此,我们的经验是体外循环很少应用于左心房切除手术,有报道认为体外循环可以应用于肿瘤长入左房腔而有肿瘤栓塞风险患者,在主动脉阻断灌注至心脏停搏或低温纤颤后,体外循环可允许术中打开心房腔而避免气栓风险。左房壁部分侵犯患者不应视为手术禁忌证,手术是患者获得根治的唯一希望[7,70,86-89]。

非小细胞肺癌侵犯主动脉的报道较少,主要因为肿瘤侵犯主动脉往往无法手术根治性切除。非小细胞肺癌侵犯主动脉往往局限于动脉外膜。然而,在少数存在动脉肌层侵犯患者,手术切除侵犯管壁需钳闭动脉的近心端和远心端。建议升主动脉与降主动脉间的人工血管置换以切除侵犯动脉段并重建血运。我们认为体外循环是主动脉夹闭期间保证上下肢端血流灌注最简单有效的方法。

并发症

通过测量肺泡-动脉氧和梯度、肺内分流、肺水肿程度、肺顺应性和肺血管阻力,大量证据证实体外循环可影响肺功能。体外循环后长时间机械通气可导致更多更严重的并发症。我们的经验认为[82],T4期肺癌体外循环支持下切除后,喉返神经麻痹相关的肺水肿、急性呼吸窘迫综合征和肺不张等肺部并发症常见,出血也比较常见,体外循环支持下同期行心脏手术和肺切除患者,出血并发症发生率高达21%。

手术治疗肺动脉主干侵犯肿瘤相关报道较少,Ricci等[90]对3例非小细胞肺癌侵犯肺动脉主干患者行体外循环辅助下血管成形术,所有患者术后存活均不超过25个月。Tsuchiya等[70]体外循环辅助下行肺动脉分叉置换6例患者均在术后30个月内死亡。因此,肺动脉主干侵犯被认为是可切除但生物学上不可治愈。

主动脉和左心房切除重建被认为相对较安全,术后5年生存率高于20%(表7.4)。Fukuse等[85]行肺联合主动脉切除术后5年生存率为31%($n=15$)。Bobbio等[86]行肺联合左心房切除患者5年生存率为10%($n=23$)。最近,Ohta等[91]报道16例患者行胸主动脉联合肺切除围术期死亡率为12.5%,N0期5年生存率为70%,N2或N3期5年生存率为16.7%。

表7.4 NSCLC侵犯左心房患者手术结果

作者及发表时间	患者数量(例)	手术死亡率(%)	5年生存率(%)
Shirakusa,1991 [87]	12	8.3	NS
Martini,1994 [88]	8	NS	12.5
Tsuchiya,1994 [70]	44	NS	22
Macchiarini,1997 [7]	31	3.2	21.6
Ratto,2004 [89]	19	0	14
Bobbio,2004 [86]	23	9	10
总计	137	5.75 ± 4.2	14.0 ± 5.4

NS:原文未说明

本中心[82]体外循环辅助下行NSCLC切除患者7例无围术期死亡,并发症发生率为28%($n=2$)。7例患者中,1例术后6月死于肺栓塞,3例无术后复发,另3例复发但仍存活。

体外循环应用似乎并不增加肿瘤播散风险,研究报道证实肺癌行肺切除联合冠状动脉旁路移植尽管应用体外循环辅助但仍可获得满意的早期及长期生存。

局部晚期肺癌患者长期生存主要取决于是否根治切除。Martini 等[88]报道肺癌侵犯纵隔完全切除术后 5 年生存率为 30%,而姑息性切除仅为 14%。肺癌侵犯心脏或大血管患者,完全切除 5 年生存率分别为 23% 和 40%,而不完全切除患者生存不超过 3 年。

局部晚期 NSCLC 行体外循环辅助切除治疗效果需进一步研究证实,总的来说,局部晚期 NSCLC 患者需秉承长期生存获益最大化和治疗风险最小化原则的多学科综合治疗模式。

侵犯椎体

非小细胞肺癌直接侵犯椎体或肋脊角较上沟瘤少见。治疗方式有单纯放疗,椎骨切除及部分椎骨切除。DeMeester 等[92]的研究为肿瘤局部侵犯第三椎体以下骨膜手术切除提供证据,证实 5 年生存率达 42%,部分患者可行术前辅助放疗(30Gy)联合原发肿瘤和侵犯椎体整块切除而获得治愈。可根据术前影像学检查有无骨质破坏,术中有无肋横突侵犯评估手术切除可能性。对于侵犯范围大的肿瘤,McCormack[67]证实椎体切除联合脊柱固定术后 5 年生存率为 10%;但是对该类手术的价值尚无定论。

结论

外科手术技术的进步使局部晚期非小细胞肺癌患者的手术切除可能性及根治性大大提高。围术期管理和术后护理的进步,病人适应证优化,使手术并发症发生率和死亡率明显下降,患者预后改善。

T3 期或 T4 期肿瘤患者的预后主要取决于 N 分期已获得证实。N0 期或 N1 期患者行根治性切除可显著改善预后。而手术技术的复杂性和患者的罕见性则要求外科医生具有丰富的胸外科和血管外科经验。

我们认为,局部晚期肺癌患者应首选手术治疗,特别是对于可完整切除的患者。根治切除可改善患者的 5 年生存,特别是肺癌侵犯主气管或隆突患者(5 年生存率为 40%)。局部晚期肿瘤尝试降期后切除给外科医生带来了新的困惑:手术切除包含原病灶的所有病灶还是仅切除降期后残余病灶。

总的来说,不管局部晚期非小细胞肺癌是否能够通过手术根治,胸外科医生团队均应努力去实现局部晚期肺癌的根治性切除手术,扩大局部晚期肺癌的手术适应证。

参考文献

1. Grillo HC. Pleural and chest wall involvement. Int Trends Gen Thorac Surg. 1985;1;134-8.
2. Akay H, Cangir AK, Kutlay H, et al. Surgical treatment of peripheral lung cancer adherent to the parietal pleura. Eur J Cardiothorac Surg. 2002;22(4):615-20.

3. Rendina EA, Bognolo DA, Mineo TC, et al. Computed tomography for the evaluation of intrathoracic invasion by lung cancer. J Thorac Cardiovasc Surg. 1987;94:57-63.
4. McCaughan BC, Martini N, Bains MS, et al. Chest wall invasion in carcinoma of the lung. J Thorac Cardiovasc Surg. 1985;89:836-41.
5. Fabre D, El Batti S, Singhal S, Mercier O, Mussot S, Fadel E, Kolb F, Dartevelle PG. A paradigm shift for sternal reconstruction using a novel titanium rib bridge system following oncological resections. Eur J Cardiothorac Surg. 2012;42(6):965-70.
6. McCormack PM, Bains M, Beattie Jr EJ, Martini N. New trends in skeletal reconstruction after resection of chest wall tumors. Ann Thorac Surg. 1981;31:45-52.
7. Macchiarini P, Dartevelle P. Extended resections for lung cancer. In:Roth JA, Cox J, Hong WK, editors. Lung cancer. 2nd ed. London:Blackwell Science; 1998. p. 135-61.
8. Piehler JM, Pairolero PC, Weiland LH, et al. Bronchogenic carcinoma with chest wall invasion: factors affecting survival following en bloc resection. Ann Thorac Surg. 1982;34:684-91.
9. Patterson GA, Ilves R, Ginsberg RJ, et al. The value of adjuvant radiotherapy in pulmonary and chest wall resection for bronchogenic carcinoma. Ann Thorac Surg. 1982;34:692-7.
10. Allen MS, Mathisen DJ, Grillo HC. Bronchogenic carcinoma with chest wall invasion. Ann Thorac Surg. 1991;51:948-51.
11. Shah SS, Goldstraw P. Combined pulmonary and thoracic wall for resection for stage III lung cancer. Thorax. 1995;50:782-4.
12. Downey RJ, Martini N, Rusch VW, et al. Extent of chest wall invasion and survival in patients with lung cancer. Ann Thorac Surg. 1999;68:188-93.
13. Facciolo F, Cardillo G, Lopergolo M, et al. Chest wall invasion in non-small cell lung carcinoma:a rationale for en bloc resection. J Thorac Cardiovasc Surg. 2001;121:649-56.
14. Magdeleinat P, Alifona M, Benbrahem C, et al. Surgical treatment of lung cancer invading the chest wall:results and prognostic factors. Ann Thorac Surg. 2001;71:1094-9.
15. Burkhart HM, Allen MS, Nichols III FC, et al. Results of en bloc resection for bronchogenic carcinoma with chest wall invasion. J Thorac Cardiovasc Surg. 2002;123(4):670-5.
16. Chapelier A, Fadel E, Macchiarini P, et al. Factors affecting long-term survival after en bloc resection of lung cancer invading the chest wall. Eur J Cardiothorac Surg. 2000;18:513-8.
17. Riquet M, Lang-Lazdunski L, Le PB, et al. Characteristics and prognosis of resected T3 non-small cell lung cancer. Ann Thorac Surg. 2002;73(1):253-8.
18. Roviaro G, Varoli F, Grignani F, et al. Non-small cell lung cancer with chest wall invasion:evolution of surgical treatment and prognosis in the last 3 decades. Chest. 2003;123(5):1341-7.
19. Matsuoka H, Nishio W, Okada M, et al. Resection of chest wall invasion in patients with non small cell lung cancer. Eur J Cardiothorac Surg. 2004;26(6):1200-4.
20. Allen MS. Chest wall resection and reconstruction for lung cancer. Thorac Surg Clin. 2004;14:211-6.
21. Shaw RR, Paulson DL, Kee Jr JL. Treatment of superior sulcus tumors by irradiation followed by resection. Ann Surg. 1961;154:29-40.

22. Komaki R, et al. Superior sulcus tumors:treatment selection and results for 85 patients without metastasis (M0) at presentation. Int J Radiat Oncol Biol Phys. 1990;19:31.
23. Shahian DM, Neptune WB, Ellis Jr FH. Pancoast tumors:improved survival with preoperative and postoperative radiotherapy. Ann Thorac Surg. 1987;43:32.
24. Dartevelle P, Chapelier A, Macchiarini P, et al. Anterior transcervical-thoracic approach for radical resection of lung tumors invading the thoracic inlet. J Thorac Cardiovasc Surg. 1993;105:1025.
25. Hilaris BS, Martini N, Wong GY, et al. Treatment of superior sulcus tumors (Pancoast tumor). Surg Clin North Am. 1987;67:965-77.
26. Rusch VW, Giroux DJ, Kraut MJ, et al. Induction chemoradiation and surgical resection for non-small cell lung carcinomas of the superior sulcus:initial results of Southwest Oncology Group Trial 9416 (Intergroup Trial 0160). J Thorac Cardiovasc Surg. 2001;121:472-83.
27. Rusch VW, Giroux D, Kraut MJ, et al. Induction chemoradiotherapy and surgical resection for non-small cell lung carcinomas of the superior sulcus (Pancoast tumors):mature results of Southwest Oncology Group trial 9416 (Intergroup 0160). Proc Am Soc Clin Oncol. 2003;22:2548.
28. Wright CD, Menard MT, Wain JC, et al. Induction chemoradiation compared with induction radiation for lung cancer involving the superior sulcus. Ann Thorac Surg. 2002;73:1541-4.
29. Kunitoh H, Kato H, Tsuboi M, et al. A phase II trial of pre-operative chemoradiotherapy followed by surgical resection in Pancoast tumors:initial report of Japan Clinical Oncology Group trial (JCOG 9806). Proc Am Soc Clin Oncol. 2003;22:2549.
30. Detterbeck FC, Jones DR, Rosenman JG. Pancoast tumors. In:Detterbeck FC, Rivera MP, Socinski MA, Rosenman JG, editors. Diagnosis and treatment of lung cancer:an evidence based guide for the practicing clinician. Philadelphia:WB Saunders; 2001. p. 233-43.
31. Detterbeck FC. Changes in the treatment of Pancoast tumors. Ann Thorac Surg. 2003;75(6):1990-7.
32. Dartevelle PG, Mussot S. Anterior approach to superior sulcus lesions. In:Shields TW, Locicero Ⅲ J, Ponn RB, Rusch VW, editors. General thoracic surgery. 6th ed. Philadelphia:Lippincott Williams and Wilkins; 2005. p. 545-53.
33. Fadel E, Missenard G, Chapelier A, Mussot S, Leroy-Ladurie F, Cerrina J, Dartevelle P. En bloc resection of non-small cell lung cancer invading the thoracic inlet and intervertebral foramina. J Thorac Cardiovasc Surg. 2002;123(4):676-85.
34. Pitz CC, de la Riviere AB, van Swieten HA, et al. Surgical treatment of Pancoast tumours. Eur J Cardiothorac Surg. 2004;26(1):202-8.
35. Paulson DL. Technical considerations in stage T3 disease:the superior sulcus lesion. In:Delarue NC, Eschapasse H, editors. International trends in thoracic surgery, vol. 1. Philadelphia:WB Saunders; 1985. p. 121.
36. Anderson TM, Moy PM, Holmes EC. Factors affecting survival in superior sulcus tumors. J Clin Oncol. 1986;4:1598.

37. Devine JW, et al. Carcinoma of the superior pulmonary sulcus treated with surgery and/or radiation therapy. Cancer. 1986;57:941.
38. Miller JI, Mansour KA, Hatcher Jr CR. Carcinoma of the superior pulmonary sulcus. Ann Thorac Surg. 1979;28:44.
39. Wright CD, et al. Superior sulcus lung tumors. Results of combined treatment (irradiation and radical resection). J Thorac Cardiovasc Surg. 1987;94:69.
40. McKneally M, Discussion of Shahian DM, Neptune WB, Ellis FH Jr. Pancoast tumors: improved survival with preoperative and postoperative radiotherapy. Ann Thorac Surg. 1987;43:32.
41. Sartori F, et al. Carcinoma of the superior pulmonary sulcus. Results of irradiation and radical resection. J Thorac Cardiovasc Surg. 1992;104:679.
42. Maggi G, et al. Combined radiosurgical treatment of Pancoast tumor. Ann Thorac Surg. 1994;57:198.
43. Ginsberg RJ, et al. Influence of surgical resection and brachytherapy in the management of superior sulcus tumors. Ann Thorac Surg. 1994;57:1440.
44. Okubo K, et al. Treatment of Pancoast tumors. Combined irradiation and radical resection. Thorac Cardiovasc Surg. 1995;43:84.
45. Dartevelle P. Extended operations for lung cancer. Ann Thorac Surg. 1997;63:12.
46. Martinod E, D'Audiffret A, Thomas P, et al. Management of superior sulcus tumors: experience with 139 cases treated by surgical resection. Ann Thorac Surg. 2002;73:1534-9.
47. Alifano M, D'Aiuto M, Magdeleinat P, et al. Surgical treatment of superior sulcus tumors: results and prognostic factors. Chest. 2003;124(3):996-1003.
48. Goldberg M, Gupta D, Sasson AR, et al. The surgical management of superior sulcus tumors: a retrospective review with long-term follow-up. Ann Thorac Surg. 2005;79(4):1174-9.
49. Dartevelle P, Macchiarini P. Carinal resection for bronchogenic cancer. Semin Thorac Cardiovasc Surg. 1996 Oct;8(4):414-25. Review.
50. Dartevelle P, Macchiarini P. Techniques of pneumonectomy. Sleeve pneumonectomy. Chest Surg Clin N Am. 1999 May;9(2):407-17, xi. Review.
51. Grillo HC, Bendixen HH, Gephart T. Resection of the carina and lower trachea. Ann Surg. 1963;158:889-93.
52. Pearson FG, Todd TRJ, Cooper JD. Experience with primary neoplasms of the trachea and carina. J Thorac Cardiovasc Surg. 1984;88:511-8.
53. Barclay RS, McSwann N, Welsh TM. Tracheal reconstruction without the use of grafts. Thorax. 1957;12:177-80.
54. dePerrot M, Fadel E, Mercier O, et al. Long-term results after carinal resection for carcinoma: does the benefit warrant the risk? J Thorac Cardiovasc Surg. 2006;131(1):81-9.
55. Jensik RJ, Faber LP, Kittle CF, Miley RW, Thatcher WC, El-Baz N. Survival in patients undergoing tracheal sleeve pneumonectomy for bronchogenic carcinoma. J Thorac Cardiovasc

Surg. 1982;84:489-96.
56. Deslauriers J, Beaulieu M, McClish A. Tracheal-sleeve pneumonectomy. In:Shields TW, editor. General thoracic surgery. 3rd ed. Philadelphia:Lea & Febiger; 1989. p. 383-7.
57. Tsuchiya R, Goya T, Naruke T, Suemasu K. Resection of tracheal carina for lung cancer. Procedure, complications, and mortality. J Thorac Cardiovasc Surg. 1990;99(5):779-87.
58. Mathisen DJ, Grillo HC. Carinal resection for bronchogenic carcinoma. J Thorac Cardiovasc Surg. 1991 Jul;102(1):16-22; discussion 22-3.
59. Roviaro GC, Varoli F, Rebuffat C, et al. Tracheal sleeve pneumonectomy for bronchogenic carcinoma. J Thorac Cardiovasc Surg. 1994;107:13-8.
60. Dartevelle P, Macchiarini P, Chapelier A. Superior vena cava resection and reconstruction. In:Faber LP, editor. Techniques of pulmonary resection. Philadelphia:WB Saunders; 1995.
61. Mitchell JD, Mathisen DJ, Wright CD, et al. Clinical experience with carinal resection. J Thorac Cardiovasc Surg. 1999;117:39-53.
62. Roviaro G, Varoli C, Romanelli A, et al. Complications of tracheal sleeve pneumonectomy:personal experience and overview of the literature. J Thorac Cardiovasc Surg. 2001;121:234-40.
63. Porhanov V, Poliakov IS, Selvaschuk AP, et al. Indications and results of sleeve carinal resection. Eur J Cardiothorac Surg. 2002;22:685-94.
64. Regnard JF, Perrotin C, Giovannetti R, et al. Resection for tumors with carinal involvement: technical aspects, results, and prognostic factors. Ann Thorac Surg. 2005;80(5):1841-6.
65. Macchiarini P, Altmayer M, Go T, et al. Technical innovations of carinal resection for nonsmallcell lung cancer. Ann Thorac Surg. 2006;82(6):1989-97.
66. Martin J, Ginsberg RJ, Abolhoda A, et al. Morbidity and mortality after neoadjuvant therapy for lung cancer:the risks of right pneumonectomy. Ann Thorac Surg. 2001;72:1149-54.
67. McCormack PM. Extended pulmonary resections. In:Pearson FG, Deslauriers J, Ginsberg RJ, et al. , editors. Thoracic surgery. New York:Churchill Livingstone; 1995. p. 897-908.
68. Spaggiari L, Regnard JF, Magdeleinat P, et al. Extended resections for bronchogenic carcinoma invading the superior vena cava system. Ann Thorac Surg. 2000;69:233-6.
69. Dartevelle P, Macchiarini P, Chapelier A. Technique of superior vena cava resection and reconstruction. Chest Surg Clin N Am. 1995;5(2):345-58.
70. Tsuchiya R, Asamura H, Kondo H, Goya T, Naruke T. Extended resection of the left atrium, great vessels, or both for lung cancer. Ann Thorac Surg. 1994;57:960-5.
71. Thomas P, Magnan PE, Moulin G, Giudicelli R, Fuentes P. Extended operation for lung cancer invading the superior vena cava. Eur J Cardiothorac Surg. 1994;8:177-82.
72. Nakahara K, Ohno K, Mastumura A, et al. Extended operation for lung cancer invading the aortic arch and superior vena cava. J Thorac Cardiovasc Surg. 1989;97:428-33.
73. Dartevelle P, Chapelier A, Navajas M, et al. Replacement of the superior vena cava with polytetrafluoroethylene grafts combined with resection of mediastinal-pulmonary malignant tumors. Report of thirteen cases. J Thorac Cardiovasc Surg. 1987;94:361-6.
74. Dartevelle PG, Chapelier AR, Pastorino U, et al. Long-term follow-up after prosthetic re-

placement of the superior vena cava combined with resection of mediastinal-pulmonary malignant tumors. J Thorac Cardiovasc Surg. 1991;102:259-65.
75. Grunenwald DH, Andre F, Le Pechoux C, et al. Benefit of surgery after chemoradiotherapy in stage ⅢB (T4 and/or N3) non-small cell lung cancer. J Thorac Cardiovasc Surg. 2001; 122:796-802.
76. Spaggiari L, Thomas P, Magdeleinat P, et al. Superior vena cava resection with prosthetic replacement for non-small cell lung cancer: long-term results of a multicentric study. Eur J Cardiothorac Surg. 2002;21:1080-6.
77. Suzuki K, Asamura H, Watanabe S, et al. Combined resection of superior vena cava for lung carcinoma: prognostic significance of patterns of superior vena cava invasion. Ann Thorac Surg. 2004;78(4):1184-9.
78. Shargall Y, de Perrot M, Keshavjee S, et al. 15 years single center experience with surgical resection of the superior vena cava for non-small cell lung cancer. Lung Cancer. 2004;45:357-63.
79. Spaggiari L, Magdeleinat P, Kondo H, et al. Results of superior vena cava resection for lung cancer. Analysis of prognostic factors. Lung Cancer. 2004;44(3):339-46.
80. Spaggiari L, Veronesi G, D'Aiuto M, et al. Superior vena cava reconstruction using heterologous pericardial tube after extended resection for lung cancer. Eur J Cardiothorac Surg. 2004;26(3):649-51.
81. DiPerna CA, Wood DE. Surgical management of T3 and T4 lung cancer. Clin Cancer Res. 2005;11(13 Pt 2):5038s-44.
82. de Perrot M, Fadel E, Mussot S, de Palma A, Chapelier A, Dartevelle P. Resection of locally advanced (T4) non-small cell lung cancer with cardiopulmonary bypass. Ann Thorac Surg. 2005;79(5):1691-6.
83. Vaporciyan AA, Rice D, Correa AM, et al. Resection of advanced thoracic malignancies requiring cardiopulmonary bypass. Eur J Cardiothorac Surg. 2002;22:47-52.
84. Wiebe K, Baraki H, Macchiarini P, et al. Extended pulmonary resections of advanced thoracic malignancies with support of cardiopulmonary bypass. Eur J Cardiothorac Surg. 2006; 29(4):571-7.
85. Fukuse T, Wada H, Hitomi S. Extended operations for non-small cell lung cancers invading great vessels and left atrium. Eur J Cardiothorac Surg. 1997;11:664-9.
86. Bobbio A, Carbognani P, Grapeggia M, et al. Surgical outcome of combined pulmonary and atrial resection for lung cancer. Thorac Cardiovasc Surg. 2004;52:180-2.
87. Shirakusa T, Kimura M. Partial atrial resection in advanced lung carcinoma with and without cardiopulmonary bypass. Thorax. 1991;46:484-7.
88. Martini N, Yellin A, Ginsberg RJ, et al. Management of non-small cell lung cancer with direct mediastinal involvement. Ann Thorac Surg. 1994;58:1447-51.
89. Ratto GB, Costa R, Vassallo G, et al. Twelve-year experience with left atrial resection in the treatment of non-small cell lung cancer. Ann Thorac Surg. 2004;78(1):234-7.
90. Ricci C, Rendina E, Venuta F, et al. Reconstruction of the pulmonary artery in patients with

lung cancer. Ann Thorac Surg. 1994;57:627-33.
91. Ohta M,Hirabayasi H,Shiono H,et al. Surgical resection for lung cancer with infiltration of the thoracic aorta. J Thorac Cardiovasc Surg. 2005;129:804-8.
92. DeMeester TR,Albertucci M,Dawson PJ,et al. Management of tumors adherent to the vertebral column. J Thorac Cardiovasc Surg. 1989;97:373-8.
93. Ratto GB, Piacenza G, Frola C, et al. Chest wall involvement by lung cancer:computed tomographic detection and results and prognostic factors. Ann Thorac Surg. 1991;51:182-8.

第8章
Ⅳ期非小细胞肺癌个体化化疗

作者：Niki Karachaliou，Rafael Rosell，Enric Carcereny
译者：程 钧

背景

转移性非小细胞肺癌的传统治疗方法为使用全身性细胞毒药物化疗。顺铂自1978年开始作为非小细胞肺癌化疗常规使用药物，但仅对15%～30%的患者有效，中位生存期也仅10～12个月，而且有部分患者出现严重毒副反应，也并无任何收益[1]。肿瘤患者个体差异性大，导致治疗转归也因人而异。化疗药物的作用效果部分是由患者体细胞癌基因及基因表达改变决定。EGFR基因野生型非小细胞肺癌患者的一线治疗方案为以铂类药物为基础的化疗。目前需要找到一种分子标志物可确定患者对铂类化疗方案耐药或敏感，从而优化非小细胞肺癌的化疗方案。自1994年开始，开始关注分子预测标志物的研究[2]。但到目前为止，仍没有找到特别有效的分子预测标记物，也未能经过随机对照试验验证。

双链断裂(DSBs)及DNA损伤反馈(DDR)：肺癌预测模型的生物学基本原理——BREC研究

顺铂可使DNA产生错误交联，而ERCC1则可修复错误交联，由此推测ERCC1可能是一种潜在的化疗反应生物标记物，但多项相关研究均未能获得阳性结果[3,4]。真核生物有两种DSB修复的方式，即同源重组(HR)和非同源末端交联(NHEJ)方式可修复化疗引起的DNA双链断裂[5]。两种方法区别在于是否使用同源DNA修复以及修复的精度。总体来说，HR方式修复使用非损伤的姐妹染色体为模板进行精确修复。另一方面，DNA末端交联使用非同源染色体末端重组进行修复。同源重组的中心反应是寻找到同源NDA，以及通过Rad51-ssDNA确定位置，自3'端通过模板进行DNA合成修复[6]。细胞对DSB的初始反应通过蛋白ATM及MRN介导。ATM蛋白为丝氨酸-苏氨酸激酶，是磷酸肌醇3激酶类似激酶(PIKK)家族成员，PIKK家族同样存在DNA蛋白激酶(DNA-PK)及ATR蛋白。这些蛋白与DNA损伤检测、细胞周期检测点调控及细胞生长相关。

ATM 蛋白可磷酸化双链断裂 DNA 周围区域 DNA 监测点 1（MDC1）信使，并触发招募 DNA 修复因子。组装过程需要一系列的 DNA 修复组件的转译期改变。特别是 E3 泛素连接酶环指蛋白 8（RNF8）可以识别磷酸化的 MDC1 并与 E3 泛素连接酶 RNF168 形成复合物。E2 泛素连接酶共扼酶 UBC13 招募 BRCA1[7]。BRCA1 在 HR 通路中有至关重要的作用[8]。最近发现 BRCA1 缺失细胞多使用 HR 修复方式，但对错链交联也高度敏感，由此推测在双链断裂修复中，BRCA1 在处理错链交联时有另一条上游通道[9]。研究模型表明 BRCA1 突变患者对铂类药物的耐药性增加 10～1000 倍，但对紫杉醇、多西他赛、长春瑞滨敏感[10-12]。BRCA1、BRCA2 在双链断裂 HR 修复过程中作用不同，BRCA2 可控制细胞内转运及 Rad51 的功能。在 BRCA2 缺失细胞中，Rad51 至细胞核内的转运效率低下，提示 BRCA2 可将 Rad51 从合成区域转运到功能区域[13]。非小细胞肺癌 BRCA1 mRNA 高表达患者使用多烯紫杉醇及吉西他滨联合化疗缓解率提高，无进展生存期（PFS）较长[14]，胃癌患者也有类似价值，胃癌患者 BRCA1 mRNA 高表达提示接受多烯紫杉醇治疗后生存期较长[15]。而西班牙肺癌协会（SLCG）Ⅱ期临床试验（NCT00883480）纳入接受顺铂联合吉西他滨、顺铂联合多烯紫杉醇治疗或者单独使用多烯紫杉醇治疗的患者，结果显示患者的生存与 BRCA1 表达无显著相关性[16]。最重要的是，在双链断裂处有很大比例的 BRCA1 形成了 BRCA1-A 复合物，该复合物由 BRCA1/BARD1 异二聚体、受体 RAP80 蛋白及因子 ABRAXAS 蛋白组成。RAP80 在 HR 修复中发挥主要作用，同时连接多个蛋白[17,18]。在 SLCG Ⅱ期试验中，生存与 RAP80 mRNA 表达相关，BRCA1 及 RAP80 均低表达的患者中位生存期长于 26 个月[16]。近期一项回顾性分析研究得出了类似结论[19]。

基于前文的结论，开展了一项Ⅲ期临床试验（NCT00617656/GECP-BREC）和Ⅱ期临床试验（BREC China, ChiCTR-TRC-12001860）正在开展以评估 BRCA1 与 RAP80 表达对于患者化疗敏感性预测的价值。两项研究均检测了患者肿瘤 BRCA1 及 RAP80 表达水平，SLCG 研究将患者按 1：1 比例随机分配到试验组与对照组，对照组患者接受多烯紫杉醇（d1）联合顺铂（d1）治疗，RAP80 低表达、BRCA1 任意表达为试验 1 组，接受吉西他滨（d1, d8）联合顺铂（d1）治疗；RAP80 高表达、BRCA1 中低表达患者为试验 2 组，接受多烯紫杉醇（d1）联合顺铂（d1）治疗；RAP80 高表达、BRCA1 高表达患者为试验 3 组，接受多西他赛治疗。中国的 BREC 研究将患者按 1：3 比例随机分配到对照组与试验组（试验组 A、B、C），治疗方案与 SLCG 研究中相同，但是剂量调整为适合中国人群的剂量，该研究由于初期结果提示试验组结果欠佳而提前终止。

Ⅳ期非小细胞肺癌化疗反应预测最佳模型

基于我们的经验，BRCA1/RAP80 模型并非晚期非小细胞肺癌标准化疗治疗预测最佳模型,其他分子也可影响 BRCA1-RAP80 预测模型。

最近一项研究显示 BRCA1 蛋白、p53 连接蛋白 1(53BP1)及 RAD51 蛋白可能在 RAP80 缺失的细胞中组装,而 BRCA1 缺失的细胞中,RAP80 及 53BP1 能在双链断裂处组装 Bonanno 等证明了 53BP1 及 BRCA1 的 mRNA 在晚期非小细胞肺癌经铂类药物化疗后有表达[21]。BRCA1 低表达患者中,若 53BP1 mRNA 低表达则提示患者对铂类药物敏感。BRCA1 缺失时,错链修复可发生在 HR 独立修复细胞中,这可能由 53BP1 影响。而若患者高表达 BRCA1,则 53BP1 表达不影响患者对铂类药物化疗的敏感性,提示 BRCA1 高表达,使肿瘤抵抗铂类药物化疗效果更强,53BP1 也可能不是确定铂剂敏感性所必需的[21]。这也能解释为什么 BRCA1 缺失细胞中,53BP1 增强非同源交联修复,而产生严重的对 PARP1 抑制因子有反应的致死性放射染色体[22]。

Rif1 存在于双链断裂与无功能的端粒位置,依赖 ATM 信号发挥功能,是 53BP1 下游主要因子,控制 5′端切除,可与 53BP1 相互反应[23]。因此,BRCA1 低表达,53BP1-Rif1 高表达可能能够更好地预测肿瘤对于铂类药物化疗的敏感性(图 8.1)。

RNF8 活性抑制可抑制 BRCA1 表达,RNF8 能在 53BP1 低表达肿瘤细胞中建立 HR 及 NHEJ 之间联系。在 RNF8/BRCA1 或 RNF8/BRCA1/53BP1 缺失细胞中,包括 53BP1,RAP80 及 RAD51 在内的其他 DNA 修复组件,不能在双链断裂处进行组装[20]。Nakada 等指出 RNF8 及 RNF168 的药理学抑制在 BRCA1 突变及 53BP1 低表达的肿瘤细胞中抑制 HR 修复,但并没有在正常细胞中抑制,联合 DNA 损伤部件及 RNF8 抑制可作为肿瘤治疗选择方案[20]。

BRCA2 的伴随蛋白 PALB2 是乳腺癌敏感性基因,由于其可辅助 BRCA2 蛋白对 DNA 损伤部位的定位的作用而被发现[24](附录彩图 8.1)。BRCA1-PALB2-BRCA2-RAD51 网络可能是一个非常重要的确定肿瘤的治疗反应程度,与 DNA 错联相关部件相对独立。通路中任何部位的缺失提示 RAD51 组件的组装失败,因此可作为一种预测肿瘤反应程度的通路。例如,我们推测 BRCA1 低表达、53BP1-RIF1 低表达、但 PALB2 高表达的肿瘤对铂类药物化疗耐药(图 8.1)。

ATM 蛋白位于 DDR 的关键部位,可调节 3 种关键 DDR 过程:细胞周期调节、DNA 修复、凋亡[25]。ATM 缺失肿瘤可通过 NHEJ 修复化疗导致的双链断裂,因此常对化疗耐药,NHEJ 在其中作为 HR 修复双链断裂失败后的备用方式[25]。NHEJ 过程中,非催化基 Ku70 和 Ku80 形成异二聚体连接游离 DNA 末端,进而招募 DNA 依赖性蛋白激酶催化亚基(DNA-PKcs)。DNA-PKcs 激酶的激活对于 NHEJ 修复中损坏末端的重新连入至关重要,可以作为 ATM 缺失肿瘤的有效治疗靶点[25]。因此,非常有必要在已测定 ATM 蛋白的患者中测定 DNA-PKcs 抑制因子。

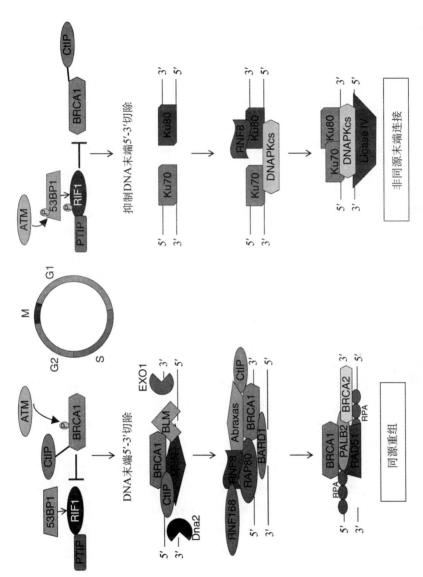

图8.1 同源重组与非同源末端连接

我们正在使用 BREC 研究患者中的残余主治标本检测 53BP1，RIF1，RNF8，ATM 及 PALB2 的 mRNA 水平，评估其是否可以作为肿瘤化疗的标记物，并阐明相关的 DNA 修复机制。

细胞凋亡、细胞自噬及细胞衰老

许多化疗药物通过内源性和外源性两种途径诱导细胞凋亡[26]。外源性细胞凋亡途径由配体与细胞表面受体形成死亡诱导信号复合物，从而激活细胞凋亡蛋白酶 8(cas-8)，进一步激活细胞凋亡蛋白酶 3(cas-3)。内源性细胞凋亡途径则由不同的凋亡刺激因子激活后促使线粒体释放细胞色素 C，从而激活细胞凋亡蛋白酶 9(cas-9)和细胞凋亡蛋白酶 3(cas-3)[26]，内源性凋亡途径由 BCL2 蛋白家族的促凋亡与抗凋亡蛋白进行调控，另有一促凋亡关键蛋白为 BH3 家族成员，即 BIM[26]。BIM 通过抑制 BCL2 蛋白家族的抗凋亡蛋白（BCL2，BCLXL，MCL1，BCL2A1)使细胞凋亡，也可通过激活促凋亡家族成员（BAX，BAK1）诱导细胞凋亡[26]。目前所知的激酶诱导肿瘤，如慢性髓系白血病、EGFR 驱动的非小细胞肺癌，可通过抑制 BIM 转录或者经 MAPK 磷酸化途径降解 BIM 蛋白而取得生存获益。化疗可通过激活 FOXO3 及其靶点（包括 BIM）诱导细胞凋亡，从而抑制肿瘤生长。

BIM 蛋白存在 BIM_s，BIM_L 及 BIM_{el} 三个亚型，三个亚型促凋亡活性存在一定差别[27]。研究表明化疗还可能通过诱导死亡诱导信号复合物启动凋亡[28]。紫杉醇诱导 BIMel 累积，从而诱导内源性和外源性细胞凋亡[29]。MAPK 通路激活可通过磷酸化和蛋白酶降解 BIM，从而抑制 BIM 激活，阻断细胞对紫杉醇的反应，这可解释化疗介导的凋亡，以及蛋白酶抑制剂联合紫杉醇可治疗 MAPK 途径激活的肿瘤。治疗前 BCL-2 家族蛋白的高度异质性可提示肿瘤对化疗的治疗反应，而化疗所诱导的细胞凋亡是一动态过程，需要进一步深入研究。

细胞死亡往往因细胞凋亡引起，但也可通过其他机制引起，如细胞自噬。研究发现多种肿瘤，包括乳腺、结肠、前列腺和脑等，经治疗后可出现细胞自噬或者细胞自噬引起的细胞死亡现象[30]。BREC 研究中，ECOG 体能状态评分(PS)及治疗方案选择存在显著相关性，PS 评分 0 分的患者中，试验组患者可获益，但差异无明显显著性，而对于 PS 评分 1 分的患者，试验组患者并无获益，反而显著增加了死亡风险。PS 评分可量化肿瘤患者的机体状态，是一项重要的预后决定指标。细胞自噬是一动态过程，伴随胞膜结构包绕细胞内蛋白及细胞器，从而降解。但细胞自噬对肿瘤细胞起杀伤作用还是保护作用，目前尚未定论。

细胞自噬是细胞新陈代谢方式，在营养或氨基酸缺乏时，或 mTOR 抑制时诱导细胞自噬流启动[31]（附录彩图 8.2）。肿瘤引起肌肉消耗及继发性肌肉减少症，使 PS 评分下降，可能就是细胞自噬障碍引起的。肿瘤细胞抑制细胞自噬的机制到底是什么？Beclin1 低表达，mTORC1 高表达，或可直接抑制 Beclin1 的 AKT 高表达，都可能是该机制的原因。Beclin1 是 Bcl2 的同源蛋白 3（BH3），是自噬体形成及溶酶体融合的关键蛋白。Beclin1 激酶的激活由 Bcl2 家族蛋白（Bcl2、Mcl1、Bcl-xL）负调控，Bcl2 家族蛋白通过结合 Beclin1，抑制自吞噬泡的形成[32]。Mst1 是丝氨酸-苏氨酸激酶，也是 Hippo 信号通路的组成部分。Mst1 可诱发 Beclin1 的磷酸化，促使 Beclin1 和 Bcl2 或者 BclxL 结合，由于该结合作用在 Mst1 活性受抑制时明显减弱，因此可推断 Mst1 激酶活性可能可以调控 Beclin1 与 Bcl2 家族蛋白之间的结合[32]。另外，ATM 在细胞质中通过 LKB1/AMPK 代谢途径激活 TSC2 肿瘤抑制因子，从而抑制 mTORC1，诱导自噬启动[33]。AMPK 可诱导自噬发生，AMPK 是主要的能量感受器，能调控细胞新生代谢，保持能量代谢，可被细胞生长因子和营养信号调节关键蛋白 mTOR 所抑制[34]（图 8.2）。

部分研究表明抗肿瘤药物可引起细胞衰老，其特征是糖酵解增强，治疗后 FDG-PET 呈高代谢，而 FLT-PET 呈低代谢[35]，虽然我们期望治疗能引起细胞衰老（TIS），特别是在凋亡信号通路受损的肿瘤细胞中，但是存活下来的衰老细胞有一定的危害性。例如，它们可以再次进入细胞周期，分泌活性因子，形成炎症[35]，因此肿瘤后续治疗需清理衰老肿瘤细胞。衰老细胞的重新代谢增加蛋白合成及衰老相关可分泌肽，随后增加蛋白压力，引起细胞自噬，阻断自噬则可以诱导衰老细胞的凋亡。

最近，Tan 等阐明了一个新的 3-磷酸肌醇依赖性蛋白激酶 1（PDK1）-Polo 样激酶 1（PLK1）-MYC 信号通路，可连接两个基本致癌机制，即磷酸肌醇 3-激酶（PI3K）和 MYC。PDK1-PLK1-MYC 通路在癌症细胞存活和肿瘤形成中有重要的功能性作用。抑制 PDK1 和 PLK1 在肿瘤药理学上了突破肿瘤中最难制作成药物的 MYC 高表达的癌蛋白。PDK1-PLK1-MYC 通路诱导的胚胎肝细胞样的基因签名与肿瘤侵袭性行为相关[36]（图 8.2）。

我们正在研究的 mTOR，BIM，BIM_{EL} 和 cas-8 和 cas-3 的 Beclin1 和 Bcl-2，Mcl-1 与 MYC 的 mRNA 水平作为分子标志物，是否可以帮助我们预测肿瘤对化疗的治疗反应，以及研究合成新型药物。

总结

以铂类为基础的联合化疗仍然是晚期非小细胞肺癌标准的一线治疗方案。肿瘤分子标志物的发现，并将这些标志物应用于预测肿瘤对于药物的治疗反应对实现晚期非小细胞肺癌的个体化治疗有着非常重要的价值。目前研究尚不能确定使用单一分子标记物来预测肿瘤对药物的治疗反应。通过分析基于 DNA 修复途径生物学研究确定的生物标志物，以及凋亡、自噬、和治疗诱导衰老等相关通路，将为肺癌治疗提供有价值的的预测模型。

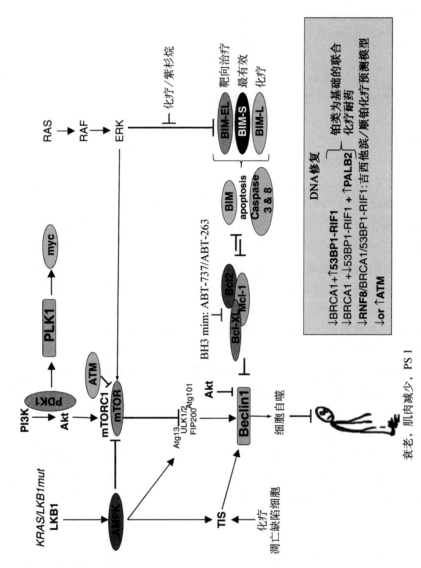

图8.2 凋亡、细胞自噬、细胞衰老交叉调节导致化疗耐药

参考文献

1. Oliver TG, Mercer KL, Sayles LC, et al. Chronic cisplatin treatment promotes enhanced damage repair and tumor progression in a mouse model of lung cancer. Genes Dev. 2010; 24(8):837-52.
2. Rosell R, Mendez P, Isla D, Taron M. Platinum resistance related to a functional NER pathway. J Thorac Oncol. 2007;2(12):1063-6.
3. Cobo M, Isla D, Massuti B, et al. Customizing cisplatin based on quantitative excision repair cross-complementing 1 mRNA expression: a phase Ⅲ trial in non-small-cell lung cancer. J Clin Oncol. 2007;25(19):2747-54.
4. Bepler G, Williams C, Schell MJ, et al. Randomized international phase Ⅲ trial of ERCC1 and RRM1 expression-based chemotherapy versus gemcitabine/carboplatin in advanced non-small- cell lung cancer. J Clin Oncol. 2013;31(19):2404-12.
5. Wei M, Zou Z, et al. Customized chemotherapy in metastatic non-small cell lung cancer (Nsclc). Transl Lung Cancer Res. 2013;2(3):180-8.
6. Li X, Heyer WD. Homologous recombination in DNA repair and DNA damage tolerance. Cell Res. 2008;18(1):99-113.
7. Shao G, Lilli DR, Patterson-Fortin J, et al. The Rap80-BRCC36 de-ubiquitinating enzyme complex antagonizes RNF8-Ubc13-dependent ubiquitination events at DNA double strand breaks. Proc Natl Acad Sci U S A. 2009;106(9):3166-71.
8. Callen E, Di Virgilio M, Kruhlak MJ, et al. 53BP1 mediates productive and mutagenic DNA repair through distinct phosphoprotein interactions. Cell. 2013;153(6):1266-80.
9. Bunting SF, Callen E, Kozak ML, et al. BRCA1 functions independently of homologous recombination in DNA interstrand crosslink repair. Mol Cell. 2012;46(2):125-35.
10. Quinn JE, James CR, Stewart GE, et al. BRCA1 mRNA expression levels predict for overall survival in ovarian cancer after chemotherapy. Clin Cancer Res. 2007;13(24):7413-20.
11. Quinn JE, Kennedy RD, Mullan PB, et al. BRCA1 functions as a differential modulator of chemotherapy-induced apoptosis. Cancer Res. 2003;63(19):6221-8.
12. Rottenberg S, Nygren AO, Pajic M, et al. Selective induction of chemotherapy resistance of mammary tumors in a conditional mouse model for hereditary breast cancer. Proc Natl Acad Sci U S A. 2007;104(29):12117-22.
13. Welcsh PL, King MC. BRCA1 and BRCA2 and the genetics of breast and ovarian cancer. Hum Mol Genet. 2001;10(7):705-13.
14. Boukovinas I, Papadaki C, Mendez P, et al. Tumor BRCA1, RRM1 and RRM2 mRNA expression levels and clinical response to first-line gemcitabine plus docetaxel in non-small-cell lung cancer patients. PLoS One. 2008;3(11):e3695.
15. Wei J, Costa C, Ding Y, et al. MRNA expression of BRCA1, PIAS1, and PIAS4 and survival after second-line docetaxel in advanced gastric cancer. J Natl Cancer Inst. 2011;103(20):1552-6.

16. Rosell R, Perez-Roca L, Sanchez JJ, et al. Customized treatment in non-small-cell lung cancer based on EGFR mutations and BRCA1 mRNA expression. PLoS One. 2009;4(5):e5133.
17. Yin Z, Menendez D, Resnick MA, French JE, Janardhan KS, Jetten AM. RAP80 is critical in maintaining genomic stability and suppressing tumor development. Cancer Res. 2012;72(19):5080-90.
18. Yan J, Kim YS, Yang XP, Albers M, Koegl M, Jetten AM. Ubiquitin-interaction motifs of RAP80 are critical in its regulation of estrogen receptor alpha. Nucleic Acids Res. 2007;35(5):1673-86.
19. Bonanno L, Costa C, Majem M, Favaretto A, Rugge M, Rosell R. The predictive value of BRCA1 and RAP80 mRNA expression in advanced non-small-cell lung cancer patients treated with platinum-based chemotherapy. Ann Oncol. 2013;24(4):1130-2.
20. Nakada S, Yonamine RM, Matsuo K. RNF8 regulates assembly of RAD51 at DNA double-strand breaks in the absence of BRCA1 and 53BP1. Cancer Res. 2012;72(19):4974-83.
21. Bonanno L, Costa C, Majem M, et al. The predictive value of 53BP1 and BRCA1 mRNA expression in advanced non-small-cell lung cancer patients treated with first-line platinumbased chemotherapy. Oncotarget. 2013;4(10):1572-81.
22. Bunting SF, Callen E, Wong N, et al. 53BP1 inhibits homologous recombination in Brca1-deficient cells by blocking resection of DNA breaks. Cell. 2010;141(2):243-54.
23. Zimmermann M, Lottersberger F, Buonomo SB, Sfeir A, De Lange T. 53BP1 regulates DSB repair using Rif1 to control 5′ end resection. Science. 2013;339(6120):700-4.
24. Zhang F, Fan Q, Ren K, Andreassen PR. PALB2 functionally connects the breast cancer susceptibility proteins BRCA1 and BRCA2. Mol Cancer Res. 2009;7(7):1110-8.
25. Riabinska A, Daheim M, Herter-Sprie GS, et al. Therapeutic targeting of a robust nononcogeneaddictionto PRKDC in ATM-defective tumors. Sci Transl Med. 2013;5(189):189ra178.
26. Rosell R, Bivona TG, Karachaliou N. Genetics and biomarkers in personalisation of lung cancer treatment. Lancet. 2013;382(9893):720-31.
27. Akiyama T, Dass CR, Choong PF. Bim-targeted cancer therapy: a link between drug action and underlying molecular changes. Mol Cancer Ther. 2009;8(12):3173-80.
28. Kaufmann SH, Earnshaw WC. Induction of apoptosis by cancer chemotherapy. Exp Cell Res. 2000;256(1):42-9.
29. Tan TT, Degenhardt K, Nelson DA, et al. Key roles of BIM-driven apoptosis in epithelial tumors and rational chemotherapy. Cancer Cell. 2005;7(3):227-38.
30. Kondo Y, Kanzawa T, Sawaya R, Kondo S. The role of autophagy in cancer development and response to therapy. Nat Rev Cancer. 2005;5(9):726-34.
31. Russell RC, Tian Y, Yuan H, et al. ULK1 induces autophagy by phosphorylating Beclin-1 and activating VPS34 lipid kinase. Nat Cell Biol. 2013;15(7):741-50.
32. Maejima Y, Kyoi S, Zhai P, et al. Mst1 inhibits autophagy by promoting the interaction between Beclin1 and Bcl-2. Nat Med. 2013;19(11):1478-88.
33. Alexander A, Cai SL, Kim J, et al. ATM signals to TSC2 in the cytoplasm to regulate

mTORC1 in response to ROS. Proc Natl Acad Sci U S A. 2010;107(9):4153-8.
34. Kim J, Kundu M, Viollet B, Guan KL. AMPK and mTOR regulate autophagy through direct phosphorylation of Ulk1. Nat Cell Biol. 2011;13(2):132-41.
35. Dorr JR, Yu Y, Milanovic M, et al. Synthetic lethal metabolic targeting of cellular senescence in cancer therapy. Nature. 2013;501(7467):421-5.
36. Tan J, Li Z, Lee PL, et al. PDK1 signaling toward PLK1-MYC activation confers oncogenic transformation, tumor-initiating cell activation, and resistance to mTOR-targeted therapy. Cancer Discov. 2013;3(10):1156-71.

第四部分
分子治疗进展

第9章
EGFR突变肺癌治疗策略

作者:Martin Früh, Qing Zhou Linda Leung, and Tony Mok
译者:曾理平

介绍

2004年表皮生长因子受体(EGFR)突变的发现是晚期非小细胞肺癌患者个体化治疗的基础[1,2]。这项发现引发了广泛的临床研究,证实了EGFR酪氨酸激酶抑制剂(TKI)对EGFR突变患者具有较高的肿瘤缓解率及持久的疾病控制[3-8]。和以铂类为基础的化疗相比,在治疗有效率、毒副反应以及生活质量等方面,EGFR-TKI的优越性是无可争议的。随着易瑞沙泛亚洲研究(Iressa Pan-Asia Study,IPASS)以及其他多项随机研究结果发表,EGFR-TKI已经成为具有EGFR突变患者的标准一线治疗。EGFR-TKI治疗肺癌的中位无疾病进展生存期(PFS)为8.4~13.6个月,中位总生存期为22~38个月。这些结果是令人鼓舞的,更重要的是,它预示了未来进一步提升的空间还很大。在本章节,我们将回顾EGFR-TKI使用的各种策略以及优化治疗效果的方法以服务将来的患者。

一线VS二线EGFR-TKI治疗

多项研究已经显示,和标准化疗相比,EGFR-TKI一线治疗可以延长PFS,但是还没有研究显示OS可显著获益。Lee等[9]的meta分析包含了23项临床试验,EGFR-TKI的一线治疗用于EGFR突变的患者和疾病进展风险降低相关(风险比=0.43,95% CI=0.38~0.49,$P<0.01$),但是对OS,EGFR-TKI没有优势。

这种现象的主要原因是化疗患者在疾病进展后转而使用 EGFR-TKI 并受益。这就产生了一个争论，EGFR-TKI 可以用作一线或者二线治疗。虽然这是一个合理的争论，但是我们必须注意到，对 EGFR 突变患者使用 EGFR-TKI 二线治疗的临床数据比较有限。西班牙胃癌研究小组报道了对 EGFR 突变阳性的患者，113 例特罗凯一线治疗和 104 例特罗凯二线/三线治疗的有效率[10]。治疗缓解率分别是 73.5%，67.4%，PFS 和 OS 是比较相近的，PFS 为 14.0 个月（95% CI，9.7~18.3 月）vs 13.0 个月（95% CI，9.7~16.3 个月），OS 为 28.0 个月（95% CI，22.7~33 个月）vs 27.0 个月（95% CI，19.9~34.1 个月）。这项研究提示 EGFR-TKI 一线治疗和二线/三线治疗对 EGFR 突变患者具有相似的有效率。但是，这项观察性的研究没有得到其他研究的支持。ISEL［以色列肺癌生存评估］[11]和 BR.21［OSI-774（特罗凯）用于治疗Ⅲ期或者Ⅳ期非小细胞肺癌的患者］研究[12]显示，EGFR 突变阳性的患者对 EGFR-TKI 二线/三线治疗的缓解率分别是 37.5%，27%。NEJSG002 研究[6]是记录了患者一线化疗失败后使用 EGFR-TKI 的肿瘤缓解率的唯一的随机分组Ⅲ期临床试验。在同样研究人群中，EGFR-TKI 二线治疗的缓解率是 58.5%，而一线吉非替尼的缓解率是 73.7%。EGFR-TKI 二线治疗缓解率低的一个可能原因是化疗对肿瘤细胞的 EGFR 突变状态或者突变数量产生了潜在的影响。Bai 等[13]报道，新辅助化疗可能会影响 EGFR 的突变状态，Zhou 等[14]也报道了 EGFR 突变的数量低和更短的 PFS 相关。对一线治疗的最强争论是源自最近的一项汇集分析，汇总了来自两项比较二代不可逆 EGFR-TKI 阿法替尼和铂类为基础化疗的姐妹研究 LUX Lung 3、6 中的 631 例常见 EGFR 突变的患者[21]。这项分析显示一线阿法替尼治疗有 3 个月的 OS 获益（27.3 个月 vs 24.3 个月，风险比=0.81，$P=0.037$）。这个 OS 获益是局限于携带 19 外显子缺失突变的亚群患者（31.7 个月 vs 20.7 个月，风险比=0.59，$P=0.0001$）。他们的分析也显示，化疗后疾病进展转而使用 EGFR-TKI，OS 减短不能被代偿。

一项正式的比较一线 EGFR-TKI 治疗后化疗和一线化疗后 EGFR-TKI 治疗的随机化研究可以最终阐明这个问题。但是，具有类似特征的唯一的研究纳入了未筛选的高加索人群。TORCH 研究（一项特罗凯或者化疗用于治疗晚期非小细胞肺癌的研究）[15]，比较了一线 EGFR-TKI 治疗后化疗和一线化疗后二线 EGFR-TKI 治疗，这项研究纳入了未筛选的来自加拿大以及意大利的人群，只有 39 个患者（14.2%）是 EGFR 突变阳性的。样本量太少不足以得到确切的结论，进过他们的数据实际也提示一线 EGFR-TKI 治疗后二线化疗的较大优势。鉴于目前的数据，可以得出合理的结论，对 EGFR 突变阳性患者，一线 EGFR-TKI 治疗应作为标准。在特殊情况下，如在等待 EGFR 突变分析结果，医生对有症状的患者有责任开始一线化疗时，二线 EGFR-TKI 治疗可以考虑。

更好的 EGFR-TKI

吉非替尼和厄洛替尼被认为是"第一代"EGFR-TKI。酪氨酸激酶是 ATP 能力转运的核心酶，而且它对细胞内 EGFR 信号的传递是必不可少的。吉非替尼和厄洛替尼都是喹唑啉类化合物，能可逆抑制 EGFR 上 ATP 结合位点，它们都是生物利用率高和半衰期长的口服药物。

埃克替尼是中国自主研发并且只能在中国使用的第三种"第一代"EGFR-TKI。这个分子具有较短的半衰期，需要每天服用 3 次。支持其有效性的唯一随机化临床试验是 ICOGEN 研究[16]。在这项研究中，对未筛选的人群，作为二线治疗，结果提示这个药物不弱于吉非替尼。对 EGFR 突变患者($n=68$)，亚组分析提示埃克替尼和吉非替尼组的中位 PFS 分别是 7.8 个月、5.3 个月。因此，埃克替尼不能被认为是"第一代"EGFR-TKI 的改进。

第二代 EGFR-TKI 显著的特点是它不可逆结合生长因子受体的 ATP 位点，以及它对 EGFR，HER-2 和 HER-4 的泛 HER 家族的抑制性。这些额外的特征可能加强了抑制 EGFR 下游功能的能力，而且原则上，可能使得第二代 TKI 的功能更强大。两种第二代 EGFR-TKI，即阿法替尼和达克米替尼，已经被广泛研究，临床前研究已经证实，阿法替尼和达克米替尼对携带 20 外显子 T790M 耐药性突变的肿瘤细胞具有潜在的抑制作用[17]。阿法替尼用于 129 例已知 EGFR 突变阳性患者的一项单臂Ⅱ期试验报道肿瘤缓解率是 61%，PFS 为 13.4 个月[18]。第二代 EGFR-TKI 的临床有效性如果不优于第一代，但也是比较好的。其他两项随机Ⅲ期研究已完成，比较了阿法替尼一线治疗和铂类为基础的化疗[19, 20]。LUX Lung 3 研究入组 345 例 EGFR 突变患者(亚裔 72%)，比较了阿法替尼和培美曲塞/顺铂化疗作为一线治疗的效果。正如预期的，PFS 有利于阿法替尼[风险比 0.58(0.43～0.78)，$P=0.0004$]。意向治疗人群的中位 PFS 是 11.1 个月，而预先计划的具有 19 外显子缺失或者 21 外显子点突变的亚组患者的中位 PFS 是 13.6 个月[19]。LUX Lung 6 是一项主要在中国完成的，使用吉西他滨/卡铂作为对照组，具有类似研究设计的姐妹研究。PFS 的主要终点分别为 11.0 个月、5.6 个月，有利于阿法替尼(风险比 0.28，$P<0.0001$)。而且，对具有常见 EGFR 突变的亚组人群，发现更长的 13.7 个月的中位 PFS[20]。在两项研究中，PFS 的延长主要是由 19 外显子缺失亚组带动的。然而，这明显的改善和 TKI 相关毒性的轻微增高是相关的，包括 3 级皮肤毒性，腹泻，黏膜炎的发生率分别为 14.6%、5.4%、5.4%。阿法替尼和第一代 TKI(吉非替尼)一线治疗直接比较的研究目前正在进行中(LUX Lung 7 NCT01466660)。

达克米替尼是另一种第二代 TKI。一项Ⅰ期研究已近帮助确定了每天服用的剂量为 45mg，而且有 EGFR 突变及不突变患者缓解的报道。基于这些，这个药物被列入一项基于要么知道或者很可能具有 EGFR 突变人群的单臂研究分析中。36

例 EGFR 突变患者的肿瘤缓解率是 76%,中位 PFS 为 18.2 个月。这项研究的主要重点,4 个月 PFS 率为 95.5%。然而,这项杰出的结果可能和患者选择偏倚有关,因此达克米替尼需要在三期随机临床试验中进行进一步分析。ARCHER 1050 是一项随机研究,比较达克米替尼和吉非替尼($n=440$)。主要重点是 PFS,目前研究正在进行中(NCT01774721)。

EGFR-TKI 耐药

EGFR-TKI 耐药可以分为原发性和继发性。20%~30% 的晚期或者转移的携带 EGFR 突变的 NSCLC 患者对 EGFR-TKI 的反应没有达到预期(原发性耐药)[3,5-8,19,20]。对那些开始就从 EGFR-TKI 获益的患者,他们最终都会出现疾病进展(继发性耐药),一般出现在 EGFR-TKI 治疗后的 1~2 年。

原发性耐药

原发性耐药也被称为内源性耐药,定义为接受 EGFR-TKI 时,没有客观反应的依据并在 3 个月之内出现疾病进展[23]。它描述了对 EGFR-TKI 敏感性的缺乏,这种缺乏和药物剂量的不足无关,潜在的机制在很大程度上还是未知的。目前描述的 EGFR 突变的 NSCLC 对 EGFR-TKI 内源性耐药的机制可以分为:①原发性 EGFR 耐药突变;②同时存在癌相关基因的基因改变;③涉及 EGFR 调节的凋亡中的促凋亡蛋白的种系改变。

1. 原发性 EGFR 耐药突变 即使是在 18~21 号外显子中,一些 EGFR 突变也和原发性耐药有关。最为第三常见的 EGFR 突变,20 号外显子插入(或者框内复制)约占所有 EGFR 突变的 4%~9%[24-26]。影响了 EGFRC-螺旋酪氨酸激酶机构域(密码子 767-775)之后氨基酸的插入突变占了大多数的所有 20 号外显子插入突变,这和临床上 EGFR-TKI 原发性耐药有关[25-27]。携带 20 号外显子突变的患者似乎可以从阿法替尼获益,虽然略差于经典的 19 号外显子缺失或者 21 号外显子 L858R 突变[28]。20 号外显子第 790 位点上的苏氨酸为蛋氨酸所取代(T790M 突变)是 EGFR-TKI 获得性耐药的最常见机制,虽然它也罕见地在 EGFR 突变肿瘤原发性耐药中被报道过[22,23,29,30]。T790M 突变通过空间位阻影响了 EGFR-TKI 结合到 EGFR 上,从而减弱了药物的疗效。T790M 突变可增加 ATP 亲和力,从而与 TKI 类药物竞争结合位点[33]。治疗前发现的 T790M 突变提示 PFS 预后较差[22],据报道,它可以在没有治疗的 EGFR 突变的肿瘤中以小克隆的形式存在,当足够的高频出现时,可能可以促进内源性耐药[30]。有学者还报道了其他罕见的 EGFR-TKI 原发性耐药突变,包括 18~21 号外显子内的 L747S 突变,19 号外显子上的 D761Y 突变以及 21 号外显子上的 T854A 突变[34]。

2. 同时存在的癌相关基因的基因改变 EGFR 下游(例如 RAS-MAPK 或者 PI3-AKT 通路)或者并行信号通路(例如 MET 信号通路)的额外基因突变可在 EGFR

抑制状况下,促进癌细胞增殖或者存活。RAS是EGFR下游的一个主要信号分子,鼠肉瘤病毒癌基因(KRAS)突变体组成性激活RAS-MARK通路。已经发现KRAS的2号外显子(密码子12-13)的突变和对EGFR-TKI的敏感性缺乏有关[31]。一般认为,EGFR和KRAS突变是互斥的,但是,已经发现在少数同时存在KRAS突变的EGFR突变肿瘤中存在对EGFR-TKI原发性耐药,而且这些患者接受EGFR-TKI治疗的预后较差[32]。同源性磷酸酶-张力蛋白基因(PTEN)负向调节PI3K-AKT通路,而且PTEN的缺失会导致对EGFR-TKI敏感性的减弱[35]。磷脂酰肌醇-3-羟激酶催化亚基α(PI3KCA)基因的体细胞突变导致组成性激活AKT,并已经被报道作为EGFR-TKI耐药的一个指标,一般和EGFR突变同时存在[34,36]。间质-上皮转化因子(MET)是一个跨膜酪氨酸激酶受体,和肝细胞生长因子(HGF)结合导致PI3-AKT通路的激活。在EGFR突变的NSCLC中,通过MET扩增或者高水平的肝细胞生长因子(HGF)激活的MET通路与对EGFR-TKI的原发性耐药有关[23,69]。其他并行通路的潜在改变与原发性耐药的相关性目前正在研究之中。

3. 涉及EGFR调节的凋亡中的促凋亡蛋白的种系改变　细胞死亡调节子(BIM)为促凋亡蛋白,可与Bcl-2相互作用,BIM含量低可导致EGFR靶向治疗介导的凋亡通路损伤,此类患者接受EGFR靶向治疗预后较差,PFS明显缩短EGFR-TKI[44]。BIM多态性缺失可使BIM蛋白失控并导致对EGFR-TKI的原发性耐药[45]。

继发性耐药

继发性耐药,又称获得性耐药,指患者对EGFR-TKI治疗初期存在反应,一段时间之后出现耐药。为了方便研究对EGFR-TKI的获得性耐药,获得性耐药(表9.1)的临床定义已经提出[46]。耐药肿瘤的再次活检可能会提高对潜在耐药机制的认识。目前,对EGFR-TKI获得性耐药机制可分为:①获得性看门基因突变;②旁路激活;③组织学转变。多重耐药机制仅见于不到5%的病例[42,43]。

表9.1　EGFR-TKIs获得性耐药的临床定义(来自Jackman等)[46]

获得性耐药的临床定义
1. 曾接受过EGFR-TKI治疗
2. 存在经典的EGFR活性突变,比如19号外显子的缺失,21号外显子L858R突变,18号外显子G719X突变,21号外显子L861Q点突变等或者 按照RECIST或者WHO标准,在接受EGFR-TKI单药治疗后部分或者完全缓解 或者 按照RECIST或者WHO标准,在接受EGFR-TKI单药治疗后病情稳定≥6个月
3. 按照RECIST或者WHO标准,在最近的30天内持续接受EGFR-TKI单药治疗,肿瘤进展
4. EGFR-TKI停用与开始新治疗之间,无其他全身治疗

缩略词:EGFR.表皮生长因子受体;TKI.酪氨酸激酶抑制剂;RECIST.实体肿瘤的疗效评价标准;WHO.世界卫生组织

1. 获得性 EGFR 看门基因突变　T790M 突变是目前已报道的获得性耐药的最常见机制,占 50%～60% 的病例[43,48,52,68]。

正如上所述,T790M 突变不仅影响 EGFR-TKI 和 EGFR 的结合,还增加 ATP 亲和力从而导致对 EGFR-TKI 耐药[33]。对大多数患者,在 EGFR-TKI 治疗期间,T790M 突变的存在到底是原发性的还是克隆选择诱导继发性的是不确定的。其他人报道了一些和 EGFR-TKI 获得性耐药有关的 EGFR 点突变,包括 19 号外显子上的 D761Y,L747S 突变还有 21 号外显子上的 T854A 突变,但它们加在一起也只占了获得性耐药机制不到 5% 的比例[39-41]。

2. 旁路激活/激酶转换　MET 扩增是第二常见的 EGFR-TKI 获得性耐药机制,占 5%～20% 的比例[17,42,43]。5% 的获得性耐药患者中检测到 PI3CA 突变[34,42]。还有很多已报道的其他比较少见的绕过 EGFR 通路的变异,例如,HER2 扩增,V-raf 鼠类肉瘤滤过性病毒致癌基因同源体 B(BRAF)突变,ERK 扩增以及 AXL 表达增加[34,43,47]。更多潜在变异正在被确认,但是鉴于它们不太常见,临床价值较小。

3. 组织学转变　腺癌转变为小细胞肺癌,上皮细胞间质转变是目前已知的 EGFR-TKI 继发耐药相关的细胞表型转变方式。

EGFR-TKI 耐药对策

EGFR-TKI 耐药患者的治疗应高度个体化的。EGFR-TKI 的过早中止可以导致疾病的快速恶化,这种"疾病爆发"现象已被公认[49]。目前一项大样本随机临床试验正在研究获得性耐药患者是否仍需使用该药物治疗[IMPRESS NCT01544179,ASPIRATION NCT01310036]。有研究显示对寡进展(即,少于或等于 4 个部位的进展)或者病程进展较慢的无症状患者,继续使用 EGFR-TKI 是合理的[50]。回顾性研究显示对出现肺癌寡进展的部位,放疗等局部治疗可提高存活[51-53]。目前认为,由于存在肿瘤异质性,耐药肿瘤也存在 EGFR-TKI 敏感和耐药肿瘤细胞混[34]。获得性耐药出现之后,继续使用 EGFR-TKI 联合化疗可以有效避免疾病爆发,并且由化疗控制耐药的肿瘤[56,57]。一项正在进行的Ⅲ期试验正在研究该治疗方案的有效性。对使用 EGFR-TKI 出现快速进展合并症状患者,特别是存在组织学转变的患者,往往需转为化疗。

T790M 突变是最常见的获得性突变,不可逆 EGFR-TKI,如已开发的第二代阿法替尼和达克米替尼,具有强化的 EGFR 抑制作用,体外实验证明具有潜在的抗 T790M 突变的活性[17,54]。阿法替尼不仅和 ATP 结合位点形成共价结合从而永久性抑制 EGFR,而且可以同时抑制人表皮生长因子 2(HER2),而达克米替尼是泛 HER 家族抑制剂。第二代药物是否可以攻克 T790M 突变引起的获得性突变目前还没有临床证实[58]。一项单臂研究显示,在 EGFR-TKI 获得性耐药的患者中,阿法替尼联合西妥昔单抗加强 EGFR 胞内和胞外的阻断可以取得很好的缓解率(>30%)[37,59]。最近,第三代 EGFR-TKI,包括可以共价或者选择性结合包括 T790M 等获得性突变的 CO-1686,AZD-9291 和 HM61713 的 I 期临床试验令人惊喜,对于 T790M 突变的亚组人群,其缓解率高达 28%~64%[60-62]。

很多新的针对不同原癌基因突变的化合物目前正在批量开发中。由于存在旁路激活,EGFR-TKI 联合旁路激酶受体抑制剂(例如,MET 抑制剂,PI3KCA 抑制剂)也是可能攻克耐药性的潜在方法[63]。

辅助 EGFR-TKI 治疗

在 EGFR 突变患者中辅助 TKI 治疗的作用目前还未明确。在 RADIANT 试验中,973 例 IB~IIIA 期的患者接受手术和标准的辅助化疗(如果需要)后,随机分成 2 组为期 2 年的特罗凯治疗组和安慰剂组。所有患者行免疫组化(IHC)或者荧光原位杂交(FISH)确定 EGFR 阳性。161 例 EGFR 突变的亚组患者接受辅助特罗凯治疗,DFS 提高 17 个月(风险比 0.61,28.5 vs 46.4 个月,风险比 0.61)[64,65]。但由于主要终点的层次测定,该结果缺少统计学意义整个研究人群的 DFS 是阴性的。除此之外,EGFR 突变的亚组人群中的初期 OS 结果与整个研究人群相近(风险比 1.09)。

美国的一项单臂试验纳入了 100 例标准化疗后接受 2 年特罗凯辅助治疗的患者,结果显示 2 年 DFS 为 76%,其中在 28 例 IIIA 期患者中,高达 91%[66]。在治疗结束之后,特罗凯治疗组出现大量复发,但是,增加药物治疗时间是否可以改善预后目前还不确切。上述结果和前期研究发现一致[37]。另有一项随机临床试验纳入了 503 例未经选择的患者,评估吉非替尼辅助治疗肺癌的价值,15 例 EGFR 突变患者探索性亚组分析显示,与安慰剂相比,辅助 TKI 治疗并不能使患者获益(DFS 风险比 1.84,$P=0.395$;OS 风险比 3.16,$P=0.15$)[67]。

总的来说,上述结果提示使用特罗凯可延迟疾病复发从而延长 DFS,但是对 OS 的作用还不确切。除此之外,特罗凯组脑转移比例更高(40% vs 12.9%),提示疾病进程以一种不利的方式被改变[65]。因此在推荐 EGFR-TKI 辅助治疗之前还需要进一步的研究。

参考文献

1. Lynch TJ, Bell DW, Sordella R, et al. Activating mutations in the epidermal growth factor receptor underlying responsiveness of non-small-cell lung cancer to gefitinib. N Engl J Med. 2004;350:2129-39.
2. Paez JG, Janne PA, Lee JC, et al. EGFR mutations in lung cancer:correlation with clinical response to gefitinib therapy. Science. 2004;304:1497-500.
3. Mok TS, Wu YL, Thongprasert S, Yang CH, Chu DT, Saijo N, Sunpaweravong P, Han

B, Margono B, Ichinose Y, Nishiwaki Y, Ohe Y, Yang JJ, Chewaskulyong B, Jiang H, Duffield EL, Watkins CL, Armour AA, Fukuoka M. Gefitinib or carboplatin-paclitaxel in pulmonary adenocarcinoma. N Engl J Med. 2009;361(10):947-57.
4. Han JY, Park K, Kim SW, Lee DH, Kim HY, Kim HT, Ahn MJ, Yun T, Ahn JS, Suh C, Lee JS, Yoon SJ, Han JH, Lee JW, Jo SJ, Lee JS. First-SIGNAL: first-line single-agent iressa versus gemcitabine and cisplatin trial in never-smokers with adenocarcinoma of the lung. J Clin Oncol. 2012;30(10):1122-8.
5. Mitsudomi T, Morita S, Yatabe Y, Negoro S, Okamoto I, Tsurutani J, Seto T, Satouchi M, Tada H, Hirashima T, Asami K, Katakami N, Takada M, Yoshioka H, Shibata K, Kudoh S, Shimizu E, Saito H, Toyooka S, Nakagawa K, Fukuoka M. West Japan Oncology Group. Gefitinib versus cisplatin plus docetaxel in patients with non-small-cell lung cancer harbouring mutations of the epidermal growth factor receptor (WJTOG3405): an open label, randomised phase 3 trial. Lancet Oncol. 2010;11(2):121-8.
6. Maemondo M, Inoue A, Kobayashi K, Sugawara S, Oizumi S, Isobe H, Gemma A, Harada M, Yoshizawa H, Kinoshita I, Fujita Y, Okinaga S, Hirano H, Yoshimori K, Harada T, Ogura T, Ando M, Miyazawa H, Tanaka T, Saijo Y, Hagiwara K, Morita S, Nukiwa T, North-East Japan Study Group. Gefitinib or chemotherapy for non-small-cell lung cancer with mutated EGFR. N Engl J Med. 2010;362(25):2380-8.
7. Zhou C, Wu YL, Chen G, et al. Erlotinib versus chemotherapy as first-line treatment for patients with advanced EGFR mutation-positive non-small-cell lung cancer (OPTIMAL, CTONG-0802): a multicentre, open-label, randomised, phase 3 study. Lancet Oncol. 2011;12:735-42.
8. Rosell R, Carcereny E, Gervais R, et al. Erlotinib versus standard chemotherapy as first-line treatment for European patients with advanced EGFR mutation-positive non-small-cell lung cancer (EURTAC): a multicentre, open-label, randomized phase 3 trial. Lancet Oncol. 2012;13:239-46.
9. Lee CK, Brown C, Gralla RJ, et al. Impact of EGFR inhibitor in non-small cell lung cancer on progression-free and overall survival: a meta-analysis. J Natl Cancer Inst. 2013;105(9):595-605.
10. Rosell R, Moran T, Queralt C, et al. Screening for epidermal growth factor receptor mutations in lung cancer. N Engl J Med. 2009;361:958-67.
11. Taron M, Ichinose Y, Rosell R, et al. Activating mutations in the tyrosine kinase domain of the epidermal growth factor receptor are associated with improved survival in gefitinib-treated chemorefractory lung adenocarcinomas. Clin Cancer Res. 2005;11:5878-85.
12. Tsao MS, Sakurada A, Cutz JC, et al. Erlotinib in lung cancer: molecular and clinical predictors of outcome. N Engl J Med. 2005;353:133-44.
13. Bai H, Wang Z, Chen K, Zhao J, Lee JJ, Wang S, Zhou Q, Zhuo M, Mao L, An T, Duan J, Yang L, Wu M, Liang Z, Wang Y, Kang X, Wang J. Influence of chemotherapy on EGFR mutation status among patients with non-small-cell lung cancer. J Clin Oncol. 2012;30(25):3077-83.

14. Zhou Q, Zhang XC, Chen ZH, et al. Relative abundance of EGFR mutations predicts benefit from gefitinib treatment for advanced non-small-cell lung cancer. J Clin Oncol. 2011;29:3316-21.
15. Gridelli C, Ciardiello F, Gallo C, et al. First-line erlotinib followed by second-line cisplatingemcitabine chemotherapy in advanced non-small-cell lung cancer:the TORCH randomized trial. J Clin Oncol. 2012;30(24):3002-11.
16. Shi Y, Zhang L, Liu X, Zhou C, et al. Icotinib versus gefitinib in previously treated advanced non-small-cell lung cancer (ICOGEN):a randomised, double-blind phase 3 non-inferiority trial. Lancet Oncol. 2013;14(10):953-61.
17. Engelman JA,Zejnullahu K, Gale CM, et al. PF00299804, an irreversible pan-ERBB inhibitor, is effective in lung cancer models with EGFR and ERBB2 mutations that are resistant to gefitinib. Cancer Res. 2007;67(24):11924-32.
18. Yang JC, Shih JY, Su WC, et al. Afatinib for patients with lung adenocarcinoma and epidermal growth factor receptor mutations (LUX-Lung 2):a phase 2 trial. Lancet Oncol. 2012;13(5):539-48.
19. Sequist LV, Yang JCH, Yamamoto N, et al. Phase Ⅲ study of afatinib or cisplatin plus pemetrexed in patients with metastatic lung adenocarcinoma with EGFR mutations. J Clin Oncol. 2013;31:3327-34.
20. Wu YL, Zhou C, Hu CP, et al. Afatinib versus cisplatin plus gemcitabine for first-line treatment of Asian patients with advanced non-small-cell lung cancer harbouring EGFR mutations (LUX-Lung 6):an open-label, randomised phase 3 trial. Lancet Oncol. 2014;15:213-22.
21. Yang JC,Sequist LV, Schuler MH, Mok T, et al. Overall survival (OS) in patients (pts) with advanced non-small cell lung cancer (NSCLC) harboring common (Del19/L858R) epidermal growth factor receptor mutations (EGFR mut):pooled analysis of two large open-label phase Ⅲ studies (LUX-Lung 3 [LL3] and LUX-Lung 6 [LL6]) comparing afatinib with chemotherapy (CT). J Clin Oncol. 2014;32(5s):abstr 8004.
22. Su KY, Chen HY, Li KC, Kuo ML, Yang JC, Chan WK, Ho BC, Chang GC, Shih JY, Yu SL, Yang PC. Pretreatment epidermal growth factor receptor (EGFR) T790M mutation predicts shorter EGFR tyrosine kinase inhibitor response duration in patients with non-small-cell lung cancer. J Clin Oncol. 2012;30(4):433-40.
23. Lee JK, Shin JY, Kim S, et al. Primary resistance to epidermal growth factor receptor (EGFR) tyrosine kinase inhibitors (TKIs) in patients with non-small-cell lung cancer harboring TKIsensitive EGFR mutations:an exploratory study. Ann Oncol. 2013;24:2080-7.
24. Arcila ME, Nafa K, Chaft JE, et al. EGFR exon 20 insertion mutations in lung adenocarcinomas:prevalence, molecular heterogeneity, and clinicopathologic characteristics. Mol Cancer Ther. 2013;12:220-9.
25. Oxnard GR, Lo PC, Nishino M, et al. Natural history and molecular characteristics of lung cancers harboring EGFR exon 20 insertions. J Thorac Oncol. 2013;8:179-84.
26. Yasuda H, Kobayashi S, Costa DB. EGFR exon 20 insertion mutations in non-small-cell lung cancer:preclinical data and clinical implications. Lancet Oncol. 2012;13:e23-31.

27. Wu JY, Wu SG, Yang CH, et al. Lung cancer with epidermal growth factor receptor exon 20 mutations is associated with poor gefitinib treatment response. Clin Cancer Res. 2008; 14(15):4877-82.
28. Yang J C-H, et al. Activity of afatinib in uncommon epidermal growth factor receptor (EGFR) mutations:findings from three trials of afatinib in EGFR mutation-positive lung cancer. Abstract O03. 05, World Congress on Lung Cancer 2013.
29. Yu HA, Arcila ME, Hellmann MD, Kris MG, Ladanyi M, Riely GJ. Poor response to erlotinib in patients with tumors containing baseline EGFR T790M mutations found by routine clinical molecular testing. Ann Oncol. 2014;25(2):423-8.
30. Inukai M, Toyooka S, Ito S, et al. Presence of epidermal growth factor receptor gene T790M mutation as a minor clone in non-small cell lung cancer. Cancer Res. 2006;66(16):7854-8.
31. Pao W, Wang TY, Riely GJ, Miller VA, et al. KRAS mutations and primary resistance of lung adenocarcinomas to gefitinib or erlotinib. PLoS Med. 2005;2(1):e17.
32. Takeda M, Okamoto I, Fujita Y, Arao T, Ito H, Fukuoka M, Nishio K, Nakagawa K. De novo resistance to epidermal growth factor receptor-tyrosine kinase inhibitors in EGFR mutationpositive patients with non-small cell lung cancer. J Thorac Oncol. 2010;5(3):399-400.
33. Yun CH, Mengwasser KE, Toms AV, et al. The T790M mutation in EGFR kinase causes drug resistance by increasing the affinity for ATP. Proc Natl Acad Sci U S A. 2008;105(6): 2070-5.
34. Ohashi K, Maruvka YE, Michor F, Pao W. Epidermal growth factor receptor tyrosine kinase inhibitor-resistant disease. J Clin Oncol. 2013;31(8):1070-80.
35. SosML, Koker M, Weir BA, et al. PTEN loss contributes to erlotinib resistance in EGFR-mutant lung cancer by activation of Akt and EGFR. Cancer Res. 2009;69(8):3256-61.
36. Ludovini V, Bianconi F, Pistola L, Chiari R, Minotti V, Colella R, Giuffrida D, Tofanetti FR, Siggillino A, Flacco A, Baldelli E, Iacono D, Mameli MG, Cavaliere A, Crinò L. Phosphoinositide -3-kinase catalytic alpha and KRAS mutations are important predictors of resistance to therapy with epidermal growth factor receptor tyrosine kinase inhibitors in patients with advanced non-small cell lung cancer. J Thorac Oncol. 2011;6(4):707-15.
37. Janjigian YY, Park BJ, Zakowski MF, Ladanyi M, Pao W, D'Angelo SP, Kris MG, Shen R, Zheng J, Azzoli CG. Impact on disease-free survival of adjuvant erlotinib or gefitinib in patients with resected lung adenocarcinomas that harbor EGFR mutations. J Thorac Oncol. 2011;6(3):569-75.
38. Wu YL, Lee JS, Thongprasert S, et al. Intercalated combination of chemotherapy and erlotinib for patients with advanced stage non-small-cell lung cancer (FASTACT-2):a randomised, double-blind trial. Lancet Oncol. 2013;14:777-86.
39. Balak MN, Gong Y, Riely GJ, et al. Novel D761Y and common secondary T790M mutations in epidermal growth factor receptor-mutant lung adenocarcinomas with acquired resistance to kinase inhibitors. Clin Cancer Res. 2006;12(21):6494-501.
40. Costa DB, Schumer ST, Tenen DG, et al. Differential responses to erlotinib in epidermal

growth factor receptor (EGFR)-mutated lung cancers with acquired resistance to gefitinib carrying the L747S or T790M secondary mutations. J Clin Oncol. 2008;26(7):1182-4.

41. Bean J, Riely GJ, Balak M. Acquired resistance to epidermal growth factor receptor kinase inhibitors associated with a novel T854A mutation in a patient with EGFR-mutant lung adenocarcinoma. Clin Cancer Res. 2008;14(22):7519-25.

42. Sequist LV, Waltman BA, Dias-Santagata D, et al. Genotypic and histological evolution of lung cancers acquiring resistance to EGFR inhibitors. Sci Transl Med. 2011;3(75):75ra26.

43. Yu HA, Arcila ME, Rekhtman N, et al. Analysis of tumor specimens at the time of acquired resistance to EGFR-TKI therapy in 155 patients with EGFR-mutant lung cancers. Clin Cancer Res. 2013;19(8):2240-7.

44. Faber AC, Corcoran RB, Ebi H, Sequist LV, et al. BIM expression in treatment-naïve cancers predicts responsiveness to kinase inhibitors. Cancer Discov. 2011;1(4):289-90.

45. Ng KP, Hillmer AM, Chuah CT, et al. A common BIM deletion polymorphism mediates intrinsic resistance and inferior responses to tyrosine kinase inhibitors in cancer. Nat Med. 2012;18(4):521-8.

46. Jackman D, Pao W, Riely GJ, et al. Clinical definition of acquired resistance to epidermal growth factor receptor tyrosine kinase inhibitors in non-small-cell lung cancer. J Clin Oncol. 2010;28(2):357-60.

47. Rho JK, Choi YJ, Kim SY, et al. MET and AXL inhibitor NPS-1034 exerts efficacy against lung cancer cells resistant to EGFR kinase inhibitors because of MET or AXL activation. Cancer Res. 2014;74(1):253-62.

48. Kuiper JL, Heideman DA, Thunnissen E, Paul MA, van Wijk AW, Postmus PE, Smit EF. Incidence of T790M mutation in (sequential) rebiopsies in EGFR-mutated NSCLCpatients. Lung Cancer. 2014;85(1):19-24.

49. Chaft JE, Oxnard GR, Sima CS, Kris MG, Miller VA, Riely GJ. Disease flare after tyrosine kinase inhibitor discontinuation in patients with EGFR-mutant lung cancer and acquired resistance to erlotinib or gefitinib: implications for clinical trial design. Clin Cancer Res. 2011;17(19):6298-303.

50. Asami K, Okuma T, Hirashima T, Kawahara M, Atagi S, Kawaguchi T, Okishio K, Omachi N, Takeuchi N. Continued treatment with gefitinib beyond progressive disease benefits patients with activating EGFR mutations. Lung Cancer. 2013;79(3):276-82.

51. Weickhardt AJ, Scheier B, Burke JM, Gan G, Lu X, Bunn Jr PA, Aisner DL, Gaspar LE, Kavanagh BD, Doebele RC, Camidge DR. Local ablative therapy of oligoprogressive disease prolongs disease control by tyrosine kinase inhibitors in oncogene-addicted non-small-cell lung cancer. J Thorac Oncol. 2012;7(12):1807-14.

52. Yu HA, Camelia S, Sima CS, Huang J, et al. Local therapy with continued EGFR tyrosine kinase inhibitor therapy as a treatment strategy in EGFR mutant advanced lung cancers that have developed acquired resistance to EGFR tyrosine kinase inhibitors. J Thorac Oncol. 2013;8(3):346-51.

53. Conforti F, Catania C, Toffalorio F, Duca M, Spitaleri G, Barberis M, Noberasco C, Delmonte A, Santarpia M, Lazzari C, De Pas TM. EGFR tyrosine kinase inhibitors beyond focal progression obtain a prolonged disease control in patients with advanced adenocarcinoma of the lung. Lung Cancer. 2013;81(3):440-4.
54. Li D, Ambrogio L, Shimamura T, Kubo S, Takahashi M, Chirieac LR, Padera RF, Shapiro GI, Baum A, Himmelsbach F, Rettig WJ, Meyerson M, Solca F, Greulich H, Wong KK. BIBW2992, an irreversible EGFR/HER2 inhibitor highly effective in preclinical lung cancer models. Oncogene. 2008;27(34):4702-11.
55. Yano S, Nakagawa T. The current state of molecularly targeted drugs targeting HGF/Met. Jpn J Clin Oncol. 2014;44(1):9-12.
56. Yoshimura N, Okishio K, Mitsuoka S, Kimura T, Kawaguchi T, Kobayashi M, Hirashima T, Daga H, Takeda K, Hirata K, Kudoh S. Prospective assessment of continuation of erlotinib or gefitinib in patients with acquired resistance to erlotinib or gefitinib followed by the addition of pemetrexed. J Thorac Oncol. 2013;8(1):96-101.
57. Goldberg SB, Oxnard GR, Digumarthy S, Muzikansky A, Jackman DM, Lennes IT, Sequist LV. Chemotherapy with Erlotinib or chemotherapy alone in advanced non-small cell lung cancer with acquired resistance to EGFR tyrosine kinase inhibitors. Oncologist. 2013;18(11):1214-20.
58. Miller VA, Hirsh V, Cadranel J, Chen YM, Park K, Kim SW, Zhou C, Su WC, Wang M, Sun Y, Heo DS, Crino L, Tan EH, Chao TY, Shahidi M, Cong XJ, Lorence RM, Yang JC. Afatinib versus placebo for patients with advanced, metastatic non-small-cell lung cancer after failure of erlotinib, gefitinib, or both, and one or two lines of chemotherapy (LUX-Lung 1):a phase 2b/3 randomised trial. Lancet Oncol. 2012;13(5):528-38.
59. Janjigian YY, Smit EF, Groen HJ, et al. Inhibition of EGFR with Afatinib and Cetuximab in Kinase Inhibitor-Resistant EGFR-Mutant Lung Cancer with and without T790M Mutations. Cancer Discov. 2014 Jul 29. [Epub ahead of print].
60. Sequist LV, Soria JC, Gadgeel SM, Wakelee HA, et al. First-in-human evaluation of CO-1686, an irreversible, highly selective tyrosine kinase inhibitor of mutations of EGFR (activating and T790M). J Clin Oncol. 2014;32(5s):abstr 8010.
61. Kim DW, Lee DH, Kang JH, Park K, Han JY, et al. Clinical activity and safety of HM61713, an EGFR-mutant selective inhibitor, in advanced non-small cell lung cancer (NSCLC) patients (pts) with EGFR mutations who had received EGFR tyrosine kinase inhibitors (TKIs). J Clin Oncol. 2014;32(5s):abstr 8011.
62. Janne PA, Ramalingam SS, Yang JCH, et al. Clinical activity of the mutant-selective EGFR inhibitor AZD9291 in patients (pts) with EGFR inhibitor-resistant non-small cell lung cancer (NSCLC). J Clin Oncol. 2014;32(5s):abstr 8009.
63. Patel MR, Dixon J, Sadiq AA, Jacobson BA, Kratzke RA. Resistance to EGFR-TKI can be mediated through multiple signaling pathways converging upon cap-dependent translation in EGFR-wild type NSCLC. J Thorac Oncol. 2013;8(9):1142-7.

64. Kelly K, Altorki NK, Eberhardt WE, O'Brien ME, et al. A randomized, double-blind phase 3 trial of adjuvant erlotinib (E) versus placebo (P) following complete tumor resection with or without adjuvant chemotherapy in patients (pts) with stage IB-ⅢA EGFR positive (IHC/FISH) non-small cell lung cancer (NSCLC): RADIANT results. J Clin Oncol. 2014;32(5s): abstr 7501.
65. Shepherd FA, Altorki NK, Eberhardt WE, O'Brien ME, et al. Adjuvant erlotinib (E) versus placebo (P) in non-small cell lung cancer (NSCLC) patients (pts) with tumors carrying EGFRsensitizing mutations from the RADIANT trial. J Clin Oncol. 2014;32(5s):abstr 7513.
66. PennellNA, Neal JW, Chaft JE, et al. SELECT:a multicenter phase II trial of adjuvant erlotinib in resected early-stage EGFR mutation-positive NSCLC. J Clin Oncol. 2014;32(5s):abstr 7514.
67. Goss GD, O'Callaghan C, Lorimer I, Tsao MS, Masters GA, Jett J, Edelman MJ, Lilenbaum R, Choy H, Khuri F, Pisters K, Gandara D, Kernstine K, Butts C, Noble J, Hensing TA, Rowland K, Schiller J, Ding K, Shepherd FA. Gefitinib versus placebo in completely resected non-small-cell lung cancer: results of the NCIC CTG BR19 study. J Clin Oncol. 2013;31(27):3320-6.
68. Arcila ME, Oxnard GR, Nafa K, et al. Rebiopsy of lung cancer patients with acquired resistance to EGFR inhibitors and enhanced detection of the T790M mutation using a locked nucleic acid-based assay. Clin Cancer Res. 2011;17:1169-80.
69. Yano S, Yamada T, Takeuchi S, et al. Hepatocyte growth factor expression in EGFR mutant lung cancer with intrinsic and acquired resistance to tyrosine kinase inhibitors in a Japanese cohort. J Thorac Oncol. 2011;6:2011-7.

第10章
ALK 重排肺癌治疗策略

作者:Fiona H. Blackhall
译者:曾理平

ALK 重排的 NSCLC

间变性淋巴瘤激酶(ALK)基因首次发现是在间变性大细胞淋巴瘤中,是2号、5染色体转位融合的一部分[1]。随后,在非小细胞肺癌(NSCLC)细胞中发现了,包含 ALK 基因的染色体 2p 段发生部分倒位或易位而形成融合基因[2,3]。ALK 融合阳性(ALK 阳性)的非小细胞肺癌约占所有肺癌的 2%~5%[4],据估计,全球每年该亚组患者超过 60 000 例。

在 NSCLC 中,ALK 最常见的融合伴侣是棘皮动物微管相关蛋白样 4(EML4)基因。根据基因融合的特定染色体位置,已经确定了至少 27 种的融合变异[5]。一个"功能性"的融合变异可以组成激活 AKK 酪氨酸激酶结构域,导致肿瘤发生。该变异在体外和体内都具有致癌作用。ALK + 的 NSCLC 靶向治疗主要通过抑制激活的 ALK 酪氨酸激酶蛋白。

治疗 ALK 阳性 NSCLC 的第一步是在诊断活检标本中确定 ALK 的融合基因。ALK 抑制剂的流行病学研究和临床试验显示有诸多临床-病理因素与 ALK 融合基因有关([6,7])。最主要的临床病理相关因素是从不或曾有轻度吸烟史,组织学为腺癌(ADC),低龄以及女性。此外,腺癌中罕见的印戒亚型与 ALK 基因融合的密切相关[8]。上述因素有助于确认 ALK 检测的"高危"人群,但 ALK 融合基因不只限于上述人群,所以仅通过上述因素不能有效识别所有 ALK 阳性的患者。如首例报道的 ALK 阳性 NSCLC 患者为有显著吸烟史男性患者[2]。

ALK 融合基因检测

用于检测基因融合的金标准方法是荧光原位杂交(FISH),也是目前 FDA 批准的 ALK +NSCLC 的检测方法。对检测 ALK 融合基因来说,FISH 是一个可靠但资源要求高的技术,需要特殊的培训和技能。ALK 融合基因的蛋白质产物也可以采用免疫组化的方法(IHC),因为 ALK 蛋白在肺组织中不是正常表达,IHC 资源要求相对低。ALK 免疫组化高表达已显示与用 FISH 检测的 ALK 融合基因的存在明显相关。IHC检测出的低表达的ALK蛋白很可能为假阳性,可通过FISH证实为阴性;IHC阴性和FISH阴性的病例已经显示出高度的一致性。迄今为止,一些抗体的可靠性和实用性已经得到证明,但何种抗体最佳,目前还存在争议。第三种方法是采用RT-PCR,随着技术改进,该方法在临床诊断实验室中的应用会越来越广泛。目前,初步共识建议如资源限制了FISH法常规筛选全部的病例,可以采用免疫组化预筛然后FISH确认。可以参考ALK检测的有循证依据的指南和建议[9]。

第一代ALK抑制剂:克唑替尼

克唑替尼(PF-02341066,辉瑞)为一种口服,小分子ALK、MET和ROS 1酪氨酸激酶的靶向抑制剂[10-12]。2011年8月FDA[13]批准了克唑替尼用于ALK+NSCLC的治疗,2012年7月欧洲药品评价局(EMEA)也批准同意[14]。FDA批准允许克唑替尼用于任何几线治疗,但EMEA仅批准用于之前经过其他治疗的ALK融合基因阳性的患者。克唑替尼最早是作为MET的一种抑制剂,但观察到对ALK有抑制作用,转而用于已经用尽了标准治疗方案的ALK阳性NSCLC患者[6]。在单臂Ⅰ期[15]和Ⅱ期试验[16]中,观察到显著的抗肿瘤活性,客观缓解率约为60%,中位无进展生存期分别为8.1个月、9.7个月。虽然是非随机对照试验结果,但与文献报道结果相比,明显优于传统单药化疗,传统单药化疗的缓解率为10%以下,中位无进展生存期仅2~3个月[17]。尽管这些统计数据是从未选择(即没有分子水平确认)的NSCLC患者中得到的,但是对晚期NSCLC,ALK融合基因不能作为预后的有利因素[18]。

FDA批准克唑替尼上市之后,开展了一项临床随机对照Ⅲ期试验(PROFILE 1007),比较克唑替尼和化疗治疗之前治疗过的ALK阳性NSCLC患者的临床效果。化疗组患者根据之前的一线化疗方案和(或)肿瘤组织学选择行多西他赛或培美曲塞治疗。结果显示,化疗组PFS为3.0个月,克唑替尼组则明显高于化疗组,其PFS为7.7个月(HR=0.49,95%CI:0.37~0.64,$P<0.001$)[19]。化疗组患者缓解率为20%[95%CI 14~26],克唑替尼缓解率明显提高,达到65%[95%CI 58~72]。该研究结果与非分子选择的历史对照组相比,化疗的缓解率略高于前期结果,但PFS的结果较前一致[17]。与化疗组相比,克唑替尼组患者咳嗽、呼吸困难、疲劳及疼痛等症状明显改善,患者体验与生活质量明显提升。对于晚期ALK+NSCLC,克唑替尼一线治疗是否优于化疗目前尚不明确。临床试验(PROFILE 1014)正在比较克唑替尼一线治疗与培美曲塞和铂类等化疗的临床效果,已完成病例招募工作,结果将于不久公布。

克唑替尼的安全性

患者对于克唑替尼耐受性良好,临床Ⅰ、Ⅱ、Ⅲ期结果都认为该药安全性良好[10,16,19]。

克唑替尼相关不良事件一般都较轻微，报道最常见不良事件为恶心，腹泻，呕吐，便秘和视力影响。很少有不良事件需药物减量或停药。克唑替尼和化疗的随机对照研究结果显示，克唑替尼患者恶心发生率较高[19]。但需要指出的是，化疗患者往往多常规给予预防性止吐药，而克唑替尼患者一般不常规予以预防性止吐处理。另外比较常见的毒副反应一般都比较轻微，包括外周性水肿，头晕，乏力和食欲下降，内分泌的影响，特别是睾酮耗竭相对较常见，克唑替尼治导致的转氨酶升高一般发生在前 2 个月（平均发病 40 天）的治疗内。在 PROFILE 1001 和 1005 研究[15,16]的 1054 例患者中，ALT 升高超过正常值上限的 3 倍、5 倍和 10 倍的发生率分别为 15%、7.4% 和 3%，ALT 升高多为 3~4 级不良反应事件，但多不伴总胆红素升高。目前推荐克唑替尼治疗患者应每月至少检测一次肝功能，若结果异常，则应增加检测频率，减量予以较低剂量的克唑替尼治疗使肝功能恢复正常。

部分克唑替尼患者初期可出现总睾酮水平迅速降低[21,22]，推测有可能是由于下丘脑或垂体效应发生的，该效应也可导致患者出现乏力等症状。克唑替尼停药可使睾酮水平恢复正常。目前尚缺乏晚期肺癌患者睾酮水平的临床数据，也缺乏化疗以及其他治疗方法对于睾酮水平影响的数据。期待包括 PROFILE 1014 试验等前瞻性随机对照试验结果，可以进一步明确克唑替尼相关的睾酮缺乏的原因，以及可能导致的后遗症[20]。

治疗耐药

ALK 阳性 NSCLC 患者对克唑替尼初始缓解率约为 60%，这表明在部分患者存在原发性耐药。体外细胞和分子研究发现 EGFR 通路激活可导致克唑替尼耐药[23,24]，治疗前的细胞促凋亡蛋白 BIM 的水平也可影响肿瘤对克唑替尼的反应[25]。总的来说，原发性耐药的原因和机制目前研究还不充分。而获得性耐药的研究进展相对较快。但克唑替尼初始治疗有反应的患者往往最后出现耐药，导致疾病进展。体外实验以及检测疾病进展患者活检标本发现，克唑替尼治疗导致的多种分子改变是其主要原因。对于药物研发研究最关键的改变是与克唑替尼结合的 ALK 基因突变的发生。检测发现，约 1/3 的获得性耐药患者发生了以下位点的突变，看门区域的 ALKL1196M 突变，核糖结合口区附近的 ALK 1206 突变，DFG 模体的 ALKG1269A 突变，以及 ALKC1156Y 突变，ALKL1152R 突变，ALKF1174L 突变，ALK1151Tins 突变和 ALKG1202R 突变等（参考综述[26,27],[6]）。其他获得性耐药的机制包括 ALK 基因拷贝数增加，ALK 融合基因的丢失，EGFR 通路的激活及突变，KRAS 基因突变和 KIT 扩增[28]。除了介导耐药性的分子机制，克唑替尼透过血脑屏障并进入中枢神经系统（CNS）的能力较差。因此，该药对于控制中枢神经系统的转移灶效果欠佳[29]。

第二代 ALK 抑制剂临床研发

正在开发的第二代 ALK 抑制剂，很大程度上旨在克服和（或）减少 ALK 抑制时出现获得性耐药的发生率,并对中枢神经系统转移具有更佳的疗效。

LDK 378(诺华)

LDK378 是一种选择性 ALK 抑制剂,可有效抑制看门基因 C1156Y 突变、对克唑替尼耐药的 ALK 融合基因。在Ⅰ期临床试验评估[30]中,总缓解率为 70%,克唑替尼治疗时已经进展或者对克唑替尼耐药的患者,缓解率为 73%。该药对未治疗的中枢神经系统转移的患者也有一定效果。该项研究发现,所有 NSCLC 患者($n=123$)的 PFS 是 8.6 个月,最常见的不良反应为恶心(72%)、腹泻(69%)、呕吐(50%)和疲劳(31%)。患者对 LDK378 耐受性良好。Ⅰ期临床试验中,最常见的 3 级和 4 级不良事件 ALT 升高,腹泻和 AST 升高,发生率分别为 12%、7%和 6%。LDK 378 的一些研究正在进行中,以评估其在克唑替尼治疗后患者,未曾使用克唑替尼患者,合并 CNS 转移患者中的价值。

目前正在开展一项临床Ⅱ期多中心单臂研究,拟招募 137 例曾接受化疗或克唑替尼后出现疾病进展的患者,评估患者对 LDK 378 治疗反应,主要终点为缓解率[31]。另有一类似研究拟招募未曾使用克唑替尼治疗的患者[32]。还有两项Ⅲ期随机对照试验已经启动,分别评估 LDK378 与一线化疗[33]和二线化疗[34]的临床效果。

AP26113(阿瑞雅德)

AP26113(阿瑞雅德)是一种有效的 ALK 抑制剂,对已知的克唑替尼耐药突变有对抗作用,同时还可抑制 ROS1 酪氨酸激酶和突变的表皮生长因子受体(EGFR),包括 EGFR T790M 耐药突变。第一个人体研究结果已报道[35],该研究纳入合并 ALK 突变的未曾使用 ALK 抑制剂治疗患者,克唑替尼耐药患者,活动性脑转移患者,结果发现曾行克唑替尼治疗的患者的缓解率为 61%(19/31),克唑替尼耐药合并脑转移的患者也观察到应答。AP26113 的毒副反应和克唑替尼类似,多表现为轻度恶心、乏力、腹泻。尽管对 EGFR 突变有抑制活性,但皮疹等并发症罕见。治疗早期阶段,约 10%的患者会出现呼吸困难、缺氧和肺炎等严重的肺部症状,多在患者刚开始接受 AP26113 治疗的前几天内发生,经过 AP26113 中断治疗以及类固醇等抗炎支持治疗,多可逆转肺部症状。因此,需重新评估 AP26113 的治疗剂量(90~180mg,QD)是否合理,同时严格控制该药治疗的适应证,选择一般状况好,治疗前无须氧气支持治疗的患者,无间质性肺病,ECOG PS 评分为 0~1 分得患者行 AP26113 治疗,可以明显减少肺部不良事件的发生。临床Ⅱ期试验推荐剂量为每日 1 次,1 次 180 mg,需要评估该剂量的合理性,目前尚有几项临床试验正在进行中,其结果将有助于全面了解该药的安全性及临床疗效。

Alectinib[CH5424802(日本中外/罗氏)]

Alectinib[CH5424802(日本中外/罗氏)]是一种有效 ALK 选择性抑制剂,对大多数 ALK 获得性耐药突变有抑制活性,活性较克唑替尼提高[36]。来自日本的小样本研究纳入 46 例未曾使用克唑替尼的患者使用 Alectinib 治疗,患者客观缓解率为 93.5%,中位缓解时间超过 14 个月[37]。由于其治疗肿瘤具有高缓解率,因此很有必要开展临床研究对比克唑替尼和 Alectinib 的效果。

PF-06463922(辉瑞)

PF-06463922(辉瑞)是 ALK 和 ROS-1 的新型小分子 ATP 抑制剂,体外实验表明其具有抑制所有已知克唑替尼获得性耐药突变的活性。动物模型研究表明 PF-06463922 可通过血-脑屏障。体外和临床初期研究表明该药针对 ALK 非突变或突变肿瘤细胞均有效。目前有相关研究正在进行,拟评估该药对于未曾使用克唑替尼治疗的患者和曾使用克唑替尼治疗患者的临床效果,PF-06463922 与克唑替尼的临床随机对照试验也正在进行中[38]。

TSR-011(Tesaro)

TSR-011(Tesaro)是一种强效 ALK 和 TRK 双重抑制剂,目前正在进行相关的早期临床试验。NTRK-A 基因重排存在于 3% 的其他原癌基因驱动突变阴性的 NSCLC 中,TRK 激酶作为 NTRK-A 的组成部分而同时激活[39]。临床 I 期试验表明,TSR-011 的不良反应主要为可逆性 DLTS,包括感觉迟钝和 QT 间期延长等,该药对 3 例携带 ALK 突变、克唑替尼治疗之后出现疾病进展的患者中至少 2 例存在抗肿瘤活性,而在 17 例可评估患者中,8 周时的疾病控制率(疾病稳定和部分缓解)是 65%。

HSP-90 抑制剂

热休克蛋白(HSPs)是引导异常表达的 ALK 融合基因到它们的亚细胞位点和亚基的分子伴侣蛋白的一个家族。体外实验表明即使在克唑替尼耐药情况下,抑制 HSP 也可诱导肿瘤 ALK 融合蛋白降解,抑制 ALK 融合基因活性[6]。临床早期试验表明两种 HSP 90 抑制剂,retaspimycin(IPI-504)和 ganetespib(STA-9090)对 ALK 阳性 NSCLC 患者具有临床治疗活性[40-42]。一些评估单用 HSP-90 抑制剂或者联合其他药物,包括化疗、ALK 抑制剂治疗 ALK 阳性 NSCLC 的临床试验正在进行中。

总结与展望

第一代 ALK 抑制剂克唑替尼,由于临床早期试验显示治疗 ALK 阳性 NSCLC 的患者效果良好,其临床应用推广比较迅速。目前最主要的问题是,克唑替尼和(或)其他 ALK 靶向抑制剂比一线化疗相比,治疗晚期 ALK 阳性 NSCLC 是否更有效,目前正在进行相关的临床试验(PROFILE 1014),该试验结果将于近期公布。

ALK 靶向治疗的原发耐药和继发耐药是另一个亟需解决的关键问题。目前已将部分 EGFR-TKIs 耐药性研究经验转化到 ALK 靶向治疗耐药的研究上。通过对克唑替尼治疗后出现进展的患者行多次标本活检,证实存在可影响克唑替尼与靶点有效结合的新突变。多种第二代 ALK 靶向抑制剂有着一定的前景,可暂时克服 ALK 突变有关的克唑替尼耐药机制,但最好的 ALK 抑制剂是否会从这些抑制剂中出现还为时尚早。值得注意的是,目前关于第二代 ALK 抑制剂和克唑替尼的对比研究较少,而这类研究对于确定二代靶向抑制剂的有效性至关重要,可确保 ALK 融合基因阳性的 NSCLC 患者在下一个十年能得到最好的治疗,获得最佳预后。

除了第二代 ALK 抑制剂,另一种针对耐药患者的治疗策略是克唑替尼联合针对潜在耐药突变和旁路激活的药物。例如,泛 HER 家族抑制剂达克米替尼,目前正在评估其与克唑替尼联合治疗的临床效果[43]。而合并中枢神经系统转移,特别是脑转移,全脑放疗(WBRT)可破坏血-脑屏障,提高药物渗透到脑组织内,从而增加脑转移瘤对克唑替尼的治疗反应。另单次大剂量 500mg 克唑替尼治疗对脑转移患者也有一定效果[44]。与全脑放射治疗后行克唑替尼治疗相比,克唑替尼联合全脑放射治疗的优势尚不明确。脑转移患者行 ALK 靶向治疗的临床试验正在进行中[45]。

另外还有一些其他问题,包括克唑替尼在局部晚期 ALK 阳性 NSCLC 综合治疗中的价值,手术切除的 ALK 阳性 NSCLC 患者是否需行克唑替尼辅助治疗。因为 ALK 阳性 NSCLC 患者相对较少,因此开展上述临床研究比较困难。ALK 靶向治疗的研究发展迅速,克唑替尼可能会被第二代 ALK 抑制剂所取代,但由于其是第一个 ALK 抑制剂,其临床发展过程在未来几十年仍具有重要历史参考意义。

参考文献

1. Morris SW, et al. Fusion of a kinase gene, ALK, to a nucleolar protein gene, NPM, in non-Hodgkin's lymphoma. Science. 1994;263(5151):1281-4.
2. Soda M, et al. Identification of the transforming EML4-ALK fusion gene in non-small-cell lung cancer. Nature. 2007;448(7153):561-6.
3. Rikova K, et al. Global survey of phosphotyrosine signaling identifi es oncogenic kinases in lung cancer. Cell. 2007;131(6):1190-203.
4. Camidge DR, Doebele RC. Treating ALK-positive lung cancer-early successes and future challenges. Nat Rev Clin Oncol. 2012;9(5):268-77.
5. Sasaki T, et al. The biology and treatment of EML4-ALK non-small cell lung cancer. Eur J Cancer. 2010; 46(10):1773-80.
6. Ou SH, et al. Crizotinib for the treatment of ALK-rearranged non-small cell lung cancer: a success story to usher in the second decade of molecular targeted therapy in oncology. Oncologist. 2012;17(11):1351-75.
7. Peters S, et al. Treatment and detection of ALK-rearranged NSCLC. Lung Cancer. 2013; 81(2):145-54.

8. Popat S, et al. ALK translocation is associated with ALK immunoreactivity and extensive signet-ring morphology in primary lung adenocarcinoma. Lung Cancer. 2012;75(3):300-5.
9. Lindeman NI, et al. Molecular testing guideline for selection of lung cancer patients for EGFR and ALK tyrosine kinase inhibitors:guideline from the College of American Pathologists, International Association for the Study of Lung Cancer, and Association for Molecular Pathology. J Thorac Oncol. 2013;8(7):823-59.
10. Kwak EL, et al. Anaplastic lymphoma kinase inhibition in non-small-cell lung cancer. N Engl J Med. 2010; 363 (18):1693-703.
11. Ou SH, et al. Activity of crizotinib (PF02341066), a dual mesenchymal-epithelial transition (MET) and anaplastic lymphoma kinase (ALK) inhibitor, in a non-small cell lung cancer patient with de novo MET amplification. J Thorac Oncol. 2011;6(5):942-6.
12. Bergethon K, et al. ROS1 rearrangements define a unique molecular class of lung cancers. J Clin Oncol. 2012;30 (8):863-70.
13. FDA Approval for crizotinib. http://www.cancer.gov/cancertopics/druginfo/fda-crizotinib.
14. Crizotinib european public assessment report. http://www.ema.europa.eu/ema/index.jsp?curl=pages/medicines/human/medicines/002489/human_med_001592.jsp&mid=WC0b01ac058001d124.
15. Camidge DR, et al. Activity and safety of crizotinib in patients with ALK-positive non-small-cell lung cancer:updated results from a phase 1 study. Lancet Oncol. 2012;13(10):1011-9.
16. Crinò L, Kim D,Riely GJ, Janne PA, Blackhall FH, Camidge DR, Hirsh V, Mok T, Solomon BJ, Park K, Gadgeel SM, Martins R, Han J, De Pas TM, Bottomley A, Polli A, Petersen J, Tassell VR, Shaw AT. Initial phase II results with crizotinib in advanced ALK-positive nonsmall cell lung cancer (NSCLC):PROFILE 1005. J Clin Oncol. ASCO Annual Meeting Abstracts. 2011;29(15_Suppl (May 20 Supplement) 7514).
17. Hanna N, et al. Randomized phase Ⅲ trial of pemetrexed versus docetaxel in patients with nonsmall-cell lung cancer previously treated with chemotherapy. J Clin Oncol. 2004;22(9):1589-97.
18. Shaw AT, et al. Pemetrexed-based chemotherapy in patients with advanced, ALK-positive nonsmall cell lung cancer. Ann Oncol. 2013;24(1):59-66.
19. Shaw AT, et al. Crizotinib versus chemotherapy in advanced ALK-positive lung cancer. N Engl J Med. 2013;368(25):2385-94.
20. A study of crizotinib versus chemotherapy in previously untreated alk positive east asian nonsmall cell lung cancer patients. NCT01639001. www.clinicaltrials.gov.
21. Weickhardt AJ, et al. Rapid-onset hypogonadism secondary to crizotinib use in men with metastatic nonsmall cell lung cancer. Cancer. 2012;118(21):5302-9.
22. Weickhardt AJ, et al. Symptomatic reduction in free testosterone levels secondary to crizotinib use in male cancer patients. Cancer. 2013;119(13):2383-90.
23. Lovly CM, Pao W. Escaping ALK inhibition:mechanisms of and strategies to overcome resistance. Sci Transl Med. 2012;4(120):120ps2.

24. Sasaki T, et al. A novel ALK secondary mutation and EGFR signaling cause resistance to ALK kinase inhibitors. Cancer Res. 2011;71(18):6051-60.
25. Takezawa K, et al. Role of ERK-BIM and STAT3-survivin signaling pathways in ALK inhibitor induced apoptosis in EML4-ALK-positive lung cancer. Clin Cancer Res. 2011;17(8):2140-8.
26. Choi YL, et al. EML4-ALK mutations in lung cancer that confer resistance to ALK inhibitors. N Engl J Med. 2010; 363(18):1734-9.
27. Katayama R, et al. Mechanisms of acquired crizotinib resistance in ALK-rearranged lung cancers. Sci Transl Med. 2012;4(120):120ra17.
28. Doebele RC, et al. Mechanisms of resistance to crizotinib in patients with ALK gene rearranged non-small cell lung cancer. Clin Cancer Res. 2012;18(5):1472-82.
29. Gainor JF, et al. The central nervous system as a sanctuary site in ALK-positive non-small-cell lung cancer. J Thorac Oncol. 2013;8(12):1570-3.
30. Shaw AT, Camidge R, Felip E, Sharma S, Tan DSW, Kim D, De Pas T, Vansteenkiste JF, Santoro A, Liu G, Goldwasser M, Dai D, Boral AL, Mehra R. Results of a first-in-human phase I study of the ALK inhibitor LDK378 in advanced solid tumors. Ann Oncol. 2012; 23(Supplement 9):53.
31. LDK378 in adult patients with alk-activated NSCLC previously treated with chemotherapy and crizotinib. NCT01685060. www.clinicaltrials.gov.
32. LDK378 in crizotinib naïve adult patients with alk-activated non-small cell lung cancer. NCT01685138. www.clinicaltrials.gov.
33. LDK378 versus chemotherapy in previously untreated patients with alk rearranged non-small cell lung cancer. NCT01828099. www.clinicaltrials.gov.
34. LDK378 versus chemotherapy in ALK rearranged (ALK positive) patients previously treated with chemotherapy (platinum doublet) and crizotinib. NCT01828112. www.clinicaltrials.gov.
35. Camidge DR, Bazhenova L, Salgia R, et al. First-in-human dose-finding study of the ALK/EGFR inhibitor AP26113 in patients with advanced malignancies:updated results. J Clin Oncol. 2013;31(Suppl):Abstr 8031.
36. Sakamoto H, et al. CH5424802, a selective ALK inhibitor capable of blocking the resistant gatekeeper mutant. Cancer Cell. 2011;19(5):679-90.
37. Nakagawa K, Kiura K, NishioA M et al. A phase I/II study with a highly selective ALK inhibitor CH5424802 in ALK-positive non-small cell lung cancer (NSCLC) patients:Updated safety and efficacy results from AF-001JP. J Clin Oncol 2013;(Suppl):Abstract 8033.
38. Targeting resistance in lung cancer. Cancer Discov. 2013;3(12):OF9.
39. Doebele R, Vaishnani A, Capeletti M, et al. NTRK1 gene fusions as a novel oncogene target in lung cancer. JCO. 2013;31:Abstract 8023.
40. Socinski MA, et al. A multicenter phase II study of ganetespib monotherapy in patients with genotypically defined advanced non-small cell lung cancer. Clin Cancer Res. 2013;19(11):

3068-77.

41. Sequist LV, et al. Activity of IPI-504, a novel heat-shock protein 90 inhibitor, in patients with molecularly defined non-small-cell lung cancer. J Clin Oncol. 2010;28(33):4953-60.
42. Normant E, et al. The Hsp90 inhibitor IPI-504 rapidly lowers EML4-ALK levels and induces tumor regression in ALK-driven NSCLC models. Oncogene. 2011;30(22):2581-6.
43. A study of combined C- MET inhibitor and PAN-HER inhibitor (PF-02341066 and PF-00299804). In patients with non- small cell lung cancer. NCT01121575. www. clinicaltrials. gov.
44. Peled N, et al. Effective crizotinib schedule for brain metastases in ALK rearrangement metastatic non-small-cell lung cancer. J Thorac Oncol. 2013;8(12):e112-3.
45. Dziadziuszko R, Jassem J. Beneath the blood brain barrier: the challenge of diagnosis and management of central nervous system involvement in ALK-positive lung cancer. J Thorac Oncol. 2013;8(12):1465-6.

第11章
KRAS突变肺癌治疗策略

作者：Celine Mascaux，Frances A. Shepherd
译者：袁小帅

简介

近数十年来，在非小细胞肺癌（non-small cell lung cancer，NSCLC）中如表皮生长因子受体（the epidermal growth factor receptor，EGFR）和间变性淋巴瘤激酶（the anaplastic lymphoma kinase，ALK）等致癌基因突变的发现促进了分子靶向治疗的发展。然而，作为最古老和最常见的肺癌癌基因之一，大鼠肉瘤（rat sarcoma，RAS）基因因其对预后和预测的影响尚存较大争议，而仍旧未被国内外学者们得到完全深刻的认识，同时RAS突变癌症的试验性靶向治疗结果并不令人满意。Jennifer Harvey和Werner Kirsten分别于1964和1967年在白血病大鼠诱导的小鼠肉瘤病毒中首次发现了原癌基因RAS家族的两个基因[1,2]。起初这些基因被认为与人类肿瘤并无关联，但它们的人类细胞变体被Weindberg等[3]于1981年发现和研究。3个高度同源性、编码21 kDa蛋白且密切相关的RAS基因在人类基因组中被发现[4]：HRAS和KRAS，分别与Harvey和Kirsten在大鼠肉瘤病毒中发现的RAS基因同源；NRAS，首次经由人神经母细胞瘤细胞中分离出来[5,6]。RAS基因的编码蛋白p21是一个具有内源性GTP酶活性的GTP/GDP双向开关（附录彩图11.1）[8]。RAS蛋白以两种状态存在：一种是活化状态，此时与GTP相连接；另一种是非活化状态，此时GTP已被水解为GDP。在其生理状态下，RAS蛋白的活化形式可激活多个下游通路从而启动细胞增殖，生长，运动和存活。同时因RAS蛋白具有内源性GTP酶活性，它们会自发性回归到其非活化形态，从而控制细胞生长与增殖。RAS突变激活可导致内源性GTP酶活性的丧失，从而阻止GTP水解为GDP以及RAS蛋白的失活。随后，突变的RAS蛋白将被永久激活，致使下游因子的持续活化以及细胞生长、增殖和存活状态的失控[8]。

在RAS原癌基因突变中最常见的为NSCLC，突变率为15%～30%。大多数NSCLC的RAS突变都发生在KRAS中，然而HRAS和NRAS在肺癌中的突变也偶有发生[4]。在本章节中，除了KRAS突变的流行病学分析之外，我们还将回

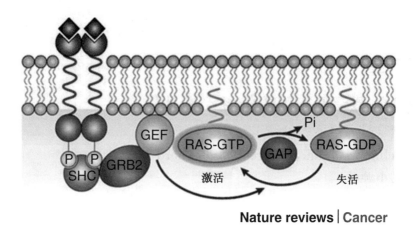

图 11.1　RAS 蛋白 GTP 酶激活与失活[7]

顾:①NSCLC 中 KRAS 突变对预后的影响;②KRAS 突变在标准化治疗(化疗和靶向治疗)中的预测价值;③针对 KRAS 突变及下游通路的治疗策略。

KRAS 突变的流行病学分析

KRAS 突变在肺腺癌中发生的概率较高(约 20%～30%)而在鳞状细胞癌中相对发生概率偏低(约 5%)[4]。而根据不同种族 KRAS 突变率也有不同变化:高加索血缘的患者为 25%～50%,而亚细亚人种的患者则为 5%～15%[9]。已有很多研究证实了 KRAS 突变和烟草消费之间存在显著相关,KRAS 突变在现今或过往吸烟人群中较终生非吸烟人群更为常见[4]。而且,烟草烟雾导致的 DNA 损伤可引起某些类型的突变。在 KRAS 和 p53 中,碱基颠换(取代嘧啶为嘌呤或嘌呤为嘧啶,如 G→T 或 G→C)更常见于现今或过往吸烟人群,而碱基转换(取代嘧啶为嘧啶或嘌呤为嘌呤,如 G→A)则更常见于终生非吸烟人群[10,11]。通常 NSCLC 中的 KRAS 突变为外显子 2 密码子 12 区域的单氨基酸替换,外显子 2 密码子 13 区域的替换则不太常见(约 10%),极少见于外显子 3 密码子 61 区域[3]。碱基颠换 GGT＞TGT(甘氨酸-半胱氨酸替代,密码子 12,G12C)和 GGT＞GTT(甘氨酸-缬氨酸替代,密码子 12,G12V)是 NSCLC 中最常见的 KRAS 突变(G12C 和 G12V 上分别为 39%～40% 和 20%～21%)[12,13];然后是碱基转换 GGT＞GAT(甘氨酸-天冬氨酸替代,密码子 12,G12D)和 GGT＞GCT(甘氨酸-丙氨酸替代,密码子 12,G12A),突变率分别为 17% 和 6%～10%[12,13];最后是最为少见的突变 GGC＞TGC(甘氨酸-缬氨酸替代,密码子 13,G13V)和 GGT＞AGT(甘氨酸-丝氨酸置换,密码子 12,G12S),约占 3%。

近年来广谱突变分析研究结果表明,NSCLC 中的 KRAS 突变可与其他基因突变同时发生。即便通常认为 EGFR 和 KRAS 突变是互相排斥的,但仍有罕见案例报道了 EGFR 和 KRAS 伴随突变的现象[14]。在法国,由 28 个中心进行的常规全国性的 EGFR、KRAS、HER2、BRAF、PI3K 基因突变和 ALK 基因重排检测得到全球范围内最大队列的分子数据。在第一个经测试的 10 000 例非小细胞肺癌患者中,47% 的样本发现了一个已知的目标,同时 56.9% 的患者接受了生物引导治疗。KRAS 突变在 27% 的患者中被检测到,并且在吸烟人群(37.1%)较非吸烟人群(9.6%)发生频率更高。99 例患者检测到共突变,其中 44 例患者检测到 KRAS 和其他基因的共突变,其中 5 例伴随 EGFR 突变,10 例伴随 ALK 基因重排,6 例伴随 BRAF 突变以及 33 例伴随 PI3k 突变[14]。在美国,肺癌突变联盟(the Lung Cancer Mutation Consortium,LCMC)对 1000 例进展期肺腺癌患者肿瘤标本的 10 种致癌基因出现频率进行了评估。1007 例患者中,63% 出现一个已知致癌基因,其中 28% 可从靶向治疗中获益。共有 25% 的患者出现 KRAS 突变,3% 有两个致癌基因的突变(具体基因并未报道)。发生基因突变的患者接受靶向治疗与为接受靶向治疗的患者相比有更好的预后[15]。

KRAS 基因突变的预后价值

预后因素指的是可预测患者结果(通常为存货)的患者或肿瘤因素,通常与实施的治疗相独立。NSCLC 的最主要临床预后因素包括分期、性别、年龄及体力状态等[16]。20 年前一个小型外科研究首次报道了 KRAS 是作为肺腺癌负性预后因素的肿瘤基因[17]。自此,KRAS 的预后意义被国内外学者在 NSCLC 中进行了广泛研究,但尚未获得一致的结果(表 11.1),可能原因为由不同研究发现突变采用了不同实验室技术以及针对不同患者群体,从而产生了较大的异质性。

测试辅助治疗的随机对照试验提供了大型前瞻性队列以评估早期 NSCLC 中 KRAS 突变的预后价值。东部肿瘤协作组(the Eastern Cooperative Oncology Group,ECOG)E4592 随机试验评估了手术切除的 Ⅱ～ⅢA 期 NSCLC 患者的辅助胸部放疗+/-四周期的顺铂/依托泊苷化疗[21]。184 例被评估的肿瘤中,44 例(24%)发现 KRAS 突变,分别为鳞状细胞癌组织学的 4%,和非鳞状细胞癌组织学的 33%($P<0.05$)。尽管多变量分析发现存在 KRAS 突变的预后作用趋势($P=0.066$),存在 KRAS 突变的患者中位总生存期(OS)并无统计学差异(30 个月 vs 42 个月,KRAS 突变患者 vs 野生型患者,$P=0.38$)[21]。

北美组间试验 JBR.10 纳入了 482 例手术切除的 ⅠB～Ⅰ期 NSCLC,根据 KRAS 或随机基因进行分层并分别进行四周期的辅助顺铂/长春瑞滨或仅作观察,检测到 113(26%)例 RAS 基因突变的患者。观察组中再次得到了 RAS 突变并非 OS 的重要预后因素($P=0.40$)[22]。

表 11.1 NSCLC KRAS 突变患者预后情况

作者/临床试验	试验纳入患者数量/KRAS检测患者数量	KRAS突变情况(%) 突变型	KRAS突变情况(%) 野生型	PFS (HR;95% CI)	PFS p-value	OS (HR;95% CI)	OS p-value
Capelletti 等(2%)(2010)[18] CALGB9633	344/258	71(27%)	187(73%)	NR	NR	1.1	0.747
Scoccianti 等(2012)[19] EUELC	762/249	46(18%)	203(81%)	1.30(0.82~2.06)	0.26	NR	NR
Ma 等(2008)[20] IALT	1867/718	98(14%)	620(86%)	NR	0.03	NR	0.31
Schiller 等(2001)[21] ECOG 4592	217/184	44(24%)	140(76%)	NR	NR	NR	0.38
Tsao 等(2007)[22] JBR.10	482/450	117(26%)	333(74%)	NR	NR	1.23(0.76~1.97)	0.40
合并分析以及 meta 分析							
Mascaux 等(2005)[23]	5216/3779	695(18%)	3084(82%)	NR	NR	1.30(1.20~1.49)	0.01
Meng 等(2013)[24]	6939/6939	NR	NR	NR	NR	1.45(1.29~1.62)	NR
Shepherd 等(2013)[25] LACE-BIO	1718/1543	300(19.4%)	1243(81.6%)	1.05(0.80~1.36)	0.73	1.04(0.78~1.38)	0.79
Shepherd 等(2013)[25] LACE-BIO ADC	813/605	204(33.7%)	401(66.3%)	0.98(0.78~1.24)	0.87	1.00(0.78~1.29)	0.97

HR:风险比;CI:置信区间;PFS:无进展生存期;OS:总生存期;NR:原文未说明;ADC:腺癌

欧洲早期肺癌研究(the European Early Lung Cancer,EUELC)762例手术切除的NSCLC研究队列以及国际癌症研究署(the International Agency for Research on Cancer,IARC)的研究中检测到的KRAS突变率为18.5%,腺癌相较鳞状细胞癌更易发生KRAS基因突变(分别为30.6%和4.3%)。结论为KRAS突变对无进展生存(progression-free survival,PFS)并非显著的预后标志物[19]。

国际辅助肺癌试验(the International Adjuvant Lung Cancer Trial,IALT)中1867例患者随机接受术后顺铂辅助化疗或观察,KRAS突变检出率仅为14%。研究观察到了KRAS在无病生存期(disease-free survival,DFS)中存在显著的不利影响($P=0.03$),而在OS中则无($P=0.31$)。然而在小的非鳞状细胞/非腺癌的亚群中,KRAS突变则在DFS和OS中均存在显著的负性预后影响(分别为$P=0.04$和$P=0.006$)[20]。

肿瘤和白血病B组-9633(the Cancer and Leukemia Group B-9633,CALGB-9633)Ⅲ期临床试验中ⅠB期NSCLC患者随机接受观察或四周期卡铂/紫杉醇治疗,KRAS突变检出率为27%,但并不具有显著的预后价值($P=0.747$)[18]。

由于单独的研究结果意见并不一致,因而2005年报道了一个大型汇总了28项研究和3620例患者的meta分析,以评估KRAS突变对肺癌患者生存是否具有预后意义[23]。总体来讲,KRAS突变的出现是OS的负性预后因素(HR 1.30,95% CI 1.20~1.49,$P=0.01$)。在肺腺癌患者($n=1436$)亚组中,KRAS突变对OS是具有预后意义的(HR 1.52,95% CI 1.30~1.78,$P=0.02$),而对鳞癌患者则无意义($n=280$,HR 1.49,95% CI 0.88~2.52,$P=0.48$)。而应用聚合酶链式反应(polymerase chain reaction,PCR)检测得到的结果则表明KRAS突变是显著的预后标记物($n=2631$,HR 1.40,95% CI 1.18~1.65,$P=0.03$)。当进行早期和晚期疾病对比分析时可知,KRAS突变并无显著预后影响[23]。

2013年一个更大型的meta分析研究发表,囊括了41项临床试验总计6939例患者[24]。该研究证实KRAS突变对NSCLC患者生存的不利影响(HR 1.45,95% CI 1.29~1.62),亚洲患者($n=1524$,HR 1.97,95% CI 1.58~2.44)和非亚洲患者($n=4856$,HR 1.37,95% CI 1.25~1.5)得到了相似的结果,且KRAS突变对肺腺癌患者的显著影响($n=3502$,HR 1.39,95% CI 1.24~1.55)得到了证实,而鳞状细胞癌患者受到的影响则并未进行汇总分析。生存的负性显著影响体现在早期患者(Ⅰ期,$n=535$,HR 1.81,95% CI 1.36~2.39;Ⅰ~ⅢA期,$n=474$,HR 1.68,95% CI 1.11~2.55),而非进展期患者(ⅢB~Ⅳ期,$n=975$,HR 1.3,95% CI 0.99~1.71)。结果并非采用PCR来检测KRAS突变,而是基于突变特异性寡核苷酸探针(mutation-specific oligonucleotide probe,MSOP)、变性梯度凝胶电泳(denaturating gradient gel eletrophoresis,DGGE)、RLFP以及直接测序法等。13项关于密码子12位点的突变其总HR也证实在该亚研究组中其作为负性预后因素的存在($n=1665$,HR 1.71,95% CI 1.44~2.04)[24]。

2013年肺辅助顺铂化疗评估（Lung Adjuvant Cisplatin Evaluation-Bio,LACE-Bio)研究组公布了一项汇总分析的研究结果,该研究由4项随机临床试验(ANITA,IALT,JBR.10,CALBG-9633)1718例患者组成,意图比较辅助化疗组(ACT)和观察组(OBS)之间KRAS突变的差异[25]。该研究组通过限制性片段长度多态性(restriction fragment length polymorphism,RFLP)、等位基因特异性寡核苷酸杂交、等位基因突变系统分析以及质谱法等技术手段在三家研究所以盲法开展分析研究,而这些方法均被大量文献证实比直接测序法的灵敏度更高。研究样本大小为1543例,其中763例OBS,780例ACT;KRAS突变检出率为19%(300例),其中密码子12突变275例,密码子13突变13例,密码子14突变1例。类似的,KRAS突变在腺癌中较鳞癌中更易出现(34% vs 6%,$P<0.001$);而女性相较男性也更易发生KRAS突变(27% vs 17%,$P=0.001$);另外更年轻的肺癌患者也更倾向于存在KRAS突变($P=0.0003$)。在多因素变量分析中,仅有年龄($P=0.044$)和组织学类型($P<0.001$)存在统计学意义。在OBS组中,KRAS突变对OS(HR 1.04,95% CI 0.78~1.38,$P=0.79$)和DFS(HR 1.05,95% CI 0.80~1.36,$P=0.73$)均无显著预后影响,而试验也不存在显著异质性($P=0.47$);值得注意的是,KRAS突变和腺癌亚组的OS(HR 1.04,95% CI 0.78~1.38,$P=0.79$)和PFS(HR 1.05,95% CI 0.80~1.36,$P=0.73$)均无显著相关性;非腺癌肿瘤与KRAS突变之间的相关性反而呈现出突变出现伴随预后更差的趋势(鳞状细胞癌:HR 1.41,95% CI 0.89~2.23,其他非腺癌肿瘤:HR 1.86,95% CI 1.22~2.82);而OBS中密码子12(突变型 vs 野生型,HR 1.04,CI 0.77~1.40)和密码子13(突变型 vs 野生型,HR 1.01,CI 0.47~2.17)突变对OS的预后并无显著差异[25]。同样,密码子12突变的各个亚组在OS(G12C/G12V vs 野生型,HR 1.04,95% CI 0.74~1.46;G12D/G12S vs 野生型,HR 0.95,95% CI 0.50~1.81;G12A/G12R vs 野生型,HR 1.08,95% CI 0.49~2.37,interaction $P=0.99$)和PFS(G12C/G12V vs 野生型,HR 1.04,95% CI 0.76~1.42;G12D/G12S vs 野生型,HR 1.03,95% CI 0.57~1.85;G12A/G12R vs 野生型,HR 1.15,95% CI 0.55~2.39,interaction $P=0.98$)的预后上也并无统计学差异。研究组还对KRAS联合p53的双突变进行了分析,结果证实其并无显著预后价值,但考虑到双突变人群较少(24例,9例死亡),缺乏足够的统计学说服力。

KRAS突变状态对治疗反应的预测作用

预测因素是可预测肿瘤对治疗反应(肿瘤缩小或治疗可使生存获益)的临床因素、细胞和分子生物标记物等。与预后因素能确定肿瘤特征对患者的影响相反,预测因素可确定治疗对肿瘤的影响。这些措施并非总是相似,这是由于肿瘤反应并不一定能够转变为更好的生存获益[26]。

KRAS 突变状态对 EGFR 抑制剂治疗反应的预测作用

KRAS 是 EGFR 下游的效应因子,当 EGFR 的胞内酪氨酸激酶结合配体被活化后,同源序列 2(sequence homology 2,SH2)结合蛋白质生长因子受体结合蛋白 2 并诱导 SOS1、SOS2 以及 RAS 鸟嘌呤核苷酸交换因子的聚集和 GDP 的解离,并使得 GTP 结合到 RAS 上从而被活化[27]。因此,或许因为突变的 KRAS 蛋白的组成性激活可激活其下游通路及细胞增殖,而这独立于上游 EGFR 抑制效应之外,故可诱导 EGFR 抑制剂的拮抗。KRAS 基因突变检测的价值已在转移性结肠癌的相关研究中被报道,EGFR 单克隆抗体在 KRAS 野生型患者中可获得更好的效果[28,29]。多项临床试验已对 KRAS 突变在 NSCLC 患者 EGFR 抑制剂敏感性中的预测价值进行了评估(表 11.2)。

EGFR 酪氨酸激酶抑制剂(Tyrosine Kinase Inhibitor,TKI)

已有 5 项临床试验(TRIBUTE,BR.21,SATURN,BR.19 和 TOPICAL),以厄洛替尼/吉非替尼组(单独或连用)与安慰剂组作对比,来研究 KRAS 突变作为 EGFR 抑制剂预后的预测标记物。TRIBUTE III 期随机临床试验比较并评估了一线化疗药物辅助厄洛替尼组和安慰剂组在晚期 NSCLC 中的作用[30]。274 例受试患者中 KRAS 突变检出率为 21%,而突变被认为与一线化疗药物辅助厄洛替尼患者相较单纯化疗药物患者存在明显更短的 TTP(3.4 个月 vs 6 个月,$P=0.03$)有相关性;同样,突变为 OS 的显著相关因素(4.4 个月 vs 13 个月,$P=0.019$)[30]。加拿大国立癌症研究所临床试验组的 BR.21 III 期随机安慰剂对照试验评估了厄洛替尼在晚期 NSCLC 标准化疗失败患者中的效用[31]。KRAS 突变在 206 名肿瘤患者中进行了评估,其中 30 例患者(15%)为阳性。KRAS 野生型肿瘤患者采用厄洛替尼治疗方案对 OS 有显著获益(HR 0.69,95% CI 0.49~0.97,$P=0.03$),而 KRAS 突变型肿瘤患者则无(HR 1.67,95% CI 0.62~4.50,$P=0.31$),而 KRAS 野生型和突变型肿瘤患者的响应率分别为 10% 和 5%。然而在 Cox 模型中,KRAS 突变状态和治疗方案之间的统计学关系则仅是近乎显著($P=0.09$);尽管单因素分析有明显的趋势,在多变量分析中则毫无统计学差异($P=0.13$)[31]。在特罗凯于不可切除 NSCLC(the Sequential Tarceva® in unresectable NSCLC,SATURN)临床试验中,IIIB/IV 期 NSCLC 经四周期铂类药物化疗后并无疾病进展的患者,被随机分配到厄洛替尼维持治疗组或安慰剂组[32]。在 889 例中进行 KRAS 突变检测,阳性检出率为 18%。野生型 KRAS 组患者的厄洛替尼治疗针对 OS 有一定程度的获益(HR 0.70,95% CI 0.57~0.87,$P<0.001$),而在突变型 KRAS 组患者中则无显著趋势(HR 0.77,95% CI 0.50~1.19)。然而在 KRAS 突变状态和治疗方案的交互检测中则并无统计学意义($P=0.95$)[32]。BR.19 随机

表 11.2　KRAS 突变情况作为预测 EGFR 酪氨酸酶抑制剂治疗 NSCLC 效果的临床研究

作者/研究	研究设计	试验纳入患者数量/KRAS检测患者数量	KRAS突变情况（%） WT	KRAS突变情况（%） Mut	PFS WT	PFS Mut	OS WT	OS Mut
Eberhard 等（2005）[30] TRIBUTE	紫杉醇/卡铂+厄洛替尼/安慰剂 1070/264	209 (79.2%)	55 (20.8%)	E-TTP 5.3 mo (CI 4.4~6.1 mo) P-TTP 5.4 mo (CI 4.4~6.1)	E-TTP 3.4mo (CI 1.5~6.3 mo) P-TTP 6 mo (CI 4.9~7.1)	E-12.1 mo (CI 9.2~15.6 mo) P-11.3 mo (CI 9.1~NR)	E-4.4 mo (CI 3.4~12.9mo) P-13.5 mo (CI 11.1~15.9)	
				原文中未列出多组间 P 值		原文中未列出多组间 P 值		
Zhu 等（2008）[31] BR.21	厄洛替尼与安慰剂治疗晚期非小细胞肺癌比较 731/206	176 (85%)	30 (15%)	NR		HR=0.69 (CI 0.49~0.97) P=0.03	HR 1.67 (0.62~4.50) P=0.31	
						Interaction P=0.0059		
Brugger 等（2011）[32] SATURN	对铂类为基础一线联合化疗有良好反应的患者，使用厄洛替尼或安慰剂维持治疗 889/493	403 (82%)	90 (18%)	HR=0.70; (CI 0.59~0.87) P<0.001	HR=0.77, (CI 0.50~1.19) P=0.2246	HR=0.86 (CI 0.68~1.08) P=NR	HR=0.79 (CI 0.49~1.27) P=NR	
				Interaction P=0.886		Interaction P=0.891		
Goss 等（2013）[33] BR.19	吉非替尼与安慰剂治疗完整切除的非小细胞肺癌患者比较 503/350	382 (72.6%)	96 (27.4%)	HR=1.08 (CI 0.74~1.59) P=0.69	HR=1.77 (CI 1.00~3.13) P=0.05	HR=1.13 (CI 0.78~1.65) P=0.51	HR=1.51 (CI 0.84~2.70) P=0.16	
				Interaction P=0.15		Interaction P=0.36		

续表

作者/研究	研究设计 试验纳入患者数量/KRAS检测患者数量	KRAS突变情况(%) WT	KRAS突变情况(%) Mut	PFS WT	PFS Mut	OS WT	OS Mut
Lee 等(2012)[34] TOPICAL	厄洛替尼与安慰剂一线治疗不适宜化疗的非小细胞肺癌患者比较 670/390	317 (81%)	73 (19%)	E-2.7 mo (CI 2.2~2.9) P-2.6 mo (CI 2.3~2.9) P=NR	E-3.5 mo (CI 1.7~4.8) P-2.7 mo (CI 1.8~3.9) P=NR	E-3.7 mo (CI 2.8~4.2) P-3.4 mo (CI 2.7~4.3) P=NR	E-4.2 mo (CI 1.8~6.2) P-3.6 mo (CI 1.9~4.4) P=NR
Johnson 等(2013)[35] ATLAS	晚期非小细胞肺癌经贝伐单抗一线治疗之后,使用贝伐单抗联合或不联合厄洛替尼用于维持治疗比较 1145/332	239 (72.0%)	93 (28%)	HR=0.67 (CI 0.49~0.91) P=0.01	HR=0.93 (CI 0.55~1.56) P=0.77	NR	原文中未列出多组间P值
				原文中未列出多组间P值			
Sequist 等(2011)[36] ARQ-197-209	厄洛替尼联合tivantinib与安慰剂比较用于治疗先前有其他治疗的非小细胞肺癌患者 167/65%	NR	15	HR=1.01 (CI 0.63~1.60) P=0.977 Interaction P<0.006	HR=0.18 (CI 0.05~0.70) P=0.13	NR	HR=0.43 (CI 0.12~1.50) P=0.17
Scagliotti 等(2013)[37] MARQUEE	厄洛替尼联合tivantinib与安慰剂用于晚期肺非鳞癌患者的二线或三线治疗的比较 1048/986	764 (72.9%)	284 (27.1%)	HR=1.01	HR=0.18	HR=0.94 (CI 0.77~1.14)	HR=1.04 (CI 0.78~1.40)
				原文中未列出多组间P值		原文中未列出多组间P值	

续表

作者/研究	研究设计 试验纳入患者数量/KRAS检测患者数量	KRAS突变情况(%)		PFS		OS	
		WT	Mut	WT	Mut	WT	Mut
Douillard 等(2009)[38] INTEREST	吉非替尼与多西他赛用于非小细胞肺癌二线治疗的比较 1466/275	226 (82%)	49 (18%)	HR=1.23 (CI,0.90~1.68) $P=0.20$	HR=1.16 (CI,0.56 v 2.41) $P=0.68$	HR=1.03 (CI,0.77~1.37) $P=0.86$	HR=0.81 (CI,0.44~1.49) $P=0.50$
				原文中未列出多组间 P 值		Interaction $P=0.51$	
Garassino 等(2012)[39] TAILOR	厄洛替尼与多西他赛用于EGFR野生型非小细胞肺癌二线治疗的比较 222/219	167 (76.3%)	52 (23.7%)	HR=0.65 (CI 0.46~0.90)	HR=0.84 (CI 0.47~1.52)	NR	
				Interaction $P=0.237$		原文中未列出多组间 P 值	

E:厄洛替尼,P:安慰剂,HR:风险比,CI:置信区间,PFS:无进展生存期,OS:总生存期,Mo:月,TPP:肿瘤进展时间,WT:野生型,Mut:突变型,NR:原文中未说明,ADC:腺癌

对照Ⅲ期临床试验则评估了 NSCLC 患者术后辅助吉非替尼的效用,研究者在 350 位肿瘤患者(厄洛替尼治疗方案人数为 169 例,安慰剂治疗组方案人数为 181 例)中进行了 KRAS 突变状态的检测[33]。254 例 KRAS 野生型肿瘤患者的厄洛替尼治疗并不能使 DFS(HR 1.08,95% CI 0.74~1.59,$P=0.69$)和 OS(HR 1.13,95% CI 1.13 95% CI 0.78~1.65,$P=0.51$)获益,而 96 例 KRAS 突变型肿瘤患者的厄洛替尼治疗则在 DFS(HR 1.77 95% CI 1.00~3.13,$P=0.05$)上存在显著的有害效应,尽管 OS(HR 1.51,95% CI 0.84~2.70,$P=0.16$)并非如此。Cox 回归模型在 KRAS 突变状态和治疗方案上并未表现出显著的交互(DFS,$P=0.15$;OS,$P=0.36$),同时多变量分析证实对预后并无显著影响(DFS,$P=0.12$;OS,$P=0.5$)[33]。TOPICAL 试验是一项双盲、安慰剂对照的Ⅲ期临床试验,针对不适合传统化疗的 NSCLC 病人以厄洛替尼为一线治疗方案[34]。纳入 670 例患者参与试验,共 390 例患者进行了基因检测,而 KRAS 突变检出率为 19%(70 例)。这些 KRAS 突变阳性的患者经厄洛替尼治疗后其中位 OS 为 4.2 个月($n=35$,95% CI 1.8~6.2),中位 PFS 为 3.5 个月(95% CI 1.7~4.8));安慰剂组患者中位 OS 则为 3.6 个月($n=38$,95% CI 1.9~4.4),中位 PFS 为 2.7 个月(95% CI 1.8~3.9)。而野生型 KRAS 患者中,厄洛替尼治疗组($n=210$)和安慰剂组($n=180$)在中位 OS(3.7 个月,95% CI 2.8~4.2;vs 3.4 个月,95% CI 2.7~4.3)和中位 PFS(2.7 个月,95% CI 2.2~2.9;vs 2.6 个月,95% CI 2.3~2.9)上均无明显差异[34]。

ATLAS 和 MARQUEE 试验评估的则是厄洛替尼联用其他靶向治疗药物的效用。ATLAS 是一项采用随机、双盲、安慰剂对照方法的Ⅲb 期临床试验,纳入了经一线铂类化疗辅助贝伐单抗联合治疗后病情稳定或伴随反应的局部晚期、复发或转移性 NSCLC 患者,比较贝伐单抗治疗有或无厄洛替尼的效用评估[40]。93 例 KRAS 突变阳性的患者中,额外应用厄洛替尼并无显著 PFS 获益(HR 0.93,95% CI 0.55~1.56;$P=0.7697$);而在 KRAS 野生型患者中,贝伐单抗额外辅助厄洛替尼治疗则可获益(HR 0.67,CI 0.49~0.91;$P=0.01$)[35]。ARQ-197-209 的Ⅱ期临床试验中,对患者随机采用厄洛替尼辅助或不辅助 tivantinib(一类 MET 抑制剂)治疗,结果表明,两类靶向药物联用可使 PFS(HR 0.18,95% CI 0.05~0.70;$P<0.01$, interaction $P=0.006$)和 OS(HR,0.43;95% CI,0.12~1.50;interaction $P=0.17$)均显著获益[36]。根据此Ⅱ期临床试验的结果,MARQUEE Ⅲ期随机临床试验评估了厄洛替尼联合 tivantinib 或二三线化疗药物安慰剂在非鳞状组织学的晚期 NSCLC 患者中的效用。522 例安慰剂组患者的 KRAS 突变检出率为 28.4%(148 例),而 526 例 tivantinib 治疗组患者的 KRAS 突变检出率为 25.9%(136 例)。研究结果表明,tivantinib 治疗组和安慰剂组患者相比,KRAS 野生型和突变型肿瘤患者的 OS 都无显著差异(野生型,HR 0.94,95% CI 0.77~

1.14；突变型，HR 1.04，95% CI 0.78~1.40)[37]。

有2项临床试验评估了EGFR TKI和多西他赛两类药物对KRAS突变状态下肿瘤的治疗效用。INTEREST(The Iressa Non-Small-Cell Lung Cancer Trial Evaluating Response Against Taxotere)试验在进展期NSCLC患者中比较评估了吉非替尼和多西他赛作为二线治疗方案孰优孰劣[38]。275例NSCLC进行了KRAS突变检测，阳性检出率为18%[41]。KRAS突变的生存获益在吉非替尼和多西他赛两类药物中不完全一致(KRAS突变，HR 0.81，95% CI 0.44~1.49，$P=0.50$；KRAS野生型，HR 1.03，95% CI 0.77~1.37，$P=0.86$, interaction $P=0.51$)，因而其并不具有预测性价值[38]。TAILOR(Tarceva Italian Lung Optimization Trial)为一项Ⅲ期随机临床试验，通过在野生型EGFR的NSCLC患者中比较评估了厄洛替尼和多西他赛作为二线治疗方案的效用。219例NSCLC进行了KRAS突变检测，52例阳性。同样的，KRAS突变生存获益在厄洛替尼和多西他赛两类药物中亦不具有预测性价值(KRAS突变，HR 0.84，95% CI 0.47~1.52；KRAS野生型，HR 0.65，95% CI 0.46~0.90，$P=0.237$)[39]。

有2个meta分析研究了NSCLC中就KRAS突变状态和其对EGFR TKI治疗的反应间的关系，均表明KRAS突变对生存预后无预测性价值。其中2008年的研究包含17项临床试验共计1008例NSCLC患者，其中165例患者检出KRAS突变。研究结果表明突变与EGFR TKI的反应缺失之间存在显著相关性(阳性似然比 LR=3.52；-LR=0.84)，低汇总灵敏度(0.21，95% CI 0.16~0.28)提示其抗性也发生在一部分野生型KRAS肿瘤中，对EGFR TKI的抵抗或许存在其他机制。然而，检测很有具体性(0.94，95% CI 0.89~0.97)，这提示EGFR TKI完全或部分的反应与KRAS突变并存的可能性极低[42]。另一项2010年的研究包含22项NSCLC研究共计1470例患者，其中231例患者检出KRAS突变。野生型KRAS肿瘤相较突变型KRAS肿瘤的客观反应率(the objective response rates, ORR)增高(分别为26% and 3%)，ORR的总汇集相对风险为0.29(95% CI 0.18~0.47，$P<0.01$)。KRAS突变与ORR间具显著的统计学相关性，同时这也与厄洛替尼(RR 0.28，95% CI 0.12~0.63，$P<0.01$)、吉非替尼(RR 0.30，95% CI 0.16~0.57，$P<0.01$)在亚洲人群(RR 0.22，95% CI 0.07~0.63；$P=0.01$)、高加索人群(RR 0.31，95% CI 0.17~0.54；$P<0.01$)两个亚组中的研究结果一致[43]。

若干最新研究证实，KRAS突变在EGFR TKI反应性中的预测价值或许因不同突变类型而有所差异。一项仅纳入14例患者，其中密码子12和13位点突变各有4例的小型研究评估了KRAS突变状态和其野生型EGFR的晚期NSCLC患者对EGFR TKI的反应状况。密码子13位点突变患者相较密码子12位点突变患者表现为更差的PFS($P=0.04$)和OS($P=0.005$)[44]。就在最近由Fiala等开展了一项研究,证实不同的 KRAS 突变类型或许针对 EGFR TKI 治疗的反应具有不同的预测影响[45]。研究者们对 488 例ⅢB 期 NSCLC 患者进行了 KRAS 突变检测,阳性检出率为 15.4%(69 例),其中有 3 例为 KRAS 和 EGFR 的共突变。研究结果表明,KRAS 突变在吸烟人群较非吸烟人群更为常见(17.9% vs 5.8%,$P=0.0048$),在腺癌患者较鳞状细胞癌患者更为常见(21% vs 4.4%,$P=0.0004$),但在不同性别间并无显著统计学差异。KRAS 突变常见类型依次为 G12C(52.2%)、G12V(11.6%)和 G12D(7.2%)。一个 38 人组成的亚组给予厄洛替尼或吉非替尼治疗,结果表明,发生 G12C 位点突变的 24 例患者较非 G12C 位点突变的 14 位患者,其 PFS 发生明显缩短(中位 PFS 4.3 周 vs 9.0 周,HR 2.7,$P=0.009$)而 OS 仅发生轻微缩短(中位 OS 9.3 周 vs 12.1 周,HR 2.0,$P=0.068$)。未来仍需进行 NSCLC 患者的独立队列研究以证实上述数据的准确性[45]。

EGFR 单克隆抗体

以往研究证实阳性 KRAS 突变的结肠癌患者采用 EGFR 单克隆抗体西妥昔单抗和帕尼单抗疗法可使获益下降[28,29],或许 NSCLC 中存在类似的结果。然而,KRAS 在 NSCLC 中 EGFR 单克隆抗体治疗并无预测价值(表 11.3)。BMS099 Ⅲ期随机临床试验在晚期 NSCLC 患者中比较了紫杉醇/卡铂联合或不联合西妥昔单抗的化疗方案[46]。202 例可评估肿瘤中 KRAS 突变发生率为 17%(35 例),结果表明 KRAS 状态与 ORR 之间并无显著相关性($P=0.19$),KRAS 野生型(HR 1.07,95% CI 0.77~1.30,$P=0.69$)或突变型(HR 0.64,95% CI 0.27~1.50,$P=0.30$)患者的化疗方案中加入西妥昔单抗治疗并不能提高 PFS,OS 分析也得到类似的结果(野生型:HR 0.93,95% CI 0.67~1.30,$P=0.68$;突变型:HR 0.97,95% CI 0.45~2.07,$P=0.93$)[46]。Ⅲ期一线爱必妥(First-Line ErbituX,FLEX)研究比较了在 EGFR 蛋白表达的晚期 NSCLC 患者中采用顺铂/长春瑞滨联合或不联合西妥昔单抗治疗方案,KRAS 突变在西妥昔单抗反应中的作用在此研究中被进行了评估[47]。研究队列中 395 例肿瘤中 75 例(19%)发现 KRAS 突变,根据 KRAS 状态分组的治疗结果比较结果证实并无 OS(野生型:HR 0.96,95% CI 0.75~1.23,$P=0.74$;突变型:HR 1.00,95% CI 0.60~1.66,$P=1.00$,interaction $P=0.88$)、PFS(野生型:HR 0.97,95% CI 0.76~1.24,$P=0.80$;突变型:HR 0.84,95% CI 0.50~1.40,$P=0.50$,interaction $P=0.38$)以及 ORR(野生型:RR 1.50,95% CI 0.94~2.41,$P=0.088$;突变型:RR 2.11,95% CI 0.76~5.88,$P=0.14$,interaction $P=0.5$)的预测价值[47]。

表11.3 KRAS突变用于妻妥昔单抗治疗非小细胞肺癌效果预测

作者/研究	研究设计 试验纳入患者数量/ KRAS检测患者数量	KRAS突变情况(%)		PFS			OS		
		WT	Mut	WT	Mut		WT	Mut	
Khambata-Ford 等 (2010)[46] BMS099 Trial	紫杉烷/卡铂+/-妻妥昔 单抗治疗晚期非小细胞 肺癌比较 676/202	167 (82.7%)	35 (17.3%)	HR=1.07 (CI 0.77~1.5) P=0.69	HR=0.64 (CI 0.27~1.5) P=0.3		HR=0.93 (CI 0.67~1.3) P=0.68	HR=0.97 (CI 0.45~2.07) P=0.93	
				原文中未列出多组间 P 值			原文中未列出多组间 P 值		
O'Byrne 等(2011) [47] FLEX	顺铂/长春瑞滨+/-塞妥 昔单抗治疗晚期非小细 胞肺癌比较 1861/395	320 (81%)	75 (19%)	HR=0.97 (CI 0.76~1.24) P=0.80	HR=0.84 (CI 0.50~1.40) P=0.50		HR=0.96 (CI 0.75~1.23) P=0.74	HR=1.00 (CI 0.60~1.66) P=1.00	
				Interaction P=0.38			Interaction P=0.88		

HR:风险比;CI:置信区间;PFS:无进展生存期;OS:总生存期;Mo:月;WT:野生型;Mut:突变型;NR:原文中未说明

KRAS 突变状态对化疗反应的预测价值

已有若干研究评估了 KRAS 突变在经化疗的 NSCLC 患者中的预测价值(表 11.4)。

ECOG4592 临床试验中,患者被随机分配进行术后放疗或放疗同时化疗的治疗方案。KRAS 突变检出率为 24%(44/197),接受化疗的患者其 KRAS 突变状态具有轻微统计学差异。化疗组中 70 为野生型 KRAS 患者相较突变型 KRAS 患者具有更长的生存期(RR 0.59,95% CI 0.32~1.075,$P=0.09$),然而基于治疗方案分组的 KRAS 野生型或突变型肿瘤的生存期并无显著统计学差异,野生型患者接受单纯化疗和联合放化疗的生存期分别为 43 个月和 42 个月,而突变型患者接受单纯化疗和联合放化疗的生存期则分别为 37 个月和 25 个月。统计学差异不明显(interaction $P=0.2$)的原因可能为每个分组的样本量偏小[21]。

NCIC CTG JBR.10 试验则是进行了ⅠB 期和Ⅱ期 NSCLC 术后辅助长春瑞滨/顺铂治疗方案和观察两组的比较,将 KRAS 作为分层变量进行了前瞻性分析研究。KRAS 突变检出率为 24.3%(117/451),结果显示野生型 KRAS 的肿瘤患者接受化疗后 DSS 有一定获益(HR 0.72,95% CI 0.51~1.02,$P=0.06$),而突变型患者则无(HR 1.07,95% CI 0.61~1.88,$P=0.82$),DSS 交互并无意义(interaction $P=0.2$)。试验结果证实化疗组存在显著性总生存期获益,然而在野生型 KRAS 的肿瘤患者(HR 0.84,95% CI 0.63~1.12,$P=0.24$)和突变型患者(HR 0.82,95% CI 0.50~1.35,$P=0.44$)之间并无显著差异(interaction $P=0.97$)[48]。

LACE-BIO 汇总分析结果表明,KRAS 突变对辅助化疗的 OS 和 DFS 并无显著获益影响[25]。KRAS 野生型和突变型对 OS 均无显著获益(野生型:治疗组 vs 对照组 HR 0.89,95% CI 0.76~1.05,$P=0.15$;突变型:HR 1.05,95% CI 0.76~1.46,$P=0.77$),交互性检测亦无统计学意义(interaction $P=0.50$),甚至在腺癌亚组内亦是如此(interaction $P=0.99$);KRAS 突变亚型的分析结果也证实密码子 12 位点的突变患者 OS 无获益(HR 0.95,CI 0.67~1.35,$P=0.77$),辅助化疗对密码子 13 位点的突变患者则是有害的(HR 5.78,CI 2.06~16.2,$P<0.001$),然而该亚组仅有 24 位患者,仍需更大样本量数据支持。同时研究在 49 位患者的亚组中评估了 KRAS/p53 双突变对于辅助化疗中的预测价值,结果表明,化疗组相较观察组而言对患者有害无益(HR 2.49 CI 95% 1.10~5.66,$P=0.03$)。同时,化疗对 KRAS 野生型 p53 野生型、KRAS 突变型 p53 野生型、KRAS 野生型 p53 突变型以及 KRAS 突变型 p53 突变型 4 个分组的影响均无统计学差异($P=0.06$)[25],而该项研究由于样本量偏小,未来尚需其他数据库的验证。

表 11.4 KRAS 突变用于非小细胞肺癌化疗效果预测

作者/研究	研究设计 试验纳入患者数量/ KRAS检测患者数量	KRAS突变情况(%) WT	KRAS突变情况(%) Mut	PFS WT	PFS Mut	OS WT	OS Mut
Schiller 等（2001）[21] ECOG 4592	Ⅱ～ⅢA期非小细胞肺癌行术后放疗+/-化疗比较 217/184	140（76%）	44（24%）	NR		Chemo/XRT median 42 mo XRT median 43 mo	Chemo/XRT median 25 mo XRT median 37 mo
				原文中未列出多组间 P 值	原文中未列出多组间 P 值	Interaction $P=0.2$	
Butts 等（2010）[48] JBR.10	辅助化疗与临床观察比较 482/450	333（74%）	117（26%）	HR=0.72 (CI 0.51~1.02) $P=0.06$	HR 1.07 (CI 0.61~1.88) $P=0.82$	HR=0.84 (CI 0.63~1.12) $P=0.24$	HR=0.82 (CI 0.50~1.35) $P=0.44$
				Interaction $P=0.2$		Interaction $P=0.97$	
Shepherd 等（2013）[25] LACE-Bio	辅助化疗与临床观察比较 1718/1536	1243（81.6%）	300（19.4%）	HR 0.86 (CI 0.74~1.00) $P=0.04$	HR=0.93 (CI 0.68~1.27) $P=0.65$	HR=0.89 (CI 0.76~1.05) $P=0.15$	HR=1.05 (CI 0.76~1.46) $P=0.77$
				Interaction $P=0.63$		Interaction $P=0.50$	
Shepherd 等（2013）[25] LACE-Bio ADC	辅助化疗与临床观察比较 813/605	204（33.7%）	401（66.3%）	NR		HR=0.88 (CI 0.66~1.17) $P=0.37$	HR=0.92 (CI 0.61~1.37) $P=0.67$
				原文中未列出多组间 P 值		Interaction $P=0.86$	

HR：风险比；CI：置信区间；PFS：无进展生存期；OS：总生存期；Mo：月；WT：野生型；Mut：突变型；NR：原文中未说明；Chemo：化疗；XRT：放疗

KRAS 突变 NSCLC 治疗

到目前为止,针对 NSCLC 中 KRAS 突变的治疗尚无推荐方案,关于为何有关 KRAS 突变治疗性抑制剂的探索至今仍无重大进展,可能的原因有以下几点。首先,RAS 突变产生的癌基因蛋白已丧失功能,例如 GTP 酶活性的丧失,从而使抑制剂发挥作用更加困难。其次,KRAS 突变的依赖性相较其他驱动基因的突变更弱一些[12]。再次,KRAS 蛋白激活多重下游通路从而调控必要的细胞功能如细胞生长、增殖、迁移、血管生成以及凋亡等(附录彩图 11.2)[9],因此 KRAS 活性的抑制或许需要一个针对多种被激活的下游效应因子的联合治疗策略。最后,KRAS 突变的不同亚型可激活不同的下游通路且对药物敏感度的影响不同[49,50]。因此个体患者的 KRAS 活性抑制或许需要一个基于具体突变类型、肿瘤内其他分子变化以及不同公有药物等的联合治疗方案。现已开展了相当多的研究,致力于寻找可使 KRAS 突变蛋白失活的癌基因特异性综合破坏作用的靶向治疗。下一部分将阐述针对各类发生 KRAS 突变的 NSCLC 患者迄今为止已评估或正在评估的治疗方案的选择。靶向抑制 KRAS 蛋白可采用多种方式,包括通过防止 RAS 附着到膜上以抑制其活化,针对其下游效应蛋白,以及直接抑制 RAS 等。针对 KRAS 突变 NSCLC 的已完成和正在进行中的临床试验分别见于表 11.5 和表 11.6。

RAS 活化的抑制

1. 法尼基转移酶抑制剂 已经过实验的 KRAS 突变 NSCLC 治疗方法之一为法尼基转移酶抑制剂(Farnesyl Transferase Inhibitors,FTIs)。KRAS 在细胞质中比较被蛋白法尼基转移酶异戊二烯化从而激活其活性,15 碳链的增加可使 RAS 蛋白疏水性增加从而有利于将蛋白质掺入细胞内膜[27]。FTIs 通过抑制法尼基转移酶活性从而阻断 RAS 蛋白活化,而已有若干临床试验针对未经选择的晚期 NSCLC 患者采用 FTIs 联合化疗药物的治疗方案,然而并未有疗效比单独应用化疗方案的报道[55,56]。遗憾的是,数项研究均无前瞻性的集成肿瘤资料库,故而针对 KRAS 野生型和突变型肿瘤人群潜在预后进行评论是不现实的。

2. 其他 Saralisib (S-trans, trans-farnesyl thiosalicylic acid)可破坏 KRAS 的膜定位,从而阻断 RAS 信号转导。由于替代膜结合机制的缘故,FTIs 无法抑制 KRAS 和 NRAS 的功能。与 FTIs 不同,Saralisib 可抑制所有类型的 RAS。一项 Ⅱ 期临床试验则针对 KRAS 突变的晚期肺腺癌患者单独使用 Saralisib 治疗并对结果进行评估。研究结果显示 30 位接受治疗的患者均无良好效果,其中还包括 11 例病情稳定的患者[57]。

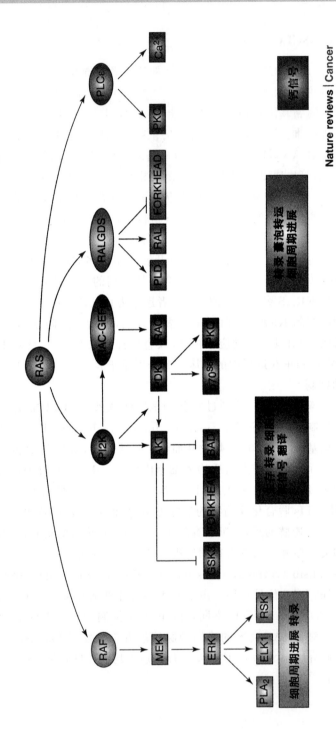

图11.2 RAS下游信号通路

表 11.5 KRAS 突变非小细胞肺癌治疗药物临床试验

试验	临床试验分期	试验设计	作用靶点	患者选择	KRAS WT	KRAS mut	PFS WT	PFSmut	OS WT	OSmut
Hainsworth 等(2010)[51]	II	司美替尼与培美曲塞治疗晚期非小细胞肺癌比较	MEK-1/2	未经选择					HR 1.08 (CI 0.75～1.54) P=0.79	
Janne 等(2013)[52]	II	多西他赛+/-司美替尼治疗局部进展期或转移性肺癌	MEK-1/2	KRAS突变		87		HR 0.58 (CI 0.42～0.79) P=0.01		HR 0.80 (CI 0.56～1.14) P=0.21
Bennouma 等(2013)[53]	I	曲美替尼	MEK-1/2	未经选择	8	22	2.1 mo (CI 1.8～5.2)	3.8 mo (CI 1.9～5.5)		
Riely 等(2012)[54]	II	地磷莫司单药二线治疗非小细胞肺癌后稳定期使用地磷莫司或安慰剂治疗对照	mTOR	KRAS突变		7936 例稳定期患者随机分组		R-median 4 mo P-median 2 mo HR 0.36 P=0.013		R-median 8 mo P-median 5 mo HR 0.46 P=0.09

HR:风险比;CI:置信区间;PFS:无进展生存期;OS:总生存期;Mo:月;WT:野生型;Mut:突变型;NR:原文中未说明;R:地磷莫司;P:安慰剂

表 11.6　正在进行的 KRAS 突变非小细胞肺癌的相关临床试验

试验	临床试验分期	试验 ID	治疗	作用靶点	治疗分线	患者选择
SELECT-1	Ⅲ	NCT01933932	多西他赛＋司美替尼与安慰剂对比	MEK1/MEK2	2nd line	KRAS 突变晚期非小细胞肺癌
	Ⅱ	NCT01229150	司美替尼＋/－厄洛替尼比较	MEK1/MEK2	2nd or more	晚期非小细胞肺癌，根据 KRAS 突变情况进行分层
	Ⅱ	NCT01362296	曲美替尼与多西他赛比较	MEK1/MEK2	2nd line	KRAS 突变晚期非小细胞肺癌
IPI-504-15	ⅠB/Ⅱ	NCT01427946	依维莫司联合瑞他霉素	mTOR 与内质网应激诱导剂	Any	KRAS 突变非小细胞肺癌
	Ⅱ	NCT01395758	Tivantinib/厄洛替尼与单药化疗对比	MET	2nd or more	KRAS 突变晚期非小细胞肺癌
Galaxy-2	Ⅲ	NCT01798485	多西他赛联合 ganetespib 与安慰剂对比	Hsp90	2nd or more	晚期非小细胞肺癌
	Ⅱ	NCT01951690	Defactinib	FAK	Any	KRAS 突变晚期非小细胞肺癌
	Ⅱ	NCT01833143	硼替佐米	蛋白体	Any	不吸烟的 KRAS 突变非小细胞肺癌或者 KRAS G12D 突变型非小细胞肺癌

异戊烯基结合蛋白PDEδ可通过促进KRAS在细胞质中的扩散维持其空间结构调控法尼基化KRAS正确的定位和信号转导[58]。一类可抑制KRAS-PDEδ互作的小分子已被证实可于体内和体外影响KRAS信号转导,而目前为止尚未开展人类的临床试验[59]。

靶向下游效应因子

1. MEK抑制剂 RAS下游通路中最具特征性的是RAF/丝裂原活化蛋白激酶(mitogen-activated protein kinase,MAPK)/胞外信号调节激酶激酶(extracellular signal-regulated kinase kinase,MEK)/细胞外信号调节激酶(extracellular signal-regulated kinase,ERK)的级联反应(图11.2)。RAF激活MEK1和MEK2,进而激活ERK1和ERK2蛋白活性,最终磷酸化包括调控G1-S期节点蛋白等转录因子在内的若干胞浆和核蛋白。现已有针对MEK的药物被应用于KRAS突变的肿瘤治疗[27]。

Selumetinib(AZD6244)是一类MEK1/2的有效非竞争性抑制剂。在一项Ⅱ期临床试验中,未经选择的晚期NSCLC患者接受每日2次口服100mg的Selumetinib或每3周1次培美曲塞500 mg/m² IV[51],结果显示两者OS(HR 1.08, 80% CI 0.75~1.54;$P=0.79$)和针对治疗方案的反应均无显著差异。另一项Ⅱ期临床试验中,针对发生KRAS突变的局部晚期或转移(ⅢB~Ⅳ期)NSCLC患者采用了多西他赛联合($n=44$)或不联合($n=43$)Selumetinib的治疗方案,结果显示多西他赛联用Selumetinib组表现为显著的临床获益[52],PFS显著延长(HR 0.58;80% CI 0.42~0.79;$P=0.01$)并伴有明显高反应率(0 vs 37%;$P<0.0001$),而OS则并无显著延长驱使(HR 0.80,95% CI 0.56~1.14,$P=0.21$)[52]。一项Ⅲ期临床试验(SELECT-1,NCT01933932)评估了针对已证实KRAS突变的NSCLC患者采用化疗联用Selumetinib的治疗方案的效用。

已有一项针对既往治疗过的晚期NSCLC患者采用Selumetinib与MK-2206(一类AKT抑制剂)联用方案的生物标记物靶向治疗研究(BATTLE 2,NCT01248247)。另一项以KRAS状态分层的Ⅱ期临床试验(NTC01229150)则是针对某些对标准化疗不敏感的NSCLC患者采用Selumetinib与或不与厄洛替尼联用进行治疗从而进行评估。

IND.215 NCIC CTG试验为ⅠB期临床试验,针对既往治疗或未经治疗的晚期/转移性NSCLC患者,采用Selumetinib联用培美曲塞、培美曲塞联用顺铂以及紫杉醇联用卡铂等3种治疗方案进行治疗,而试验中仅KRAS突变的患者方采用培美曲塞联用Selumetinib的治疗方案。当推荐Ⅱ期剂量被用于其他化疗方案时,研究者将招募一个扩展队列,同时这些患者也将参与KRAS突变的研究(NCT01783197)。

曲美替尼(GSK1120212)是一类MEK1/2抑制剂。30例曾经经过其他治疗的

NSCLC患者（22例存在KRAS突变）在应用GSK1120212治疗后，1例患者症状得到部分缓解，10例患者疾病趋于稳定；突变型KRAS亚组患者的中位PFS为3.8个月（95% CI 1.9～5.5），而野生型KRAS亚组患者的中位PFS则为2.1个月（95% CI 1.8～5.2）[60]。另一项Ⅰ/ⅠB期临床试验中，针对22例KRAS野生型肿瘤患者和25例KRAS突变型肿瘤患者采用曲美替尼联用多西他赛的方案进行治疗，结果显示ORR分别为36%（8PR和7SD）和28%（1CR，6PR和8SD），而OS和PFS并未报道[53]。一项Ⅱ期随机临床试验（NCT01362296）开展了针对KRAS突变型NSCLC患者分别采用GSK1120212与多西他赛进行治疗的药效研究。初步结果显示，129例KRAS突变型肿瘤患者达到12%的ORR；然而中期分析表明曲美替尼相较多西他赛并不能提高PFS（HR 1.14，95% CI 0.75～1.75，$P=0.52$）[61]。而另一项针对晚期NSCLC的Ⅰ/ⅠB期临床试验则是对曲美替尼和培美曲塞的药效进行了比较，结果显示20例KRAS突变型肿瘤患者中有3PR和10SD，而22例KRAS野生型肿瘤患者中则有3PR和12SD。该研究结果尚需进一步数据验证[62]。

2. PI3K抑制剂　　KRAS也可激活磷脂酰肌醇(-3)激酶（phosphatidylinositol 3-kinase，PI3K）通路，同时PI3K通路和RAS-RAF-MEK通路存在广泛串话。2条通路均为RAS激活，且均可调节雷帕霉素靶蛋白（mammalian target of rapamycin，mTOR）的活性[9,27]。若干体内体外实验结果表明未来在KRAS突变的NSCLC治疗中PI3K抑制剂和MEK抑制剂的联用将有广阔前景[41,63,64]，而至今尚未有关于两类药物联用的报道。

3. mTOR抑制剂　　mTOR是PI3K/AKT信号通路和MEK信号通路的下游中介蛋白，现已研发出若干mTOR抑制剂如依维莫司（RAD001）、替西罗莫司（CCI-779）和ridaforolimus（AP23573/MK-8669）等。基于Ⅰ期试验中NSCLC的SD和PR，现已有Ⅱ期临床试验对进行重度系统性治疗的晚期NSCLC患者采用依维莫司进行治疗的效用进行评估。42例既往化疗的患者中3例观察到药物反应，而43例既往化疗联用EGFR TKIs的患者中1位观察到药物反应，这表明依维莫司在NSCLC治疗中存在一定临床活性[66]。2008年曾有NSCLC治疗中ridaforolimus具有anectodal活性的相关报道[67]，之后一项Ⅱ期随机研究评估了既往化疗失败的晚期KRAS突变NSCLC患者应用ridaforolimus单药的效用。共79例患者开始ridaforolimus单药的治疗，8周后1位出现局部反应，36例疾病维持稳定；ridaforolimus继续应用，但36例维持稳定的患者随机给予ridaforolimus或安慰剂。结果显示，随机队列中应用ridaforolimus组中位PFS明显增长（4个月 vs 2个月，HR 0.36，$P=0.013$）；而ridaforolimus组OS为18个月，安慰剂组则为5个月（HR 0.46，$P=0.09$）[54]。尽管由于ridaforolimus组相较安慰剂组的PFS显著增长，该研究结果应考虑为"正性"，但KRAS突变型NSCLC患者总体群的低反应率大大降低了该项研究结果的意义。

近期临床前数据表明,当内质网应激诱导剂 retaspamycin(IPI-504)与 mTOR 抑制剂联用时可促进 KRAS 驱动肿瘤的衰退[68],ⅠB/Ⅱ期临床研究(NCT01427946)正在进行针对 KRAS 突变型 NSCLC 患者采用 retaspamycin 和依维莫司联用的效用评估。

4. MET 抑制剂　MET 基因编码一类肝细胞生长因子(hepatocyte growth factor,HGF)的高亲和力跨膜受体蛋白,HGF 和 MET 受体的结合可导致酪氨酸激酶结构域的磷酸化以及包括 RAS 通路在内的下游信号通路的激活[69,70]。MET 的扩增是 EGFR 阳性突变 NSCLC 患者拮抗 EGFR TKIs 的机制之一[70],tivantinib 是一类 ATP 独立的口服 MET 抑制剂。ARQ-197-209 Ⅱ期临床试验将有过往治疗的 NSCLC 患者随机分组接受厄洛替尼(150mg,1 日 1 次)+/- tivantinib (360 mg,1 日 2 次)治疗,结果显示厄洛替尼联用 tivantinib 组 PFS 适度延长(HR 0.81,95% CI 0.57~1.16,$P=0.24$)[36],而 KRAS 突变亚组患者($n=15$)经联用治疗后明显获益(PFS HR 0.18,95% CI 0.05~0.70;$P<0.01$,interaction $P=0.006$);OS HR,0.43;95% CI,0.12~1.50;$P=0.17$)[36]。基于上述结果,验证性 MARQUEE 试验将 1048 例晚期 NSCLC 患者(不包含鳞癌)随机分组并给予厄洛替尼联用 tivantinib 治疗或安慰剂治疗,患者根据 EGFR 和 KRAS 的突变进行分层[37]。结果显示,尽管联用组的 PFS 有所提高(HR 0.74,95% CI 0.64~0.85,$P<0.001$),但其 OS 相较安慰剂组并无获益(HR 0.98,95% CI 0.84~1.15,$P=0.81$)。该临床研究的结果也不能被完全认可,由于在 KRAS 突变亚组患者中应用 tivantinib 治疗并无无 OS 获益(HR 1.04,95% CI 0.78~1.40)[37]。另一项进行中的随机临床试验(NCT01395758)针对 KRAS 突变型 NSCLC 患者采用 tivantinib/厄洛替尼或单药化疗(吉西他滨、多西他赛或培美曲塞等)的治疗方案并进行比较评估。

5. Hsp90 抑制剂　热休克蛋白 80(heat shock protein 90,Hsp90)是一类协助其他蛋白完成折叠、抵抗热应力、降解等功能的伴侣蛋白,同时它也可维持部分肿瘤生长所需蛋白的稳定性,故而现如今 Hsp90 抑制剂被应用于抗肿瘤药物的研究[71]。体内和体外的临床前研究表明 Hsp90 抑制剂或可在 KRAS 突变肿瘤中发挥功能[72,73],并促进 ganetespib(STA-9090,一类 Hsp90 抑制剂)的临床试验开展。一项Ⅱ期临床试验针对晚期 NSCLC 患者采用 ganetespib 进行单药治疗并评估其效用,其中 14 例患者为野生型 EGFR 和突变性 KRAS,1 例 PR 患者,7 例 SD 患者[74]。另一项进行中的Ⅲ期临床试验(Galaxy 2,NCT01798485)针对晚期 NSCLC 采用多西他赛联用 ganetespib 的治疗方案或多西他赛单药治疗并进行比较评估,但该研究对象并不局限于发生 KRAS 突变的患者。

6. CDK4/6 抑制剂　CDK4 和 6 是一类细胞周期蛋白依赖性激酶,主要功能为调控细胞周期中 G1 期过渡至 S 期的节点蛋白[75]，KRAS 和 CDK4 间的人为致死相互作用为 KRAS 突变的 NSCLC 提供了一个潜在的治疗策略[76]。LY2835219 是一类 CDK4/6 的 ATP 竞争性小分子抑制剂，可在包括 NSCLC 在内的多种人类肿瘤异种移植模型中发挥作用[77]。一项包含 75 例晚期且有既往治疗 NSCLC 患者的 I 期临床研究结果表现出有趣的反应率。在中期分析时于治疗前后进行病变测量的 47 例患者中，34 例存在 SD 或 PR，且其中 9 例存在肺癌；同时，这 9 例肺癌患者中 4 例被发现位 KRAS 突变型肿瘤，且 4 例全部存在 PR 或 SD[77]。

RAS 的直接抑制

至今尚无此类药物，但随着技术的发展未来会出现直接针对 RAS 的抑制剂。一种 G12C RAS 不可逆的变构抑制剂已于近期被报道[78]。这类化合物依赖于突变的半胱氨酸进行结合反应，故而不会影响到野生型蛋白。

结论

NSCLC 中 KRAS 突变的预后价值尽管经历了 20 年之久的研究，至今仍未有定论。根据两项大型 meta 分析的结果，KRAS 突变似乎是 NSCLC 中的一个较弱的负性预后因子，但在 LACE-BIO 汇总研究中并未得到确认。多变的结果究其原因可能是研究来自于全球不同地区，甚至包含部分患者人群 EGFR 突变发生率更高的地区，且 EGFR 突变可能提高野生型 KRAS 肿瘤患者的生存率。此外，不同类型的 KRAS 突变其预后价值也不尽相同，当然这都需要未来的进一步研究来证实。

KRAS 突变的预测性价值已在 NSCLC 的不同治疗策略中得到了证实。2 项 meta 分析认为 KRAS 突变为 NSCLC 中 EGFR TKIs 反应的负性预测生物标记物，然而目前尚未有文献或研究能证实 KRAS 状态与生存获益间存在确定性关联。汇总分析，特别是安慰剂对照的临床试验，对获取足够统计学的确定性数据有极大帮助。而此时 KRAS 不能用于选择 NSCLC 患者进行 EGFR TKIs 治疗，且并无证据表明 KRAS 突变可预测 NSCLC 中抗 EGFR 单克隆抗体的敏感度。并无强力证据证实 KRAS 突变在化疗预后中的任何预测价值，因此 KRAS 突变并不能用来选择合适的病人进行化疗。近期数据显示化疗对密码子 13 突变的患者是不利的，但此项研究结果尚需进一步研究来证实其真实性。LACE-BIO 最近的一项汇总分析结果表明，KRAS/p53 双突变患者相较双野生型患者采用辅助化疗的预后更差，然而此项研究双突变数据样本量过小，尚需未来体外实验的确认以及独立数据集。

尽管对 KRAS 研究持续了 20 年，现如今针对 KRAS 突变型肿瘤仍无有效的靶向治疗方案，靶向针对 KRAS 尚处于实验室阶段。KRAS 突变型 NSCLC 患者采用化疗联合 MEK 抑制剂的治疗方案获得了若干有趣的数据，而该研究的 III 期临床试验正在进行中。其他临床试验中也测验了若干药物。由于 KRAS 蛋白可激活多种下游信号通路，KRAS 活性的抑制或许需要靶向若干活化的下游效应因子进行联合治疗，抑或基于突变的具体类型，甚至于肿瘤的分子特性。寻找癌基因特异性合成致死作用导致 KRAS 突变蛋白失活的靶向治疗的大型研究正在进行中。新技术使新药的开发成为可能。由于现今广泛开展的针对 KRAS 基因突变的研究以及各类选定 KRAS 突变 NSCLC 患者评估单药或联用效应的临床试验，均使我们相信抑制 KRAS 活性的治疗选择必将诞生于不远的将来。

参考文献

1. Harvey JJ. An unidentified virus which causes the rapid production of tumours in mice. Nature. 1964;204;1104-5.
2. Kirsten WH, Mayer LA. Morphologic responses to a murine erythroblastosis virus. J Natl Cancer Inst. 1967;39;311-35.
3. Shih C, Padhy LC, Murray M, Weinberg RA. Transforming genes of carcinomas and neuroblastomas introduced into mouse fibroblasts. Nature. 1981;290;261-4.
4. Rodenhuis S, Slebos RJ. The ras oncogenes in human lung cancer. Am Rev Respir Dis. 1990;142;S27-30.
5. Shimizu K, Goldfarb M, Perucho M, Wigler M. Isolation and preliminary characterization of the transforming gene of a human neuroblastoma cell line. Proc Natl Acad Sci U S A. 1983;80;383-7.
6. Hall A, Marshall CJ, Spurr NK, Weiss RA. Identification of transforming gene in two human sarcoma cell lines as a new member of the ras gene family located on chromosome 1. Nature. 1983;303;396-400.
7. Downward J. Targeting RAS, signalling pathways in cancer therapy. Nat Rev Cancer. 2003;3;11-22.
8. Karnoub AE, Weinberg RA. Ras oncogenes;split personalities. Nat Rev Mol Cell Biol. 2008;9;517-31.
9. Karachaliou N, Mayo C, Costa C, et al. KRAS mutations in lung cancer. Clin Lung Cancer. 2013;14;205-14.
10. Riely GJ, Kris MG, Rosenbaum D, et al. Frequency and distinctive spectrum of KRAS mutations in never smokers with lung adenocarcinoma. Clin Cancer Res. 2008;14;5731-4.
11. Lee YJ, Kim JH, Kim SK, et al. Lung cancer in never smokers;change of a mindset in the molecular era. Lung Cancer. 2011;72;9-15.
12. Mitsudomi T. The RAS biology. WCLC proceedings 2013;Abstract E10. 11.
13. Yu HA, Sima CS, Shen R, et al. Comparison of the characteristics and clinical course of 677 patients with metastatic lung cancers with mutations in KRAS codon 12 and 13. ASCO proceedings 2013;Abstract 8025.
14. Barlesi F, Blons H, Beau-Faller M, et al. Biomarkers（BM）France;results of routine EG-

FR, HER2, KRAS, BRAF, PI3KCA mutations detection and EML4-ALK gene fusion assessment on the fi rst 10 000 non-small cell lung cancer (NSCLC) patients (pts). In ASCO, edition 2013.

15. Kris MG, Johnson BE, Berry L, et al. Treatment with therapies matched to oncogenic drivers improves survival in patients with lung cancers: results from the Lung Cancer Mutation Consortium (LCMC). In WCLC, edition 2013.

16. Paesmans M, Sculier JP, Libert P, et al. Prognostic factors for survival in advanced non-small cell lung cancer: univariate and multivariate analyses including recursive partitioning and amalgamation algorithms in 1052 patients. The European Lung Cancer Working Party. J Clin Oncol. 1995;13:1221-30.

17. Slebos RJ, Kibbelaar RE, Dalesio O, et al. K-ras oncogene activation as a prognostic marker in adenocarcinoma of the lung. N Engl J Med. 1990;323:561-5.

18. Capelletti M, Wang XF, Gu L. Impact of KRAS mutations on adjuvant carboplatin/paclitaxel in surgical resected stage IB NSCLC:CALBG 9633. J Clin Oncol. 2010;28:Abstract 7008.

19. Scoccianti C, Vesin A, Martel G, et al. Prognostic value of TP53, KRAS and EGFR mutations in nonsmall cell lung cancer: the EUELC cohort. Eur Respir J. 2012;40:177-84.

20. Ma X, Vataire AL, Sun H. TP53 AND KRAS Mutations as markers of outcome of adjuvant cisplatin-based chemotherapy in completely resected non-small cell lung cancer (NSCLC): the International Adjuvant Lung Cancer Trial (IALT) biological program. Ann Oncol. 2008; 19:61.

21. Schiller JH, Adak S, Feins RH, et al. Lack of prognostic significance of p53 and K-ras mutations in primary resected non-small-cell lung cancer on E4592: a Laboratory Ancillary Study on an Eastern Cooperative Oncology Group Prospective Randomized Trial of Postoperative Adjuvant Therapy. J Clin Oncol. 2001;19:448-57.

22. Tsao MS, Aviel-Ronen S, Ding K, et al. Prognostic and predictive importance of p53 and RAS for adjuvant chemotherapy in non small-cell lung cancer. J Clin Oncol. 2007;25:5240-7.

23. Mascaux C, Iannino N, Martin B, et al. The role of RAS oncogene in survival of patients with lung cancer: a systematic review of the literature with meta-analysis. Br J Cancer. 2005; 92:131-9.

24. Meng D, Yuan M, Li X, et al. Prognostic value of K-RAS mutations in patients with non-small cell lung cancer: a systematic review with meta-analysis. Lung Cancer. 2013;81:1-10.

25. Shepherd FA, Domerg C, Hainaut P, et al. Pooled analysis of the prognostic and predictive effects of KRAS mutation status and KRAS mutation subtype in early-stage resected non-small- cell lung cancer in four trials of adjuvant chemotherapy. J Clin Oncol. 2013;31:2173-81.

26. Mok T, Wu Y, Thongprasert S, et al. Gefitinib vs carboplatin-placlitaxel in pulmonary adenocarcinoma. N Engl J Med. 2009;361(10):947-57.

27. Malumbres M, Barbacid M. RAS oncogenes: the first 30 years. Nat Rev Cancer. 2003;3:459-65.

28. Karapetis CS, Khambata-Ford S, Jonker DJ, et al. K-ras mutations and benefit from cetuximab in advanced colorectal cancer. N Engl J Med. 2008;359:1757-65.

29. Amado RG, Wolf M, Peeters M, et al. Wild-type KRAS is required for panitumumab efficacy in patients with metastatic colorectal cancer. J Clin Oncol. 2008;26:1626-34.
30. Eberhard DA, Johnson BE, Amler LC, et al. Mutations in the epidermal growth factor receptor and in KRAS are predictive and prognostic indicators in patients with non-small-cell lung cancer treated with chemotherapy alone and in combination with erlotinib. J Clin Oncol. 2005;23:5900-9.
31. Zhu CQ, da Cunha Santos G, Ding K, et al. Role of KRAS and EGFR as biomarkers of response to erlotinib in National Cancer Institute of Canada Clinical Trials Group Study BR. 21. J Clin Oncol. 2008;26:4268-75.
32. Brugger W, Triller N, Blasinska-Morawiec M, et al. Prospective molecular marker analyses of EGFR and KRAS from a randomized, placebo-controlled study of erlotinib maintenance therapy in advanced non-small-cell lung cancer. J Clin Oncol. 2011;29:4113-20.
33. Goss GD, O'Callaghan C, Lorimer I, et al. Gefitinib versus placebo in completely resected non-small-cell lung cancer: results of the NCIC CTG BR19 study. J Clin Oncol. 2013;31:3320-6.
34. Lee SM, Khan I, Upadhyay S, et al. First-line erlotinib in patients with advanced non-small cell lung cancer unsuitable for chemotherapy (TOPICAL): a double-blind, placebo-controlled, phase 3 trial. Lancet Oncol. 2012;13:1161-70.
35. Johnson B, Miller V, Amler LC, et al. Biomarker evaluation in the randomized, double-blind, placebo-controlled, phase Ⅲb ATLAS trial, comparing bevacizumab (B) therapy with or without erlotinib (E), after completion of chemotherapy with B for the treatment of locally advanced, recurrent, or metastatic non-small cell lung cancer (NSCLC). Eur J Cancer. 2009;7:5.
36. Sequist LV, von Pawel J, Garmey EG, et al. Randomized phase II study of erlotinib plus tivantinib versus erlotinib plus placebo in previously treated non-small-cell lung cancer. J Clin Oncol. 2011;29:3307-15.
37. Scagliotti G, Novello S, Ramlau R, et al. Results of the phase 3 study: MET inhibitor Tivantinib (ARQ 197) Plus Erlotinib versus Erlotinib plus Placebo in NSCLC. ESMO/ECCO proceedings 2013.
38. Douillard JY, Shepherd FA, Hirsh V, et al. Molecular predictors of outcome with gefitinib and docetaxel in previously treated non-small-cell lung cancer: data from the randomized phase Ⅲ INTEREST trial. J Clin Oncol. 2010;28:744-52.
39. Garassino MC, Martelli O, Bettini A, et al. A phase Ⅲ trial comparing erlotinib versus docetaxel as second-line treatment of NSCLC patients with wild-type EGFR. ASCO proceedings 2012.
40. Johnson BE, Kabbinavar F, Fehrenbacher L, et al. ATLAS: randomized, double-blind, placebo-controlled, phase ⅢB trial comparing bevacizumab therapy with or without erlotinib, after completion of chemotherapy, with bevacizumab for first-line treatment of advanced non-small-cell lung cancer. J Clin Oncol. 2013;31:3926-34.

41. Engelman JA, Chen L, Tan X, et al. Effective use of PI3K and MEK inhibitors to treat mutant Kras G12D and PIK3CA H1047R murine lung cancers. Nat Med. 2008;14:1351-6.
42. Linardou H, Dahabreh IJ, Kanaloupiti D, et al. Assessment of somatic k-RAS mutations as a mechanism associated with resistance to EGFR-targeted agents: a systematic review and meta-analysis of studies in advanced non-small-cell lung cancer and metastatic colorectal cancer. Lancet Oncol. 2008;9:962-72.
43. Mao C, Qiu LX, Liao RY, et al. KRAS mutations and resistance to EGFR-TKIs treatment in patients with non-small cell lung cancer: a meta-analysis of 22 studies. Lung Cancer. 2010; 69:272-8.
44. Metro G, Chiari R, Duranti S, et al. Impact of specific mutant KRAS on clinical outcome of EGFR-TKI-treated advanced non-small cell lung cancer patients with an EGFR wild type genotype. Lung Cancer. 2012;78:81-6.
45. Fiala O, Pesek M, Finek J, et al. The dominant role of G12C over other KRAS mutation types in the negative prediction of efficacy of epidermal growth factor receptor tyrosine kinase inhibitors in non-small cell lung cancer. Cancer Genet. 2013;206:26-31.
46. Khambata-Ford S, Harbison CT, Hart LL, et al. Analysis of potential predictive markers of cetuximab benefit in BMS099, a phase III study of cetuximab and first-line taxane/carboplatin in advanced non-small-cell lung cancer. J Clin Oncol. 2010;28:918-27.
47. O'Byrne KJ, Gatzemeier U, Bondarenko I, et al. Molecular biomarkers in non-small-cell lung cancer: a retrospective analysis of data from the phase 3 FLEX study. Lancet Oncol. 2011;12:795-805.
48. Butts CA, Ding K, Seymour L, et al. Randomized phase III trial of vinorelbine plus cisplatin compared with observation in completely resected stage IB and II non-small-cell lung cancer: updated survival analysis of JBR-10. J Clin Oncol. 2010;28:29-34.
49. Ihle NT, Byers LA, Kim ES, et al. Effect of KRAS oncogene substitutions on protein behavior: implications for signaling and clinical outcome. J Natl Cancer Inst. 2012;104:228-39.
50. Garassino MC, Marabese M, Rusconi P, et al. Different types of K-Ras mutations could affect drug sensitivity and tumour behaviour in non-small-cell lung cancer. Ann Oncol. 2011; 22:235-7.
51. Hainsworth JD, Cebotaru CL, Kanarev V, et al. A phase II, open-label, randomized study to assess the efficacy and safety of AZD6244 (ARRY-142886) versus pemetrexed in patients with non-small cell lung cancer who have failed one or two prior chemotherapeutic regimens. J Thorac Oncol. 2010;5:1630-6.
52. Janne PA, Shaw AT, Pereira JR, et al. Selumetinib plus docetaxel for KRAS-mutant advanced non-small-cell lung cancer: a randomised, multicentre, placebo-controlled, phase 2 study. Lancet Oncol. 2013;14:38-47.
53. Bennouma J, Leighl NB, Kelly K, et al. Oral MEK1/MEK2 inhibitor trametinib (GSK1120212) in combination with docetaxel in a phase 1/1b trial involving KRAS-mutant and wild-type (WT) advanced non-small cell lung cancer (NSCLC): efficacy and biomarkers

results. WCLC proceedings 2013:Abstract 2411.
54. Riely G, Brahmer JR, Planchard D. A randomized discontinuation phase II trial of ridaforolimus in non-small cell lung cancer (NSCLC) patients with KRAS mutations. J Clin Oncol. 2012;30:Abstract 7531.
55. Adjei AA, Mauer A, Bruzek L, et al. Phase II study of the farnesyl transferase inhibitor R115777 in patients with advanced non-small-cell lung cancer. J Clin Oncol. 2003;21:1760-6.
56. Eder Jr JP, Ryan DP, Appleman L, et al. Phase I clinical trial of the farnesyltransferase inhibitor BMS-214662 administered as a weekly 24 h continuous intravenous infusion in patients with advanced solid tumors. Cancer Chemother Pharmacol. 2006;58:107-16.
57. Riely GJ, Johnson ML, Medina C, et al. A phase II trial of Salirasib in patients with lung adenocarcinomas with KRAS mutations. J Thorac Oncol. 2011;6:1435-7.
58. Chandra A, Grecco HE, Pisupati V, et al. The GDI-like solubilizing factor PDEdelta sustains the spatial organization and signalling of Ras family proteins. Nat Cell Biol. 2012;14:148-58.
59. Zimmermann G, Papke B, Ismail S, et al. Small molecule inhibition of the KRAS-PDEdelta interaction impairs oncogenic KRAS signalling. Nature. 2013;497:638-42.
60. Gilmartin AG, Bleam MR, Groy A, et al. GSK1120212 (JTP-74057) is an inhibitor of MEK activity and activation with favorable pharmacokinetic properties for sustained in vivo pathway inhibition. Clin Cancer Res. 2011;17:989-1000.
61. Blumenschein GR, Smit EF, Planchard D, et al. MEK114653:a randomized, multicenter, phase II study to assess efficacy and safety of trametinib (T) compared with docetaxel (D) in KRAS-mutant advanced non-small cell lung cancer (NSCLC). ASCO proceedings 2013:Abstract 8029.
62. Kelly K, Mazieres J, Leighl NB, et al. Oral MEK1/MEK2 inhibitor trametinib (GSK1120212) in combination with pemetrexed for KRAS-mutant and wild-type (WT) advanced non-small cell lung cancer (NSCLC):a phase I/IB trial. ASCO proceedings 2012.
63. Wee S, Jagani Z, Xiang KX, et al. PI3K pathway activation mediates resistance to MEK inhibitors in KRAS mutant cancers. Cancer Res. 2009;69:4286-93.
64. Loboda A, Nebozhyn M, Klinghoffer R, et al. A gene expression signature of RAS pathway dependence predicts response to PI3K and RAS pathway inhibitors and expands the population of RAS pathway activated tumors. BMC Med Genomics. 2010;3:26.
65. Gridelli C, Maione P, Rossi A. The potential role of mTOR inhibitors in non-small cell lung cancer. Oncologist. 2008;13:139-47.
66. Soria JC, Shepherd FA, Douillard JY, et al. Efficacy of everolimus (RAD001) in patients with advanced NSCLC previously treated with chemotherapy alone or with chemotherapy and EGFR inhibitors. Ann Oncol. 2009;20:1674-81.
67. Mita MM, Mita AC, Chu QS, et al. Phase I trial of the novel mammalian target of rapamycin inhibitor deforolimus (AP23573; MK-8669) administered intravenously daily for 5 days every 2 weeks to patients with advanced malignancies. J Clin Oncol. 2008;26:361-7.
68. De Raedt T, Walton Z, Yecies JL, et al. Exploiting cancer cell vulnerabilities to develop a

combination therapy for ras-driven tumors. Cancer Cell. 2011;20:400-13.
69. Organ SL, Tsao MS. An overview of the c-MET signaling pathway. Ther Adv Med Oncol. 2011;3:S7-19.
70. Sierra JR, Tsao MS. c-MET as a potential therapeutic target and biomarker in cancer. Ther Adv Med Oncol. 2011;3:S21-35.
71. Ciocca DR, Calderwood SK. Heat shock proteins in cancer: diagnostic, prognostic, predictive, and treatment implications. Cell Stress Chaperones. 2005;10:86-103.
72. Sos ML, Michel K, Zander T, et al. Predicting drug susceptibility of non-small cell lung cancers based on genetic lesions. J Clin Invest. 2009;119:1727-40.
73. Acquaviva J, Smith DL, Sang J, et al. Targeting KRAS-mutant non-small cell lung cancer with the Hsp90 inhibitor ganetespib. Mol Cancer Ther. 2012;11:2633-43.
74. Socinski MA, Goldman J, El-Hariry I, et al. A multicenter phase II study of ganetespib monotherapy in patients with genotypically defined advanced non-small cell lung cancer. Clin Cancer Res. 2013;19:3068-77.
75. Fernandez V, Hartmann E, Ott G, et al. Pathogenesis of mantle-cell lymphoma: all oncogenic roads lead to dysregulation of cell cycle and DNA damage response pathways. J Clin Oncol. 2005;23:6364-9.
76. Puyol M, Martin A, Dubus P, et al. A synthetic lethal interaction between K-Ras oncogenes and Cdk4 unveils a therapeutic strategy for non-small cell lung carcinoma. Cancer Cell. 2010; 18:63-73.
77. Shapiro GI, Rosen LS, Tolcher AW, et al. A first-in-human phase 1 study of the CDK4/6 inhibitor, LY2835219, for patients with advanced cancer. ASCO proceedings 2013.
78. Ostrem JM, Peters U, Sos ML, et al. K-Ras(G12C) inhibitors allosterically control GTP affinity and effector interactions. Nature. 2013;503:548-51.

# 第12章

其他分子类型突变肺癌治疗策略

作者:Manolo D'Arcangelo,Fred R. Hirsch
译者:袁小帅

简介

2004年首次在非小细胞肺癌(non-small cell lung cancer,NSCLC)中发现表皮生长因子受体(the Epidermal Growth Factor Receptor,EGFR)突变,应用EGFR酪氨酸激酶抑制剂(tyrosine kinase inhibitors,TKIs)治疗的预测价值[48,61]也开辟了一条旨在通过发现其他基因或分子变化从而开展靶向治疗的肺癌研究新道路。进而在2007年于肺癌中发现了间变性淋巴瘤激酶(anaplastic lymphoma kinase,ALK)基因的重排及其致癌特征[77]。与传统化疗相比,通过ALK和EGFR激酶抑制得到的临床结果令人振奋,这也进一步证实了在肺癌患者中针对肿瘤细胞内异常活跃的信号转导通路可得到更好的治疗效果[55,68,73,74]。然而,西方人群中仅有15%～20%的患者会发生EGFR突变和ALK易位,故而新靶点的发现十分必要,而现今胸肺部肿瘤的分子改变研究主要聚焦于生物标记物表达和肺癌中常见组织类型的特异性差异研究。腺癌(Adenocarcinoma,ADC)是肺癌中最常见的组织亚型,其分子特征也最具代表性,截至目前,50%～60%的ADC中均可发现靶向的分子改变[39]。而另一方面,作为肺癌中第二常见的组织亚型,肺鳞状细胞癌(squamous cell carcinoma,SqCC)中发现靶向分子改变的比例为25%～30%[37],而针对肺鳞状细胞癌的分子特征和治疗相关进展仍相对较少。附录彩图12.1描述了2种组织学亚型靶向癌基因的研究现状。

在本章的内容中,我们将分析晚期ADC和SqCC患者的分子改变和靶向药物的潜在作用,首先重点关注人表皮生长因子受体2(human epidermal growth factor receptor 2,HER2)、间充质上皮转化(mesenchymal epithelial transition,MET)、BRAF、基因融合等,接下来是成纤维细胞生长因子受体1(fibroblast growth factor receptor 1,FGFR1)、盘状结构域受体2(discoidin domain receptor 2,DDR2)以及PI3KCA/AKT转化等。

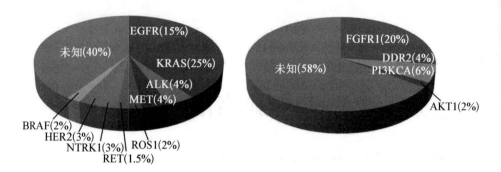

图 12.1　NSCLC 驱动基因:(a)腺癌;(b)鳞癌。

肺腺癌

近二十年来,有关肺 ADC 的基因表达、突变和其他改变以及蛋白组学的相关研究层出不穷,这些研究使大量分子改变得以发现,尽管其中许多在 NSCLC 中发生的概率不足 5%,而此类低频率的研究使评估临床特征和预后之间的关系以及开展针对特异性改变患者的靶向药物临床试验变得及其困难。为了获得更大的研究队列,通过各种途径获得支持的官方或非官方研究机构已开始在更大数据库中收集资料。美国国立癌症研究所(the National Cancer Institute,NCI)资助,由科罗拉多大学牵头成立了肺癌突变联盟(the Lung Cancer Mutation Consortium,LCMC)。联盟对 1000 例肺 ADC 中 10 个驱动突变进行了前瞻性评估,并借助 SnapShot 平台和美国食品药品管理局(the Food and Drug Administration,FDA)批准应用的荧光原位杂交(fluorescence in situ hybridization,FISH)技术对 ALK 易位和 MET 扩增进行了研究。在 1007 位具有任何基因分型的与试者中 622 位(62%)检测出可操作驱动改变,而 733 位全基因分型与试者中 465 位(63%)亦发现了可操作驱动改变[39]。KRAS 和敏化 EGFR 突变检出率分别为 25% 和 15%,ALK 重排率为 8%,其他突变包括 BRAF(2%)、HER2(2%)、PI3KCA(1%)、NRAS(1%)和 MEK1(<1%),以及 MET 扩增(1%)。值得一提的是,具有可操作突变的患者采用靶向治疗后存活时间较采用特定疗法的突变患者存活时间更久(3.5 年 vs 2.4 年,$P<0.0001$)。近期法国肿瘤中心(法国生物标记物研究)数据库收集分析的结果公布于 2013 年美国临床肿瘤协会(American Society of Clinical Oncology,ASCO)大会上[2],10 000 例肿瘤标本(76% ADC,5% SqCC)中 46% 均发现已知分子改变,其中 EGFR 占 10.2%,KRAS 占 26.8%,BRAF 占 1.8%,HER2 占 0.9%,PIK3CA 占 2.4%,ALK 重排占 3.9%。变异的频率仍较低,区位因素或许是其原因。然而,考虑到肺癌的高发病率和死亡率,发生上述变异的患者绝对数量也不容忽视,它们对治疗目的的识别价值仍相当大。

HER2 畸变

HER2，亦被称作人类 EGFR2、ERBB2/neu，是一类膜受体，和 EGFR (HER1)、HER3、HER4 一起组成 ERBB 家族。与其他家族成员不同，HER2 并无已知配体，但其仍作为包括 EGFR 在内的家族成员的首选的二聚体伴侣。考虑到 EGFR 在肿瘤发生、维持和进展[33]以及潜在的调节功能[46]中占据的中心地位，HER2 是肺癌治疗中一个极有吸引力的靶点。

HER2 功能异常可由基因拷贝数、基因序列和蛋白表达的变化引起，已知病例报道中有高达 20% 表现为 HER2 高表达[34]，而肺 ADC 中 HER2 扩增和突变的发生几率分别为 10% 和 3%[1,7,80]，HER2 最常见的突变为外显子 20 密码子 776 的框内复制/插入[1]。

HER2 预后价值已在多项研究中被报道，但结果并不一致。我们 2002 年的研究表明 HER2 蛋白表达对生存期并无影响[34]；然而近期一项 meta 分析结果则与之相反，认为肺 ADC 中 HER2 高表达具有较弱的预后价值[47]；近期由 Cappuzzo 等报道的研究中证实，HER2 扩增对 NSCLC 患者并无影响[10]；而 HER2 突变的预后影响目前尚未有文献报道[1,54]。

HER2 高表达的乳腺癌和胃癌中抗 HER2 策略是目前的治疗方案。已有若干临床试验针对 HER2 高表达或扩增的肺癌患者分别采用 2 类 HER2 靶向单克隆抗体（曲妥珠单抗，帕妥珠单抗）的效用进行评估，然而研究结果并不，无法促使在 HER2 扩增和高表达的肺癌患者中开展靶向治疗的进一步研究[23,32,43-45,93]。而另一方面，临床前研究则表明 HER2 突变存在致瘤性[63]，且存在 HER2 突变的 NSCLC 细胞系对曲妥珠单抗敏感[85]，若干病例报道亦支持上述结论，而最近 Mazières 等发表了一项研究，对 16 例 HER2 突变阳性的患者开展抗 HER2 治疗（曲妥珠单抗、拉帕替尼、阿法替尼和 masatinib）的疗效进行了回顾，结果令人满意，总反应率（overall response rate，ORR）达到 50%，疾病控制率（disease control rate，DCR）达到 82%，其中效果最佳的药物为曲妥珠单抗（$n=15$，DCR$=96\%$）和阿法替尼（$n=4$，DCR 100%）。针对 HER2 突变肺癌患者的另一类正在研发的药物为不可逆泛 HER2 抑制剂家族，包括拉帕替尼、阿法替尼、达克米替尼、来那替尼等。拉帕替尼是一类用于 HER2 阳性突变乳腺癌治疗的可逆的泛 ErbB 抑制剂，在 NSCLC 治疗中表现出极少的活性[76]。一项比利时的试验性 II 期试验结果证实阿法替尼在 HER2 突变的 NSCLC 治疗中存在较强活性，5 位突变患者均出现治疗反应[16]。研究亦评估了达克米替尼被用于 HER2 扩增或突变 NSCLC 患者的治疗，22 位 HER2 阳性突变患者仅有少量出现治疗反应（ORR 17%）[42]，另外，基因扩增患者对治疗并无反应。另一方面，一项 I 期试验结果表明来那替尼对 HER2 突变肺癌患者存在一定活性[22]；而一项 II 期随机试验（NCT01827267）针对 84 例 HER2 突变 NSCLC 患者采用来那替尼单药治疗或联用 mTOR 抑制剂治疗的比较分析正在进行中。

综上,HER2 高表达或扩增似乎并不能影响该类病人开展抗 HER2 治疗的反应,而出现 HER2 突变则可选择合适的 NSCLC 亚型患者可采用单克隆抗体或小分子抑制剂进行抗 HER2 治疗。未来继续更深入研究和更大型 Ⅱ、Ⅲ 期临床试验的开展。

MET 扩增

MET 原癌基因位于染色体 7q21,编码肝细胞生长因子(hepatocyte growth factor,HCF)的酪氨酸激酶受体蛋白,蛋白过表达、基因扩增和突变可导致 MET 异常。MET 蛋白在肺癌中广泛表达,通常表达率范围可达 25%～75%[35]。已知 MET 过表达是肺癌的负性预后因素,已有数项研究表明,4% 的肺癌中可出现 MET 基因拷贝数增加,这被认为与患者预后较差存在相关性[9,56],但也有研究持相反意见[20]。MET 基因突变可发生于约 5% 的肺癌样本中,有关 MET 突变的预后价值及其和肿瘤发生发展之间的关系尚未得到充分阐述[17,49],而近期研究则认为其在疾病进展中起一定作用[24]。

20% 的 EGFR 阳性突变肺癌患者进行 EGFR TKIs 治疗时发生抵抗,MET 扩增被认为是发生抵抗的机制,因此开发抗 MET 药物与 EGFR TKIs 联用是延缓或客服其治疗抵抗的有效手段。onartuzumab(METMab)是一类人源单克隆 MET 抗体,尽管一项 Ⅱ 期研究表明其在 MET 免疫组化(immunohistochemistry,IHC)阳性患者的治疗中可有效延长无进展生存期(progression free survival,PFS)[78],另一项 Ⅲ 期试验(METLung)开展了针对有过既往治疗的 MET IHC 阳性 NSCLC 患者采用 onartuzumab 联用 EGFR TKIs 厄洛替尼作为治疗方案的研究却因缺乏足够的临床治疗意义而于近期被叫停(http://www.gene.com/media/press-releases/14562/2014-03-02/genentech-provides-update-on-phase-Ⅲs)。该项研究的具体数据尚未发布,而另 2 项正在进行中的 Ⅲ 期试验(NCT01519804,NCT01496742)中 onartuzumab 联用化疗药物分别在 SqCC 和 ADC 的治疗数据仍未公布。类似情况发生在另一项 Ⅱ 期试验中,该研究针对非鳞癌肺癌患者采用 tivantinib 联用厄洛替尼的治疗方案,结果证实 tivantinib 作为一类非 ATP 竞争性小分子 MET 抑制剂表现出有意义的活性[72],而后续的 Ⅲ 期试验针对生物学非选择性 NSCLC 患者进行 tivantinib 联用厄洛替尼和安慰剂联用厄洛替尼 2 种治疗方案的比较,因达不到提高生存率的试验目的而于 2012 年 10 月被叫停(http://investors.arqule.com/releasedetail.cfm?ReleaseID=710618)。一项子集分析结果表明针对 IHC 阳性 2+(超过 50% 的阳性率)患者的治疗可获得更长的 PFS 和 OS,但仍需进一步研究以证实其结论。

克唑替尼是一类首先在 ALK 重排肺癌中被用作抗 ALK 药物的 MET 抑制剂,而一项比例报告中提到,1 位 MET 从头扩增不伴 ALK 重排的 NSCLC 患者发现对克唑替尼的快速反应[59]，这提示抗 MET 策略在基因从头扩增的患者中具有潜在价值。

上述提及的抗 MET 药物在治疗中的阴性结果并不等同于抗 MET 疗法的失败，截至目前，尚未有此类药物在 MET 从头扩增或突变患者中的药效评估，因而未来该亚型患者的研究就亟待开展。

BRAF 突变

BRAF 是丝氨酸/苏氨酸激酶 RAS 家族成员之一，是 KRAS 的首个下游效应因子。BRAF 突变的激活可导致激酶活性的增加并在体外进行了转化[14]。BRAF 突变作为转移性黑色素瘤中最具特征的肿瘤驱动因素，在 NSCLC 中发生的概率为 1%~5%且几乎都发生在 ADC 中[52,62]。与黑色素瘤中 80%的突变均为 V600E 突变[75]不同，肺癌中有 50%比例的 BRAF 突变为非 V600E 突变[52,62]。非 V600E 突变主要与吸烟相关，而 V600E 突变则在女性和非吸烟人群中更常见。BRAF 突变与 EGFR 突变、KRAS 突变和 ALK 重排均相互排斥，且 BRAF 突变的出现似乎使患者预后恶化。Marchetti 等的研究表明 V600E 突变和更具侵袭性肿瘤组织学类型（乳头状）之间存在相关性，且其能缩短无病生存期和总生存率（Overall survival,OS），而非 V600E 突变则无证据表明和预后影响有关联[52]。

尽管近期有几类化合物正在被研究，但有关 BRAF 抑制剂活性治疗 BRAF 突变肺癌的临床数据仍较少。其中维罗非尼是在黑色素治疗过程中开发的第一代 BRAF 抑制剂，它是经设计可特异性靶向 BRAF 蛋白的 V600E 突变氨基酸变化，而它对非 V600E 突变的蛋白是否具备抑制能力尚未可知。临床前数据和一项临床报告研究表明非 V600E 突变对维罗非尼有抵抗作用[26,91]，而相反的是若干临床报告证实维罗非尼在 BRAF V600E 突变患者中具有相当大的治疗反应[25,64]。另一种具有促进功能的 V600E BRAF 突变抑制剂为达拉菲尼。2013 年 ASCO 年会上一项Ⅱ期临床试验首次公布了单用达拉菲尼作为治疗方案的结果，13 位患者采用达拉菲尼治疗，有 5 例患者存在部分反应（ORR 54%），该研究正在已进入到下一阶段。

综上 BRAF 突变数据表明，BRAF 的分子畸变可被认作肺腺癌的靶向驱动因素。尽管临床资料较少，但唯一可参考的Ⅱ期试验数据证实 BRAF 抑制剂是一类很具前景的化合物。未来的挑战主要是开发出一种可对 V600E 和非 V600E 突变均有抑制性的 BRAF 抑制剂。

基因融合

ALK 融合一经发现后，在肺癌中陆续发现了各类杂交基因的融合。基因融合一般表现为染色体易位，反转或缺失的结果，致癌基因重排新的蛋白或与原始蛋白活性差异较大的蛋白的表达，此外，融合可是某个基因被很强的启动子操控，从而导致某个蛋白在本应不表达或低表达的正常细胞内发生异常表达。

ROS1是一类位于染色体6q22的原癌基因,而ROS1在肺癌中的重排是由Rikova等于2007年首次报道[66]。ROS1蛋白的生理作用现在仍未被完全阐明,目前已知的编码蛋白功能是一类具有酪氨酸激酶活性的跨膜受体。现已发现ROS1可进行融合的若干基因,如SLC34A2、SDC4、EZR、FIG、TPM3、CD74、KDELR2、LRIG3及其他[67,81],这些基因均是通过染色体易位并以自身5′末端融合ROS1基因的3′末端区域(包括激酶结构域)。体内和体外试验均已证实ROS1融合蛋白具有致瘤特性[12,13]。ROS1重排可在约2%的肺腺癌中发现,而在非吸烟人群中几率更高[4]。考虑到ROS1和ALK氨基酸序列的高度同源性[92],有人提出假设,ALK抑制剂如克唑替尼等对ROS1也具有抑制效果。而事实上,近期公布的PROFILE 1001研究原始数据中得到一个令人震惊的结果,克唑替尼在ROS1重排阳性患者的治疗中具有相当的抗肿瘤效果(ORR 56%)[60]。融合蛋白也是参与热休克蛋白(heat shock protein,HSP)通路,因此与ALK类似的是,ROS1融合阳性的肿瘤似乎应对HSP90抑制剂敏感[69],而目前尚未有此类治疗的相关报道。

RET基因位于10号染色体,可编码具有酪氨酸激酶活性的跨膜受体蛋白,主要参与细胞增殖、迁移、分化以及神经导航等生物过程。RET的胚系突变和体细胞突变已知可引发多发性2型内分泌肿瘤(multiple endocrine neoplasia type 2,MEN2)综合征以及与散发性甲状腺髓样癌的发生发展相关[88],另外RET重排与散发性和辐射性甲状腺乳头状癌相关。RET重排亦已被证实存在于肺ADC中,发生率约为1%~2%。一些基因如KIF5B、CCDC6、NCO4、TRIMM33等被认为可与ROS1发生融合[81,86]。RET阳性肺癌更常见于低分化肿瘤和从未吸烟者[86]。在治疗方面,若干多激酶抑制剂如凡德他尼、卡博替尼、普纳替尼、阿西替尼、舒尼替尼和索拉非尼等均可阻断RET功能。Ⅲ期试验生物学非选择NSCLC的数据包含了此类药物单用或联用的临床疗效,然而所有研究结果均为阴性,上述药物不能有效治疗肺癌的可能原因为并未进行基因型选择。另一方面,若干病例报告证实了RET阳性肺癌患者针对凡德他尼和卡博替尼治疗的反应[18,27]。特别是研究者在Ⅱ期试验(NCT01639508)中发现针对首3例RET阳性肺ADC患者采用卡博替尼进行治疗,结果显示2例患者发生部分反应,1例患者病情长期稳定。现亦有Ⅱ期试验针对RET重排阳性肺癌患者采用凡德他尼(NCT01823068)、舒尼替尼(NCT01829217)、普纳替尼(NCT01813734)进行治疗并分别评估其疗效。试验结果有望在未来几年发表,从而此类肺ADC亚型或许能有新的治疗选择。

NTRK1位于1号染色体,可编码TRKA受体酪氨酸激酶蛋白。近期,由Doebele研究组证实NTRK1存在一个全新的融合方式[83]。研究纳入了91例无其他共同致癌改变的肺ADC样本,其中3例(3.3%)发现了全新融合。临床前数据证实克唑替尼、leustartinib(CEP-701)和ARRY-470具有抗肿瘤效果。克唑替尼的抑制能力劣于另2种药物,但考虑到其已在临床上广泛应用,研究组应寻求确定针对NTRK1阳性肺癌患者采用克唑替尼治疗是否有临床获益。1位NTRK1重排患者接受克唑替尼治疗后获得了持续3个月之久的极小的治疗反应。未来,采用已存在药物或是开发新型抑制剂的临床试验将极为必要。

肺鳞状细胞癌

近年来发现了许多新的基因突变可作为肺ADC的治疗靶点,而SqCC生物学特征的认识尚停留在早期阶段,这个差距导致了晚期NSCLC患者因组织学类型不同而采用迥异的治疗方案。然而近年来,科学界对SqCC的认识产生了浓厚的兴趣,为此也发现了若干新的治疗靶点。早期的单核苷酸多态性(single-neuclotide polymorphisms,SNP)阵列研究发现了FGFR1基因作为SqCC潜在可操作靶点[3,19]。测序研究致力于发现突变的激酶[29],磷酸酪氨酸信号转导研究[66]则发现了DDR2突变可用作临床治疗靶点。癌症基因组图谱研究网络采用了SNP阵列分析、全外显子组测序、RNA和miRNA测序、甲基化谱分析等技术,绘制了178例肺SqCC的基因组和表观遗传改变图谱[6]。该研究组在96%的SqCC样本中发现了酪氨酸激酶、丝氨酸/苏氨酸激酶、PI3K的催化和调节亚基、核激素受体、G蛋白偶联受体、蛋白酶、酪氨酸磷酸酶等的突变。特别的是,他们在64%的样本中均发现了一个潜在靶基因的体细胞改变,这些数据可开辟肺SqCC个体化治疗的新途径。而且,近期将有一项意义重大的公私合伙计划将在美国拉开帷幕,即针对SqCC的"Master Protocol"计划。该计划由美国NCI和FDA牵头,目标是针对某Ⅱ期随机试验中具备疗效的药物的快速鉴定,若Ⅱ期试验结果满意,将会开展良好随机的Ⅲ期注册试验。

FGFR改变

FGFR家族包含4个具有酪氨酸激酶活性的受体,即FGFR1、FGFR2、FGFR3和FGFR4。受体激活可引起下游诸如PI3K/AKT和RAS/RAF/MEK通路的信号转导[53]。最开始关注FGFR家族是由几项研究引起,研究结果表明10%~20%的肺SqCC和不超过5%的肺ADC中出现了包含FGFR1在内的染色体8p12的扩增[19,71,87]。同时其中几项研究表明存在FGFR1扩增的肺癌细胞系对小分子FGFR1激酶阻断剂敏感[19,87],而关于此类分子事件与肿瘤预后之间是否相关则并无统一意见。一项韩国研究证实了FGFR1扩增的负性独立预后意义,而Heist等则报道基因改变与肿瘤生存并无相关性[31,87]。通过全外显子组和RNA测序可知,FGFR突变则发生于该家族的所有4个成员中[6],而FGFR2和FGFR3突变可占到SqCC的5%且具有致癌性,同时可使肿瘤细胞对FGFR激酶抑制剂变得敏感[38]。

一些临床研究对抗FGFR策略的意义进行了评估。普纳替尼是一种可有效抑制 FGFR 家族全体 4 个成员以及其他激酶的多功能抑制剂，并已被研究证实在 FGFR 扩增或突变的肺癌细胞系中存在临床前活性[28]。一项进行中的 Ⅱ 期试验（NCT01935336）评估了普纳替尼对来自科罗拉多大学的分子性选择肺癌患者的治疗效果，该研究包含一项 FGFR 改变（基因拷贝数和 mRNA 表达）的重要分析，旨在前瞻性发现每个生物标志物的患病率和重叠程度。而实际上，临床前数据表明单独的 FGFR1 扩增或许不足以决定更可能会对治疗反应的患者的类别[89]。其他针对 FGFR1 扩增的肺 SqCC 患者治疗的在研药物包括多韦替尼（TKI258，试验编号 NCT01861197），AZD4547，NVP-BGJ398 等。这些试验结果或将有力阐明 FGFR 抑制剂是否可成为 FGFR 基因或受体基因改变肺癌患者治疗的成功策略。

DDR2 突变

盘状结构域受体 2（discoidin domain receptor 2，DDR2）是一类可结合胶原蛋白并具有酪氨酸激酶活性的膜受体，当活化后可与 Src 和 Shc 发生相互作用[36]。DDR2 位于染色体 1q23.3，在 3.8% 的肺 SqCC 中可检出突变[29]。目前尚无数据证实 DDR2 突变潜在的预后意义。而在治疗方面，已有研究表明达沙替尼（BMS-354825）、伊马替尼和尼洛替尼等对 DDR2 具有高亲和力和抑制性[15]。肺癌细胞系的临床前实验显示 DDR2 是具有致癌性的，且干扰 RNA 或达沙替尼的应用可选择性抑制 DDR2 突变细胞[29]。

上述数据支持在临床上对达沙替尼的进一步研究。两项临床试验针对生物性未选择 NSCLC 采用达沙替尼单用或联用厄洛替尼为治疗方案并进行了评估[30,40]，试验结果均证实实验性治疗相比细胞毒性化疗效果更差，然而其中 1 例对厄洛替尼联用达沙替尼的治疗妨碍产生反应的患者被检出存在 DDR2 突变。一项针对 DDR2 突变阳性 SqCC 患者采用达沙替尼单一疗法治疗的 Ⅱ 期试验（NCT01514864）现正在开展中，结果将备受期待。

PI3KCA/AKT/mTOR 通路畸变

PI3KCA/AKT/mTOR 通路是一条重要的信号转导通路，参与细胞增殖、分化、运动和血管生成等现象的调控[21]。包括 EGFR、HER2、c-MET 以及 IGF1R 等在内的几种膜酪氨酸激酶可激活 PI3K，进而使 AKT 磷酸化，最终激活下游 mTOR、Bcl-2、TSC2 以及其他效应因子。PI3KCA/AKT/mTOR 通路也可与其他信号通路发生相互作用，例如 RAS 可直接激活 PI3K[84]。不同层次的通路功能失调可出现在许多恶性肿瘤中，其中就包括肺癌。癌症基因组图谱网络项目在 47% 的分析样本中发现了通路的显著改变，其中最常见的为 PI3K 点突变和扩增、PTEN 缺失和失活突变以及 AKT 过表达[6]，上述分子改变的整体频率使得阻断该通路从而达到治疗目的变得很有吸引力。另一方面，PI3K 通路的改变常与其他分子畸变共同发生，而非驱动突变的相互排斥。这提示了 PI3K 通路的改变或许是二次事件[6]。这对此通路抑制剂的研究具有极大影响。

PI3KCA 基因位于染色体 3q26.3，编码 PI3K 蛋白家族的主要催化亚基。PI3KCA 突变常见于外显子 9 和外显子 20 这 2 个热点，在鳞状组织学类型肿瘤中发生频率为 2%~9%[41,79,90]。同时 PI3KCA 扩增也见于 40% 的 NSCLC 中，在 SqCC 中更常见[57,90]。临床前研究表明，发生 PI3KCA 突变或拷贝数增加的肺癌细胞系对干扰 RNA 和小分子抑制剂治疗极其敏感[50,79,90]。包括亚型选择性抑制剂（GDC-0941）、泛 PI3K 抑制剂（BKM120、XL147）或 PI3K/mTOR 双重抑制剂（XL765）在内的 PI3K 抑制剂现均在进行临床试验，尽管目前为止获得的临床数据极其有限。考虑到其他分子畸变的共同存在，上述药物可单用或联合独行化疗药物抑或联合其他靶向治疗药物进行研究。

目前已有研究报道 PI3KCA/AKT/mTOR 通路亦可被 AKT 突变激活，这在 NSCLC 中的发生率位 0.5%~2%，在 SqCC 中更高[17,51]。E17K 突变影响 AKT1（位于染色体 14q32.32 的 AKT 亚型基因，主要功能是调控细胞凋亡），该突变具有致癌性，致使膜定位和 AKT1 磷酸化的出现[11]，且该突变似乎与 PI3KCA 突变相互排斥[5]。包括 GSK2110183、GSK2141795、AZD5363 和 GDC-0068 在内的针对所有 AKT 亚型的 ATP 竞争性抑制剂正进行早期临床研究，这些抑制剂的作用机制均很特殊，被称作"激酶活性捕获抑制剂"。这些抑制剂可使 AKT 发生高度磷酸化，随之则是非功能状态下的膜定位[58]。另一类靶向 AKT 的药物以非 ATP 竞争性变构抑制剂为代表，例如 MK2206。所有提及药物均仍处于早期临床研究，临床资料尚未可知。

结论

过去的数十年中，分子定制药物的应用彻底改变了肺癌治疗，特别是对 ADC 亚型来说 60% 的患者均能检出可操作靶点。肺癌生物学深入研究和更先进敏感的实验室技术的使用使我们对肺癌有了更深入的认识：肺癌在组织学特征和主要驱动的分子改变上均具有异质性。分子学研究结果一致认为基因组学和蛋白质组学变化（包括 HER2、BRAF 及 DDR2 的突变，若干基因的融合，MET 和 FGFR1 的扩增以及其他变化等）并非更常见，但更重要，而驱动基因异常的发现伴随了新药的研发以及已全面应用于其他疾病临床治疗药物的研究。这在各类研究中得到体现，例如：HER2 突变肺癌对曲妥珠单抗和阿法替尼治疗具有敏感性；BRAF2 突变或可帮助选择病人进行达拉菲尼治疗；ROS-1 和 MET 重排产生致瘤性融合蛋白可被克唑替尼和卡博替尼有效抑制。而对于其他生物标记物如 MET 或 PI3K/AKT 通路的改变，靶向药物的研究尚不完善。

尽管有关肺癌特别是 ADC 的分子特征研究有了极大的进步，现仍未有肿瘤患者经靶向药物治疗得到痊愈的报道，这与肿瘤的分子异质性和不可避免的治疗耐受等因素有关。一类极有前途的治疗策略为采用基于伴随分子改变或特异性通路活化的多基因驱动药物攻击肿瘤，这或许可导致肿瘤对治疗更具实质性回应从而导致持续性疾病进展的延迟。因此，旨在通过大样本人群发现生物标记物的重叠以及增加靶向治疗原发性或获得性耐药性机制知识的研究变得极为必要。同时，未来应努力开展治疗开始前和治疗中的肿瘤样本采集，从而更好地了解肿瘤分子信息的变化并据此调整治疗方案。

参考文献

1. Arcila ME, Chaft JE, Nafa K, et al. Prevalence, clinicopathologic associations, and molecular spectrum of ERBB2 (HER2) tyrosine kinase mutations in lung adenocarcinomas. Clin Cancer Res. 2012;18(18):4910-8.
2. Barlesi F, Blons H, Beau-Faller M, et al. Biomarkers (BM) France: results of routine EGFR, HER2, KRAS, BRAF, PI3KCA mutations detection and EML4-ALK gene fusion assessment on the first 10 000 non-small cell lung cancer (NSCLC) patients (pts). J Clin Oncol. 2013;31 Suppl 15:8000.
3. Bass AJ, Watanabe H, Mermel CH, et al. SOX2 is an amplified lineage-survival oncogene in lung and esophageal squamous cell carcinomas. Nat Genet. 2009;41(11):1238-42.
4. Bergethon K, Shaw AT, Ignatius Ou SH, et al. ROS1 rearrangements define a unique molecular class of lung cancers. J Clin Oncol. 2012;30:863-70.
5. Bleeker FE, Felicioni L, Buttitta F, et al. AKT1(E17K) in human solid tumours. Oncogene. 2008;27(42):5648-50.
6. Cancer Genome Atlas Research Network. Comprehensive genomic characterization of squamous cell lung cancers. Nature. 2012;489(7417):519-25.
7. Cappuzzo F, Varella-Garcia M, Shigematsu H, et al. Increased HER2 gene copy number is associated with response to gefitinib therapy in epidermal growth factor receptor-positive non small-cell lung cancer patients. J Clin Oncol. 2005;23(22):5007-18.
8. Cappuzzo F, Bemis L, Varella-Garcia M. HER2 mutation and response to trastuzumab therapy in non-small-cell lung cancer. N Engl J Med. 2006;354(24):2619-21.
9. Cappuzzo F, Marchetti A, Skokan M, et al. Increased MET gene copy number negatively affects survival of surgically resected non-small-cell lung cancer patients. J Clin Oncol. 2009;27(10):1667-74.
10. Cappuzzo F, Cho YG, Sacconi A, et al. p95HER2 truncated form in resected non-small cell lung cancer. J Thorac Oncol. 2012;7(3):520-7.
11. Carpten JD, Faber AL, Horn C, et al. A transforming mutation in the pleckstrin homology domain of AKT1 in cancer. Nature. 2007;448(7152):439-44.
12. Charest A, Kheifets V, Park J, et al. Oncogenic targeting of an activated tyrosine kinase to the Golgi apparatus in a glioblastoma. Proc Natl Acad Sci U S A. 2003;100:916-21.
13. Charest A, Wilker EW, McLaughlin ME, et al. ROS fusion tyrosine kinase activates a SH2 domain-containing phosphatase-2/phosphatidylinositol 3-kinase/mammalian target of rapam-

ycin signaling axis to form glioblastoma in mice. Cancer Res. 2006;66:7473-81.
14. Davies H,Bignell GR, Cox C, et al. Mutations of the BRAF gene in human cancer. Nature. 2002;417(6892):949-54.
15. Day E, Waters B, Spiegel K, et al. Inhibition of collagen-induced discoidin domain receptor 1 and 2 activation by imatinib, nilotinib and dasatinib. Eur J Pharmacol. 2008;599(1-3):44-53.
16. De Grève J,Teugels E, Geers C, et al. Clinical activity of afatinib (BIBW 2992) in patients with lung adenocarcinoma with mutations in the kinase domain of HER2/neu. Lung Cancer. 2012;76(1):123-7.
17. Ding L,Getz G, Wheeler DA, et al. Somatic mutations affect key pathways in lung adenocarcinoma. Nature. 2008;455(7216):1069-75.
18. Drilon A, Wang L, Hasanovic A, et al. Response to Cabozantinib in patients with RET fusionpositive lung adenocarcinomas. Cancer Discov. 2013;3(6):630-5.
19. Dutt A, Ramos AH, Hammerman PS, et al. Inhibitor-sensitive FGFR1 amplification in human non-small cell lung cancer. PLoS One. 2011;6(6):e20351.
20. Dziadziusko R, Wynes M, Singh S, et al. Correlation between MET gene copy number by silver in situ hybridization and protein expression by immunohistochemistry in non-small cell lung cancer. J Thorac Oncol. 2012;7(2):340-7.
21. Engelman JA, Luo J,Cantley LC. The evolution of phosphatidylinositol 3-kinases as regulators of growth and metabolism. Nat Rev Genet. 2006;7(8):606-19.
22. Gandhi L,Bahleda R, Tolaney SM, et al. Phase I study of neratinib in combination with temsirolimus in patients with human epidermal growth factor receptor 2-dependent and other solid tumors. J Clin Oncol. 2014;32(2):68-75.
23. Gatzemeier U, Groth G, Butts C, et al. Randomized phase II trial of gemcitabine-cisplatin with or without trastuzumab in HER2-positive non-small-cell lung cancer. Ann Oncol. 2004;15(1):19-27.
24. Gherardi E, Birchmeier W, Birchmeier C, et al. Targeting MET in cancer:rationale and progress. Nat Rev Cancer. 2012;12(2):89-103.
25. Gautschi O, Pauli C, Strobel K, et al. A patient with BRAF V600E lung adenocarcinoma responding to vemurafenib. J Thorac Oncol. 2012;7(10):e23-4.
26. Gautschi O, Peters S, Zoete V, et al. Lung adenocarcinoma with BRAF G469L mutation refractory to vemurafenib. Lung Cancer. 2013;82(2):365-7.
27. Gautschi O, Zander T, Keller FA, et al. A patient with lung adenocarcinoma and RET fusion treated with vandetanib. J Thorac Oncol. 2013;8(5):e43-4.
28. Gozgit JM, Wong MJ, Moran L, et al. Ponatinib (AP24534), a multitargeted pan-FGFR inhibitor with activity in multiple FGFR-amplified or mutated cancer models. Mol Cancer Ther. 2012;11(3):690-9.
29. Hammerman PS, Sos ML, Ramos AH, et al. Mutations in the DDR2 kinase gene identify a novel therapeutic target in squamous cell lung cancer. Cancer Discov. 2011;1(1):78-89.
30. Haura EB, Tanvetyanon T, Chiappori A, et al. Phase I/II study of the Src inhibitor dasatinib

in combination with erlotinib in advanced non-small-cell lung cancer. J Clin Oncol. 2010; 28(8):1387-94.

31. Heist RS, Mino-Kenudson M, Sequist LV, et al. FGFR1 amplification in squamous cell carcinoma of the lung. J Thorac Oncol. 2012;7(12):1775-80.

32. Herbst RS, Davies AM, Natale RB, et al. Efficacy and safety of single-agent pertuzumab, a human epidermal receptor dimerization inhibitor, in patients with non small cell lung cancer. Clin Cancer Res. 2007;13(20):6175-81.

33. Hirsch FR, Franklin WA, Veve R, et al. HER2/neu expression in malignant lung tumors. Semin Oncol. 2002;29(1 Suppl 4):51-8.

34. Hirsch FR, Varella-Garcia M, Franklin WA, et al. Evaluation of HER-2/neu gene amplification and protein expression in non-small cell lung carcinomas. Br J Cancer. 2002;86(9):1449-56.

35. Ichimura E, Maeshima A, Nakajima T, et al. Expression of c-met/HGF receptor in human non small cell lung carcinomas in vitro and in vivo and its prognostic significance. Jpn J Cancer Res. 1996;87(10):1063-9.

36. Ikeda K, Wang LH, Torres R, et al. Discoidin domain receptor 2 interacts with Src and Shc following its activation by type I collagen. J Biol Chem. 2002;277(21):19206-12.

37. Liao RG, Watanabe H, Meyerson M, Hammerman PS. Targeted therapy for squamous cell lung cancer. Lung Cancer Manag. 2012;1(4):293-300.

38. Liao RG, Jung J, Tchaicha J, et al. Inhibitor-sensitive FGFR2 and FGFR3 mutations in lung squamous cell carcinoma. Cancer Res. 2013;73(16):5195-205.

39. Johnson BE, Kris MG, Berry L, et al. A multicenter effort to identify driver mutations and employ targeted therapy in patients with lung adenocarcinomas: the Lung Cancer Mutation Consortium (LCMC). J Clin Oncol. 2013;31(Suppl):8019.

40. Johnson FM, Bekele BN, Feng L, et al. Phase II study of dasatinib in patients with advanced non-small-cell lung cancer. J Clin Oncol. 2010;28(30):4609-15.

41. Kawano O, Sasaki H, Endo K, et al. PIK3CA mutation status in Japanese lung cancer patients. Lung Cancer. 2006;54(2):209-15.

42. Kris MG, Mok T, Ou SH, et al. First-line dacomitinib (PF-00299804), an irreversible pan-HER tyrosine kinase inhibitor, for patients with EGFR-mutant lung cancers. J Clin Oncol. 2012;30(Suppl):7530.

43. Krug LM, Miller VA, Patel J, et al. Randomized phase II study of weekly docetaxel plustrastuzumab versus weekly paclitaxel plus trastuzumab in patients with previously untreated advanced nonsmall cell lung carcinoma. Cancer. 2005;104(10):2149-55.

44. Langer CJ, Stephenson P, Thor A, et al. Trastuzumab in the treatment of advanced non-small- cell lung cancer: is there a role? Focus on Eastern Cooperative Oncology Group study 2598. J Clin Oncol. 2004;22(7):1180-7.

45. Lara Jr PN, Laptalo L, Longmate J, et al. Trastuzumab plus docetaxel in HER2/neu-positive non-small-cell lung cancer: a California Cancer Consortium screening and phase II trial. Clin Lung Cancer. 2004;5(4):231-6.

46. Lenferink AE, Pinkas-Kramarski R, van de Poll ML, et al. Differential endocytic routing of homo- and hetero-dimeric ErbB tyrosine kinases confers signaling superiority to receptor heterodimers. EMBO J. 1998;17(12):3385-97.
47. Liu L, Shao X, Gao W, et al. The role of human epidermal growth factor receptor 2 as a prognostic factor in lung cancer: a meta-analysis of published data. J Thorac Oncol. 2010; 5(12):1922-32.
48. Lynch TJ, Bell DW, Sordella R, et al. Activating mutations in the epidermal growth factor receptor underlying responsiveness of non-small-cell lung cancer to gefitinib. N Engl J Med. 2004;350(21):2129-39.
49. Ma PC, Kijima T, Maulik G, et al. c-MET mutational analysis in small cell lung cancer: novel juxtamembrane domain mutations regulating cytoskeletal functions. Cancer Res. 2003; 63(19):6272-81.
50. Maira SM, Pecchi S, Huang A, et al. Identification and characterization of NVP-BKM120, an orally available pan-class I PI3-kinase inhibitor. Mol Cancer Ther. 2012;11(2):317-28.
51. Malanga D, Scrima M, De Marco C, et al. Activating E17K mutation in the gene encoding the protein kinase AKT1 in a subset of squamous cell carcinoma of the lung. Cell Cycle. 2008;7(5):665-9.
52. Marchetti A, Felicioni L, Malatesta S, et al. Clinical features and outcome of patients with non-small-cell lung cancer harboring BRAF mutations. Clin Oncol. 2011;29(26):3574-9.
53. Mason I. Initiation to end point: the multiple roles of fibroblast growth factors in neural development. Nat Rev Neurosci. 2007;8(8):583-96.
54. Mazières J, Peters S, Lepage B, et al. Lung cancer that harbors an HER2 mutation: epidemiologic characteristics and therapeutic perspectives. J Clin Oncol. 2013;31(16):1997-2003.
55. Mok TS, Wu YL, Thongprasert S, et al. Gefitinib or carboplatin-paclitaxel in pulmonary adenocarcinoma. N Engl J Med. 2009;361(10):947-57.
56. Okuda K, Sasaki H, Yukiue H, et al. Met gene copy number predicts the prognosis for completely resected non-small cell lung cancer. Cancer Sci. 2008;99(11):2280-5.
57. Okudela K, Suzuki M, Kageyama S, et al. PIK3CA mutation and amplification in human lung cancer. Pathol Int. 2007;57(10):664-71.
58. Okuzumi T, Fiedler D, Zhang C, et al. Inhibitor hijacking of Akt activation. Nat Chem Biol. 2009;5(7):484-93.
59. Ou SH, Kwak EL, Siwak-Tapp C, et al. Activity of crizotinib (PF02341066), a dual mesenchymalepithelial transition (MET) and anaplastic lymphoma kinase (ALK) inhibitor, in a non-small cell lung cancer patient with de novo MET amplification. J Thorac Oncol. 2011; 6(5):942-6.
60. Ou SH, Bang YJ, Camidge DR, et al. Efficacy and safety of crizotinib in patients with advanced ROS1-rearranged non-small cell lung cancer (NSCLC). J Clin Oncol. 2013;31(Suppl):8032.
61. Paez JG, Janne PA, Lee JC, et al. EGFR mutations in lung cancer: correlation with clinical

response to gefitinib therapy. Science. 2004;304(5676):1497-500.
62. Paik PK, Arcila ME, Fara M, et al. Clinical characteristics of patients with lung adenocarcinomas harboring BRAF mutations. J Clin Oncol. 2011;29(15):2046-51.
63. Perera SA, Li D, Shimamura T, et al. HER2YVMA drives rapid development of adenosquamous lung tumors in mice that are sensitive to BIBW2992 and rapamycin combination therapy. Proc Natl Acad Sci U S A. 2009;106(2):474-9.
64. Peters S, Michielin O, Zimmermann S. Dramatic response induced by vemurafenib in a BRAF V600E-mutated lung adenocarcinoma. J Clin Oncol. 2013;31(20):e341-4.
65. Planchard D, Mazières J, Riely GJ, et al. Interim results of phase II study BRF113928 of dabrafenib in BRAF V600E mutation-positive non-small cell lung cancer (NSCLC) patients. J Clin Oncol. 2013;31(Suppl):8009.
66. Rikova K, Guo A, Zeng Q, et al. Global survey of phosphotyrosine signaling identifies oncogenic kinases in lung cancer. Cell. 2007;131(6):1190-203.
67. Rimkunas VM, Crosby KE, Li D, et al. Analysis of receptor tyrosine kinase ROS1-positive tumors in non-small cell lung cancer: identification of a FIG-ROS1 fusion. Clin Cancer Res. 2012;18(16):4449-57.
68. Rosell R, Carcereny E, Gervais R, et al. Erlotinib versus standard chemotherapy as first-line treatment for European patients with advanced EGFR mutation-positive non-small-cell lung cancer (EURTAC): a multicentre, open-label, randomised phase 3 trial. Lancet Oncol. 2012;13(3):239-46.
69. Sang J, Acquaviva J, Friedland JC, et al. Targeted inhibition of the molecular chaperone Hsp90 overcomes ALK inhibitor resistance in non-small cell lung cancer. Cancer Discov. 2013;3(4):430-43.
70. Scagliotti G, Novello S, Ramlau R, et al. MARQUEE: a randomized double-blind, placebo controlled, phase 3 trial of tivantinib (ARQ 197) plus erlotinib versus placebo plus erlotinib in previously treated patients with locally advanced or metastatic, non-squamous, non-small-cell lung cancer. http://www.eccamsterdam2013.ecco-org.eu/Scientific-Programme/Abstract-search? abstractid=6904.
71. Schildhaus HU, Heukamp LC, Merkelbach-Bruse S, et al. Definition of a fluorescence in-situ hybridization score identifies high- and low-level FGFR1 amplification types in squamous cell lung cancer. Mod Pathol. 2012;25(11):1473-80.
72. Sequist LV, von Pawel J, Garmey EG, et al. Randomized phase II study of erlotinib plus tivantinib versus erlotinib plus placebo in previously treated non-small-cell lung cancer. J Clin Oncol. 2011;29(24):3307-15.
73. Sequist LV, Yang JC, Yamamoto N, et al. Phase III study of afatinib or cisplatin plus pemetrexed in patients with metastatic lung adenocarcinoma with EGFR mutations. J Clin Oncol. 2013;31(27):3327-34.
74. Shaw AT, Kim DW, Nakagawa K, et al. Crizotinib versus chemotherapy in advanced ALK positive lung cancer. N Engl J Med. 2013;368(25):2385-94.

75. Shinozaki M, Fujimoto A, Morton DL, et al. Incidence of BRAF oncogene mutation and clinical relevance for primary cutaneous melanomas. Clin Cancer Res. 2004;10(5):1753-7.
76. Smylie M, Blumenschein GR, Dowlati A, et al. A phase II multicenter trial comparing two schedules of lapatinib (LAP) as first or second line monotherapy in subjects with advanced or metastatic non-small cell lung cancer (NSCLC) with either bronchioloalveolar carcinoma (BAC) or no smoking history. J Clin Oncol. 2007;25(Suppl):7611.
77. Soda M, Choi YL, Enomoto M, et al. Identification of the transforming EML4-ALK fusion gene in non-small-cell lung cancer. Nature. 2007;448(7153):561-6.
78. Spigel DR, Ervin TJ, Ramlau R, et al. Final efficacy results from OAM4558g, a randomized phase II study evaluating MetMAb or placebo in combination qith erlotinib in advanced NSCLC. J Clin Oncol. 2011;29(Suppl):7505.
79. Spoerke JM, O'Brien C, Huw L, et al. Phosphoinositide 3-kinase (PI3K) pathway alterations are associated with histologic subtypes and are predictive of sensitivity to PI3K inhibitors in lung cancer preclinical models. Clin Cancer Res. 2012;18(24):6771-83.
80. Stephens P, Hunter C, Bignell G, et al. Lung cancer: intragenic ERBB2 kinase mutations in tumours. Nature. 2004;431(7008):525-6.
81. Takeuchi K, Soda M, Togashi Y, et al. RET, ROS1 and ALK fusions in lung cancer. Nat Med. 2012;18(3):378-81.
82. Tomizawa K, Suda K, Onozato R, et al. Prognostic and predictive implications of HER2/ERBB2/neu gene mutations in lung cancers. Lung Cancer. 2011;74(1):139-44.
83. Vaishnavi A, Capelletti M, Le AT, et al. Oncogenic and drug-sensitive NTRK1 rearrangements in lung cancer. Nat Med. 2013;19(11):1469-72.
84. Vivanco I, Sawyers CL. The phosphatidylinositol 3-Kinase AKT pathway in human cancer. Nat Rev Cancer. 2002;2(7):489-501.
85. Wang SE, Narasanna A, Perez-Torres M, et al. HER2 kinase domain mutation results in constitutive phosphorylation and activation of HER2 and EGFR and resistance to EGFR tyrosine kinase inhibitors. Cancer Cell. 2006;10(1):25-38.
86. Wang R, Hu H, Pan Y, et al. RET fusions define a unique molecular and clinicopathologic subtype of non-small-cell lung cancer. J Clin Oncol. 2012;30(35):4352-9.
87. Weiss J, Sos ML, Seidel D, et al. Frequent and focal FGFR1 amplification associates with therapeutically tractable FGFR1 dependency in squamous cell lung cancer. Sci Transl Med. 2010;2(62):62ra93.
88. Wells Jr SA, Santoro M. Targeting the RET pathway in thyroid cancer. Clin Cancer Res. 2009;15(23):7119-23.
89. Wynes MW, Hinz TK, Gao D, et al. FGFR1 mRNA and protein expression, not gene copy number, predict FGFR TKI sensitivity across all lung cancer histologies. Clin Cancer Res. 2014;20(12):3299-309. doi:10.1158/1078-0432.CCR-13-3060.
90. Yamamoto H, Shigematsu H, Nomura M, et al. PIK3CA mutations and copy number gains in human lung cancers. Cancer Res. 2008;68(17):6913-21.

91. Yang H, Higgins B, Kolinsky K, et al. Antitumor activity of BRAF inhibitor vemurafenib in preclinical models of BRAF-mutant colorectal cancer. Cancer Res. 2012;72:779-89.
92. Yasuda H, de Figueiredo-Pontes LL, Kobayashi S, Costa DB. Preclinical rationale for use of the clinically available multitargeted tyrosine kinase inhibitor crizotinib in ROS1-translocated lung cancer. J Thorac Oncol. 2012;7(7):1086-90.
93. Zinner RG, Glisson BS, Fossella FV, et al. Trastuzumab in combination with cisplatin and gemcitabine in patients with Her2-overexpressing, untreated, advanced non-small cell lung cancer: report of a phase II trial and findings regarding optimal identification of patients with Her2-overexpressing disease. Lung Cancer. 2004;44(1):99-110.

第 13 章
肺癌免疫治疗

作者：David F. Heigener，Martin Reck
译者：包飞潮

前言

非小细胞肺癌是死亡率最高的恶性肿瘤[1]，因为大部分患者在诊断时已进展到晚期[2]，无法行根治性治疗[3]，而晚期肺癌的生存率极差。

150 年前，德国病理学家 Rudolf Virchow 首次描述了炎症与肿瘤的关系，他认为恶性肿瘤是基于长期慢性炎症而发生的[4]。目前认为，其分子生物学机制如下，在炎症刺激作用下，Th1 细胞首先应答后形成抗血管生成和促凋亡环境，从而杀灭病原体。而后由 Th2 细胞通过发挥促血管生成和抗凋亡作用而介导组织修复和重建，但如果炎症刺激因子持续存在，该机制会失控，从而使细胞逃脱 T 细胞的监控，形成恶性细胞[5]。由于免疫系统的复杂性，通过改变免疫系统功能治疗肺癌以前一直认为是不可行的。同一种免疫细胞在不同部位可对肿瘤发挥不同的作用，如 CD68＋巨噬细胞被认为对Ⅳ期肺癌患者治疗有益，但部位不同效果明显不同，该细胞若存在于肿瘤基质细胞则不利于预后，而若存在于肿瘤癌巢中，则可提升肿瘤患者预后，CD8＋T 细胞在不同的部位，对肿瘤的作用也明显不一样。因此通过抑制或激活某种特定免疫细胞不适用于肿瘤治疗。另外，血细胞计数，或者免疫组化等仅仅检测的是某以特定时间的情况，并不能反映整个免疫系统的动态过程。

免疫逃避是肿瘤免疫治疗的一大障碍，也可能是打开新局面的钥匙。肿瘤通过产生 TGF-β 等免疫抑制因子，抑制局部微环境免疫系统作用。而在颈部肿瘤和黑色素瘤中，全身性的免疫抑制现象已被证实，在患者的外周血中，调节性 T 细胞明显升高，下调免疫应答[7]。

通过对上述机制的深入研究，目前已有多种方法用于克服免疫逃避，如疫苗或者通过细胞调控点抑制剂抑制免疫衰减等。

疫苗治疗

1000 年前，中国就开始将天花痘通过皮肤或鼻腔接种到正常健康人群，从而使健康人群获得免疫,该方法之后被命名为疫苗。1796年,英国医师Edward Jenner观察到挤奶工很少感染天花,但常感染牛痘,尽管并不是他首次使用牛痘来预防天花,但是他首次将牛痘接种到正常健康志愿者,他对一名8岁儿童接种由感染牛痘的奶农的脓汁,并证实该儿童对天花免疫,而后,他又对一名11个月婴儿接种疫苗成功,随后Edwad Jenner医生将该法传遍欧洲。因此疫苗(Vaccination)在使用拉丁字母的语言中,皆以拉丁文中,代表"牛"的"vacca"作为字源,纪念爱德华·金纳使用牛痘作为疫苗实验的里程碑。而目前疫苗被指使用一切免疫方法来使机体获得抵抗病原体或者肿瘤细胞的能力。而肿瘤疫苗不是指可以抵抗肿瘤发生的疫苗,该疫苗不作为预防性抗肿瘤使用,仅治疗肿瘤的方法使用。

肿瘤细胞有两类可使免疫系统识别应答的抗原,一类为肿瘤特异性抗原(仅表达于肿瘤细胞),另一类为肿瘤相关性抗原(肿瘤细胞与正常细胞差异性表达)。肿瘤特异性抗原最初在致病病原体明确的肿瘤中确定,如宫颈癌中的人类乳头瘤病毒抗原,但大部分的肿瘤细胞不存在明确的病原体。

通过增殖肿瘤特异性T细胞,发现了很多肿瘤抗原,但缺乏明确的已知的病原体,如第一个通过该方法确定的肿瘤特异性抗原,即黑色素瘤特异性抗原(MAGE)[7]。

MAGE A3

MAGE A3即黑色素瘤相关抗原3,存在于35%的手术切除的非小细胞肺癌标本中,除了胚胎细胞,该抗原在其他正常细胞中无明显表达,为肿瘤疫苗治疗提供了很好的靶点。

在一双盲安慰剂对照的Ⅱ期临床试验中,纳入手术切除后的ⅠB和Ⅱ期非小细胞肺癌患者,其中122例治疗组患者接受了重组MAGE-A3联合免疫增强剂的治疗,60例对照组患者接受了安慰剂治疗,结果发现,在术后44个月的随访期内,35%的治疗组患者复发,43%的对照组患者复发,无疾病生存区间(DFI;HR 0.75;95%CI,0.46~1.23;$P=0.254$)、无疾病生存率(DFS;HR 0.76;95%CI,0.48~1.21;$P=0.248$)、总体生存率(OS;HR 0.81;95%CI,0.47~1.40;$P=0.454$)均无明显差异。所有治疗组患者体液免疫均增强,没有发现严重的毒副反应[10]。

另一项研究则使用基因检测预测肿瘤疫苗治疗的可能受益人群,将前期两项分别关于可切除黑色素瘤和转移性黑色素瘤的Ⅱ期临床试验人群作为测试人群,MAGE-A3与两种免疫增强剂(AS15和AS02)联合治疗患者[11]。可切除患者使用MAGE联合AS02治疗,以安慰剂作为对照[10]。结果发现,84种基因的表达量与临床资料效果存在相关性,使用AS15作为免疫增强剂的治疗黑色素瘤似乎可以明显提升患者总体生存期(OS;HR,0.37;95%CI,0.13~1.05;$P=0.06$),而AS02作为免疫增强剂则无法提升总体生存期(OS;HR,0.84;95%CI,0.36~1.97;$P=0.70$)。而在肺癌中,对比MAGE A3联合AS15与安慰剂治疗可切除肺癌患者的治疗效果,显示免疫治疗对于基因测定阳性患者可以提升患者预后(OS; HR,0.42;95%CI,0.17~1.03;$P=0.06$),而基因测试阴性患者则与安慰剂对照组无明显差异(OS;HR,1.17;95%CI,0.59~2.31;$P=0.65$)[12]。

一项临床Ⅲ期研究(MAGTIT,NCT00480025)纳入2278例MAGE阳性的已切除的ⅠB~ⅢA期患者目前已招募完毕,该研究使用MAGE A3联合CpG7907作为治疗组,安慰剂作为对照,也对上述84个基因进行了检测,以确定该基因检测对于治疗的预测价值,但最近该研究申明由于研究设计存在缺陷可能导致中断,但尚待进一步公布。

PRAME

PRAME即黑色素瘤优先表达抗原,该抗原在急性白血病和部分实体肿瘤如黑色素瘤和非小细胞肺癌中表达,肺癌中PRAME的表达较MAGE更普遍。该抗原仅在睾丸中表达,其余正常细胞不表达。一项纳入14例患者的小样本研究显示PRAME可诱导8例患者中的细胞毒性T细胞应答。目前还有一项临床Ⅱ期随机对照试验(NCT01853878)正在进行中,该研究纳入已切除的Ⅰ~ⅢA期患者,分别用PRAME联合AS15或安慰剂治疗,其主要研究终点为无疾病生存率。

Mucin-1

Mucin-1广泛存在于人体各个组织,其生理作用为避免细胞黏附。在腺癌、淋巴瘤、骨髓瘤等多种恶心肿瘤中过表达,Mucin-1过表达可使细胞失去极性,由于Mucin-1也存在于细胞的基底外侧,因此过表达还可以使细胞间黏附力下降,使肿瘤易发生转移[14]。Mucin-1也被称作CA15-3,为乳腺癌预后的监测指标[15]。肿瘤细胞中的Mucin-1结构与正常细胞的存在一定区别[16]。Tecemotide(商品名Stimuvax)为针对Mucin-1的肿瘤疫苗药物,在一项纳入晚期肺癌(ⅢB期和Ⅳ期)患者的临床Ⅱ期试验,171例患者经一线化疗后无进展,随机区分到疫苗治疗或普通对照组治疗,疫苗治疗组患者在为期8周的每周1次环磷酰胺治疗后每6周1次Tecemotide治疗,主要终点为总体生存期,结果发现疫苗治疗组倾向于延长患者生存期4个月左右,但缺乏统计学意义(HR,0.739;95%CI,0.509~1.073;$P=0.112$),亚组分析显示,对于局部晚期患者,延长生存的效果比较明显(HR,0.524;95%CI,0.261~1.052;$P=0.069$)。随后的进一步的Ⅲ期临床试验(START)纳入1513例不可切除的Ⅲ期非小细胞肺癌患者,经放化疗后稳定,经2∶1随机化分组到疫苗治疗组或安慰剂治疗组,每6周给药1次,共8次给药。由于安全因素,该试验已中断。274例在中断试验之前6个月纳入的患者被排除出结果分析,该研究主要研究终点为总体生存期。该研究所纳入的患者中,65%经同步放化疗治疗,35%则经序贯放化疗治疗。Tecetomide治疗组患者的中体生存期为25.6个月,而安慰剂治疗组则为22.3个月,两者缺乏显著性差异(HR,0.88;95%CI,0.75~1.03;$P=0.123$),进一步的亚组分析显示,对于经同期放化疗的患者,Tecetomide

治疗患者的中位生存期为30.8个月，而安慰剂治疗组则为20.6个月，Tecetomide显著提高患者预后（HR，0.78；95%CI，0.64～0.95；$P=0.016$），也并未发现严重毒副作用。为何同步放化疗后的患者行疫苗治疗效果好，其原因尚不明确，主要原因可能是患者选择性偏倚，同步放化疗的患者经PET和纵隔镜等检查分期准确性高，治疗多为根治性治疗；其次可能是由于紫杉醇多用于同步放化疗而较少用于序贯放化疗，该药可能有免疫刺激作用[18]，仍需进一步的研究确定该现象的具体原因。

TG4010是一种能够编码Mucin-1和IL-2的重组牛痘病毒的悬浊液。IL-2可以促进T细胞免疫应答。一项Ⅱ期临床试验纳入经免疫组化确定Mucin-1表达的148例不可切除的ⅢB和Ⅳ期肿瘤患者，随机分组到化疗联合TG4010治疗组或单纯化疗对照组，主要研究终点为6个月的无进展生存率，结果发现，治疗组的6个月无进展生存率为43.2%（32/74；95%CI，33.4%～53.5%），而对照组则为35.1%（26/74；95%CI，25.9%～45.3%）。TG4010治疗组出现注射部位疼痛较多（5.5%），对照组则为0%，治疗组发热（23.3%）、腹痛（16.4%）也明显高于对照组，分别为8.3%，2.8%，但厌食、胸腔积液的发生率明显低于对照组[19]。

Belagenpumatucel

Belagenpumatucel（商品名Lucanix）是一种非常特殊的疫苗，由四个肺癌细胞株培育出来，由于其免疫原性较差，往往需要同时使用加入TGF-β反义转基因质粒。由于肺癌患者加强免疫抑制后TGF-β水平明显升高，TGF-β反义转基因质粒可以阻断TGF-β的免疫抑制作用，从而加强免疫原性。

一项Ⅱ期临床试验，纳入75例Ⅱ～Ⅳ期肺癌患者，61例为ⅢB期或Ⅳ期患者。每月1次或隔月1次使用三种不同剂量（1.25、2.5、$5.0×10^7$个细胞/次）的Belagenpumatucel的注射治疗，最多接受16次注射治疗。检测免疫功能，毒副反应及抗肿瘤作用。在61例为ⅢB期或Ⅳ期患者，缓解率为15%，缓解的患者其细胞因子水平明显高于出现进展的患者（IFN-γ，$P=0.006$；IL-6，$P=0.004$；IL-4，$P=0.007$）。注射剂量与生存存在显著的相关性，接受2.5或$5.0×10^7$个细胞/次注射剂量治疗的患者其1年生存率和2年生存率分别为68%、52%，而接受$1.25×10^7$个细胞/次注射剂量的患者其1年生存率和2年生存率分别为39%、20%[20]。

另一项Ⅱ期临床试验纳入21例晚期肺癌患者接受16个月的$2.5×10^7$个细胞/次注射剂量的治疗，并未发现明显的毒副反应，总体生存期为562天，该研究同时测定了循环肿瘤细胞水平，结果显示循环肿瘤细胞少于2个单位的患者中位生存期为660天，明显优于循环肿瘤细胞不少于2个单位的患者，其中位生存期仅为150天（$P=0.025$）[21]。

另有一项Ⅲ期临床试验（NCT00676507），纳入曾接受过联合或不联合放疗的以铂类药物为基础化疗的ⅢA期（T3N2）、ⅢB期和Ⅳ期患者，患者每4周接受1次Belagenpumatucel或安慰剂治疗，疗程18个月，如在第21个月，第24个月无明显毒副作用则再次接受药物注射治疗,其主要研究终点为总体生存期,目前患者招募已完成,结果尚待公布。

EGF 疫苗

EGF 即表皮生长因子在非小细胞肺癌中过表达,因此针对 EGF 的疫苗似乎是可行的[22]。CIMAvaxEGF 又名古巴肺癌疫苗,系由重组了人表皮生长因子受体(EGFR)与重组奈瑟氏流脑外膜 p64k 载体蛋白经化学交联而成的耦合物,在古巴已有 18 年的应用史,2011 年的一篇报道,分析汇总了一项包含 40 例患者的临床 Ⅱ 期试验结果,以及当时正在进行的临床 Ⅲ 期试验中的 40 例患者结果,临床 Ⅱ 期试验中的 40 例患者接受单部位的注射治疗,剂量为 0.6mg,而临床 Ⅲ 期试验中得患者则接受了 4 个不同部位的注射,注射剂量为 2.4mg,该报道作者将"抗体应答优秀者"定义为抗 EGF 滴度≥1∶4000,按此标准,52.8% 的临床 Ⅱ 期试验患者和 56.4% 的临床 Ⅲ 期试验患者均达到了此标准,而将"抗体应答非常优秀者"定义为抗体滴度≥1∶64 000,10.8% 的临床 Ⅱ 期试验患者和 30.8% 的临床 Ⅲ 期试验患者均达到了此标准[23]。临床 Ⅲ 期试验尚未报道各个分期及安慰剂治疗组的相关数据,目前仍需等待其进一步结果公布。另外仍有两项临床 Ⅲ 期试验分别在英国(NCT01444118)和马来西亚(NCT00516685)进行,均已顺利完成患者招募工作,等待结果公布。

免疫检查点抑制剂

T 细胞激活是免疫应答的关键节点,受到多种抑制和刺激因素的调节,免疫检查点是一主要抑制因素[24]。目前肿瘤免疫治疗主要集中于两个免疫检查点,第一种为细胞毒性 T 淋巴细胞抗原 4,即 CTLA4,因其第一个被单克隆抗体作为靶点,因此又被称为"检查点之父"[25],CTLA4 在 T 细胞激活初期可减弱免疫应答,抑制位于淋巴结中的 T 淋巴细胞激活,其生理学功能为维持机体对自身细胞的免疫耐受,但由于肿瘤细胞可表达相关配体从而激活 CTLA4,抑制肿瘤毒性免疫应答;第二种免疫检查点位程序化细胞死亡蛋白 1(PD-1),该控点位于免疫级联瀑布反应的下游,多位于外周组织的 T 淋巴细胞中,其配体 PD-L1 和 PD-L2 位于自然杀伤细胞,但也存在于肿瘤细胞。使用上述两种检查点的抗体治疗肺癌的临床有效性及毒副作用数据列如表 13.1。

表 13.1　正在研究中的调控点抑制剂

药物	靶点	公司	临床试验
Ipilimumab	CTLA-4	Bristol-Myers Squibb	Ⅲ期试验
Nivolumab	PD-1	Bristol-Myers Squibb	Ⅲ期试验
Pembrolizumab(MK-3475)	PD-1	Merck	Ⅱ/Ⅲ期试验
MPDL3280A(RG7446)	PD-L1	Genentech	Ⅲ期试验

CTLA4

CTLA4敲除小鼠会出现致命性的自身免疫性疾病或超敏综合征,因此以往认为CTLA4阻断可能毒副作用过大,后续的实验则表明通过单克隆抗体仅部分阻断CTLA4,并未完全阻断其效应,从而可以发挥一定的临床治疗效果[25]。Ipilimumab已被批准用于治疗晚期黑色素瘤,在肺癌中目前前景也较好。在一项三臂临床Ⅱ期试验中,其中两臂为同期或分期使用该药合并卡铂和紫杉醇治疗,另一臂为卡铂和紫杉醇化疗组,主要研究终点为免疫相关性无进展生存期(ir-PFS)。该研究共纳入204例未经化疗的患者,在同期治疗组中,注射6次ipilimumab(10mg/kg),同期进行卡铂和紫杉醇联合化疗,分期治疗组化疗初期前两次则为安慰剂治疗,后续4次注射ipilimumab。6个周期之后,则同期治疗和分期治疗组均每12周给予1次ipilimumab注射治疗,而单纯化疗组则每12周给予1次安慰剂注射治疗。该研究结果显示ipilimumab治疗组患者ir-PFS优于安慰剂对照组,但统计学差异仅存在于分期治疗组与安慰剂治疗组对比中,ir-PFS分别为5.68个月,4.63个月($P=0.05$),同期治疗组与安慰剂治疗组对比则缺乏显著性差异,生存期分别为5.52个月,4.63个月($P=0.13$)。ipilimumab有趋势可以提高患者生存,分期治疗组为12.2个月,同期治疗组为9.69个月,安慰剂治疗则为6.8个月,但差异均缺乏统计学意义,目前尚不明确同期治疗与分期治疗效果存在差异的原因。亚组分析显示鳞癌患者倾向于受益,而非鳞癌患者则无明显受益,因此研究者推测可能是因为炎症细胞在鳞癌中较多[26]。

通过已发表的ipilimumab治疗黑色素瘤的研究结果来看,该药的不良反应主要是皮疹(47%～68%),往往持续3～4周,腹泻和肠炎(44%),肝炎(3%～9%),下垂体炎91%～6%)。可通过局部使用激素,必要时全身性激素治疗,对于难治性患者可以使用英夫利昔、麦考酚酯等药物治疗[27]。

PD-1/PD-L1

2011年,新英格兰医学杂志接连发表两篇文章,分别为PD-1抗体(nivolumab)和PD-L1抗体治疗肿瘤的临床疗效。两种药物均为Bristol-Myers Squibb公司研制,在多种实体肿瘤中进行验证,其中一项研究共纳入207例患者接受PD-L1抗体治疗,其中75例为肺癌患者,结果发现5例患者出现客观缓解,3例患者客观缓解时间达24周以上。不良反应主要为乏力、输液反应、腹泻、关节痛、皮疹、恶心、瘙痒、头痛等不适。39%的患者出现免疫相关并发症,多为轻到中度[28],该药的初步临床疗效尚不能使其进行商业推广。另一篇文献纳入296例患者接受PD-1抗体Nivolumab治疗,其中76例为非小细胞肺癌患者,缓解率为18%,所有296例患者中31例出现肿瘤缓解,其中20例维持到1年以上。在治疗前,对42例患者肿瘤标本进行了PD-L1表达的测定,结果发现17例患者无PD-L1表达,而这些患者没有1例出现肿瘤缓解,25例患者有PD-L1表达,其中9例患者对治疗有应答[29],因此可认为PD-L1表达可预测PD-1抗体治疗效果,但在另一项研究中则并不能重复该结果,PD-L1的表达与PD-1抗体治疗效果无相关性[30],因此目前尚不能确定免疫组化测定PD-L1表达对于PD-1抗体治疗的预测价值。Nivolumab的主要副反应为肺炎,上述研究中的3例患者出现肺炎,其他副反应包括乏力、皮疹、腹泻、瘙痒、纳差、恶心等。

正在开展多项关于Nivolumab治疗肺癌的临床试验,包括联合多种一线化疗方案的临床Ⅰ期试验(NCT01454102),以及两项以多西他赛为参照的临床Ⅲ期试验,一项针对鳞癌患者(NCT01642004),另一项针对非鳞癌患者(NCT01673867)。

MPDL3280为PD-L1抗体,一项临床Ⅰ期试验纳入85例既往接受过治疗的非小细胞肺癌患者,予以每3周注射1次MPDL3280,治疗时间为1年以上,76%的患者为非鳞癌,缓解率与肿瘤基质中PD-L1存在相关性,53例接受治疗的患者可进行缓解率评估,客观缓解率为23%,而PD-L1表达强阳性的患者,其客观缓解率为83%(5/6),在结果发表之时,所有患者均已停药,仅1例患者仍在给药。

Pembrolizumab为PD-L1的另一种抗体,38例肺癌患者接受每3周1次的抗体治疗,客观缓解率为24%,中位总生存期为51周[32]。目前正在进行一项临床Ⅱ/Ⅲ期试验,比较两种不同浓度的Pembrolizumab与多西他赛治疗既往接受过治疗的晚期肺癌的临床效果(NCT01905657)。

检查点抑制剂效果

如何评价检查点抑制剂治疗肿瘤的临床疗效目前比较困难,因为肿瘤病灶并不能在治疗之后立即缩小,甚至可以在治疗初期由于淋巴细胞涌入肿瘤病灶而出现肿瘤病灶增大,如ipilimumab治疗后可以出现T细胞浸润到肺组织中,因此,目前已开始使用免疫相关缓解标准来评价检查点抑制剂的治疗效果,该指标不同于普通的肿瘤缓解标准的主要特点是如何确定4周后肿瘤出现进展,新发病灶在接受免疫治疗的患者中并不能认为是出现进展[33],既往曾有过患者可出现治疗后期缓解(图13.1)。

抗血管生成药物的作用

抗血管生成是治疗肺癌的一种方法,贝伐单抗是针对血管内皮生长因子(VEGF)的抗体,已被批准作为与铂类基础化疗方案合用于肺癌的一线治疗。血管生成是一复杂的过程,与免疫系统存在相互作用,如VEGF可抑制免疫应答的主要细胞,树突状细胞的成熟,抗VEGF的治疗可明显增加脾脏和淋巴结肿的树突状细胞数量[36],从而诱导免疫系统杀伤肿瘤细胞,该机制也部分解释了为何抗血管生成可以用于抗肿瘤治疗。

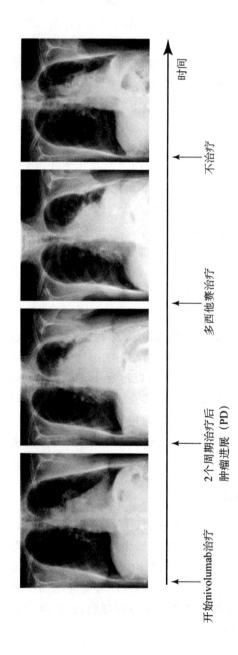

图13.1 复发肺鳞癌患者胸片,该患者接受nivolumab二线治疗,在第一次进展后给予多西他赛治疗,出现微小缓解,但因不良反应而终止化疗。但停药后可能由于延迟免疫应答而出现自发性的肿瘤缓解

VEGF抗体治疗肿瘤耐药机制在临床初期研究已得到部分证实,如髓系抑制细胞(MDSC)可促进血管生成从而致使肿瘤细胞耐受抗血管生成药物治疗[37],而非小细胞肺癌基质中髓系抑制细胞的存在也被认为是肿瘤预后差的一个因素,但由于髓系抑制细胞的功能存在异质性,因此上述理论尚不能确定其准确性。

观点

即使是Ⅰ期肺癌,也有很高的复发率,因此目前的理论认为肺癌在极早期就从局部病变进展为全身性疾病[38]。通过重建免疫监视功能,利用细胞毒性T细胞和自然杀伤细胞杀灭残存肿瘤细胞可能使肿瘤达到根治,检查点抑制剂的作用不可忽视,但仍需随机临床试验炎症其效果。

联合免疫治疗可以加强治疗的临床效果,有临床试验纳入86例转移性黑色素瘤患者使用iplimumab和nivolumab双重抑制免疫检查点,其中53例为同期用药,33例分期用药,ipilimumab后再使用nivolumab,结果显示缓解率为53%,而不良反应与ipilimumab单药治疗组相当[39],该方法是否也适用于肺癌的治疗目前尚缺乏研究结果。

免疫治疗联合化疗应用于晚期肺癌治疗,特别是维持治疗,是否可以延长患者的缓解时间仍需要研究明确。关于使用免疫抑制性化疗药物是否会减弱检查点抑制剂的效果也尚不明确,既往有研究显示化疗并不能削减ipilimumab诱导激活T细胞的作用。

综上所述,免疫治疗在肺癌中有着一定的应用前景,特别是对于晚期肺癌,可以使更多的患者获得长期的缓解。

参考文献

1. Jemal A, Bray F, Center MM, et al. Global cancer statistics. CA Cancer J Clin. 2011;61:69-90.
2. Morgensztern D, Ng SH, Gao F, et al. Trends in stage distribution for patients with non-small cell lung cancer:a National Cancer Database survey. J Thorac Oncol. 2010;5:29-33.
3. Reck M, Heigener DF, Mok T, et al. Management of non-small-cell lung cancer:recent developments. Lancet. 2013;382:709-19.
4. Virchow R. Aetiologie der neoplastischen Geschwulste. In:Die krankhaften Geschwulste. Berlin:Verlag von August Hirschwald; 1863. p. 57-101.
5. O'Callaghan DS, O'Donnell D, O'Connell F, et al. The role of inflammation in the pathogenesis of non-small cell lung cancer. J Thorac Oncol. 2010;5:2024-36.
6. Kawai O, Ishii G, Kubota K, et al. Predominant infiltration of macrophages and CD8(+) T Cells in cancer nests is a significant predictor of survival in stage IV nonsmall cell lung cancer. Cancer. 2008;113:1387-95.
7. Finn OJ. Cancer immunology. N Engl J Med. 2008;358:2704-15.
8. Riedel S. Edward Jenner and the history of smallpox and vaccination. Proc (Bayl Univ Med

Cent). 2005;18:21-5.
9. Van denEynde BJ, van der Bruggen P. T cell defined tumor antigens. Curr Opin Immunol. 1997;9:684-93.
10. Vansteenkiste J, Zielinski M, Linder A, et al. Adjuvant MAGE-A3 immunotherapy in resected non-small-cell lung cancer: phase II randomized study results. J Clin Oncol. 2013;31:2396-403.
11. Kruit WH, Suciu S, Dreno B, et al. Selection of immunostimulant AS15 for active immunization with MAGE-A3 protein: results of a randomized phase II study of the European Organisation for Research and Treatment of Cancer Melanoma Group in Metastatic Melanoma. J Clin Oncol. 2013;31:2413-20.
12. Ulloa-Montoya F, Louahed J, Dizier B, et al. Predictive gene signature in MAGE-A3 antigenspecific cancer immunotherapy. J Clin Oncol. 2013;31:2388-95.
13. Babiak A, Steinhauser M, Gotz M, et al. Frequent T cell responses against immunogenic targets in lung cancer patients for targeted immunotherapy. Oncol Rep. 2014;31:384-90.
14. Hanisch FG, Muller S. MUC1: the polymorphic appearance of a human mucin. Glycobiology. 2000;10:439-49.
15. Duffy MJ, Shering S, Sherry F, et al. CA 15-3: a prognostic marker in breast cancer. Int J Biol Markers. 2000;15:330-3.
16. Park JH, Nishidate T, Kijima K, et al. Critical roles of mucin 1 glycosylation by transactivated polypeptide N-acetylgalactosaminyltransferase 6 in mammary carcinogenesis. Cancer Res. 2010;70:2759-69.
17. Butts C, Murray N, Maksymiuk A, et al. Randomized phase IIB trial of BLP25 liposome vaccine in stage ⅢB and IV non-small-cell lung cancer. J Clin Oncol. 2005;23:6674-81.
18. Butts C, Socinski M, Mitchell P, Thatcher N. START: a phase Ⅲ study of L-BLP25 cancer immunotherapy for unresectable stage Ⅲ non-small cell lung cancer. In: ASCO annual meeting, Chicago. J Clin Oncol. 2013;31(suppl):abstr 7500.
19. Quoix E, Ramlau R, Westeel V, et al. Therapeutic vaccination with TG4010 and first-line chemotherapy in advanced non-small-cell lung cancer: a controlled phase 2B trial. Lancet Oncol. 2011;12:1125-33.
20. Nemunaitis J, Dillman RO, Schwarzenberger PO, et al. Phase II study of belagenpumatucel-L, a transforming growth factor beta-2 antisense gene-modified allogeneic tumor cell vaccine in non-small-cell lung cancer. J Clin Oncol. 2006;24:4721-30.
21. Nemunaitis J, Nemunaitis M, Senzer N, et al. Phase II trial of Belagenpumatucel-L, a TGF-beta2 antisense gene modified allogeneic tumor vaccine in advanced non small cell lung cancer (NSCLC) patients. Cancer Gene Ther. 2009;16:620-4.
22. Merlo V, Longo M, Novello S, et al. EGFR pathway in advanced non-small cell lung cancer. Front Biosci (Schol Ed). 2011;3:501-17.
23. Rodriguez PC, Neninger E, Garcia B, et al. Safety, immunogenicity and preliminary efficacy of multiple-site vaccination with an Epidermal Growth Factor (EGF) based cancer vaccine in

advanced non small cell lung cancer (NSCLC) patients. J Immune Based Ther Vaccines. 2011;9:7.

24. Champiat S, Ileana E, Giaccone G, et al. Incorporating immune-checkpoint inhibitors into systemic therapy of NSCLC. JThorac Oncol. 2014;9:144-53.

25. Pardoll DM. The blockade of immune checkpoints in cancer immunotherapy. Nat Rev Cancer. 2012;12:252-64.

26. Lynch TJ, Bondarenko I, Luft A, et al. Ipilimumab in combination with paclitaxel and carboplatin as first-line treatment in stage ⅢB/Ⅳ non-small-cell lung cancer: results from a randomized, double-blind, multicenter phase II study. J Clin Oncol. 2012;30:2046-54.

27. Weber JS, Kahler KC, Hauschild A. Management of immune-related adverse events and kinetics of response with ipilimumab. J Clin Oncol. 2012;30:2691-7.

28. Brahmer JR, Tykodi SS, Chow LQ, et al. Safety and activity of anti-PD-L1 antibody in patients with advanced cancer. N Engl J Med. 2012;366:2455-65.

29. Topalian SL, Hodi FS, Brahmer JR, et al. Safety, activity, and immune correlates of anti-PD-1 antibody in cancer. N Engl J Med. 2012;366:2443-54.

30. Antonia S, Grosso JF, Horak CE, Harbison CT, Kurland JF, Inzunza HD, Gupta A, Sankar V, Park J-S, Jure-Kunkel M, Novotny J, Cogswell J, Zhang X, Phillips T, Simmons P, Simon J. Association of tumor PD-L1 expression and immune biomarkers with clinical activity in patients with non-small cell lung cancer (NSCLC) treated with nivolumab (Anti-PD-1; BMS- 936558; ONO-4538). Presented at the world conference on Lung Cancer (abstract P2. 11-035); 2013.

31. Gettinger S, Cruz M, Gordon M, Conkling P, Fine G, Antonia S, Mokatrin A, Shen X. Molecular correlates of PD-L1 status and predictive biomarkers in patients with non-small cell lung cancer (NSCLC) treated with the anti-PD-L1 antibody MPDL3280A. In:15th world conference on Lung Cancer. Sydney; 2013.

32. Garon E, Balmanoukian A, Hamid O, Hui R, Gandhi L, Leighl N, Gubens MA, Goldman J, Lubiniecki GM, Lunceford J, Gergich K, Rizvi N. Preliminary clinical safety and activity of MK-3475 monotherapy for the treatment of previously treated patients with non-small cell lung cancer (NSCLC). Presented at the world conference on Lung Cancer (Abstract MO18. 02); 2013.

33. Wolchok JD, Hoos A, O'Day S, et al. Guidelines for the evaluation of immune therapy activity in solid tumors: immune-related response criteria. Clin Cancer Res. 2009;15:7412-20.

34. Sandler A, Gray R, Perry MC, et al. Paclitaxel-carboplatin alone or with bevacizumab for non-small- cell lung cancer. N Engl J Med. 2006;355:2542-50.

35. Reck M, von Pawel J, Zatloukal P, et al. Phase Ⅲ trial of cisplatin plus gemcitabine with either placebo or bevacizumab as first-line therapy for nonsquamous non-small-cell lung cancer: AVAil. J Clin Oncol. 2009;27:1227-34.

36. Gabrilovich DI, Ishida T, Nadaf S, et al. Antibodies to vascular endothelial growth factor enhance the efficacy of cancer immunotherapy by improving endogenous dendritic cell function.

Clin Cancer Res. 1999;5;2963-70.
37. Shojaei F, Ferrara N. Refractoriness to antivascular endothelial growth factor treatment;role of myeloid cells. Cancer Res. 2008;68;5501-4.
38. Martini N, Bains MS, Burt ME, et al. Incidence of local recurrence and second primary tumors in resected stage I lung cancer. J Thorac Cardiovasc Surg. 1995;109;120-9.
39. Wolchok JD, Kluger H, Callahan MK, et al. Nivolumab plus ipilimumab in advanced melanoma. N Engl J Med. 2013;369;122-33.
40. Chasalow SD, Wolchok, SD, Reck M, Maier S, Shahabi V. Effects of chemotherapy on ipilimumab- mediated increases in absolute lymphocyte count and activation of T-cells. ESMO congress, Vienna. Poster No. 175; 2012.

第五部分
特定类型转移性非小细胞肺癌诊治进展

第14章

肺癌寡转移

作者：Dirk De Ruysscher, Stéphanie Peeters, Christophe Dooms
译者：包飞潮

背景

目前肺癌的临床分期主要根据有无远处转移进行二分类[1]，无远处转移的肺癌患者行根治性的治疗，而合并远处转移的患者往往认为不可治愈，行全身性化疗等较姑息的治疗方式，其中位生存时间约1年。

近年来，由于PET-CT和头颅MRI广泛应用于肺癌的诊断分期，有一类肺癌合并转移患者被引起重视，该类型患者转移瘤数目有限，可以通过手术或放疗等方式行根治性治疗，获得较好的无疾病远期生存[2-15]。该肿瘤为局限性原发肿瘤与广泛性转移肿瘤之间的过渡阶段，由于转移瘤数目有限，因此被称为肺癌寡转移[16-18]。转移瘤起源于原发灶的肿瘤干细胞，通过肿瘤发生部位与微环境的相互影响而逐渐生成[16-18]。目前认为，肺癌寡转移与多发转移的分界点一般为5个远处转移灶[2]。大部分的肺癌寡转移的病例报道仅纳入1~3个远处转移灶的病例，目前尚无法确定转移受累器官数目是否影响患者预后。1~5个肺癌寡转移灶可通过VATS、SABR，调强放疗或低分割放疗等进行根治性的治疗获得较好的长期生存[2]。另外，个体化的化疗也可用于该肿瘤的治疗，提高肿瘤的控制率。多项研究显示采用化疗联合局部根治性治疗方式治疗多发性寡转移肺癌患者的中位生存期约2年，5年总体生存率为15%[2-15]。但仅1项为前瞻性单臂研究，另有1项临床Ⅰ期试验，其余13项均为回顾性研究。

本章将基于现有文献报道的基础上，介绍寡转移肺癌患者行根治性治疗的适应证，治疗方法，生存状况，毒副作用和预后相关因素。

患者选择和治疗方法

由于大多数关于寡转移肺癌的临床报道均为回顾性研究，因此如何选择行根治性局部治疗的合适适应证患者尚有困难[19]。根据报道，85%的病例仅1~3个转移灶，同时多发和异时多发的患者都被纳入，而纵隔淋巴结转移的患者则未被纳入。半数远处转移瘤行手术根治性切除，其余则行高剂量立体定向放疗，或高剂量传统分割放疗。多数同时多发肿瘤在根治性局部治疗前行化疗。同期放化疗则可用于Ⅲ期肿瘤。

生存状况

回顾性病例报道中的寡转移肺癌患者的肿瘤生物学行为存在较大的异质性，目前报道其中位生存期15个月，(6~52个月)[19]。5年中位总体生存率为23%(8%~86%)，中位数为23%。唯一的1项前瞻性Ⅱ期临床试验提示2年总体生存率仅13%，所有患者均无长期生存，中位无进展生存期则为12个月(4~24个月)。

肿瘤局部控制

系统评价报道放疗区域或手术切除区域的局部复发率为20%[19]。

毒副作用和生活质量

一项包含39例寡转移肺癌患者的Ⅱ期临床试验结果显示，仅有少部分患者出现轻微的急性或迟发性毒副作用，患者生活质量无明显下降。

预后因素

由于报道较少，目前尚不能确定根治性局部治疗的预后相关因素，从而帮助选择合适患者。相关研究纳入的患者均为全身情况较好，局部治疗的器官功能良好，可代偿切除功能的患者。最大远处转移瘤的大小与患者总体生存相关[15]。肿瘤的病理学类型与预后无明显相关性。转移部位与预后的相关性也尚未明确，有研究认为肺癌合并脑寡转移瘤预后较好，而合并肾上腺寡转移瘤则预后相对较差[15]。

讨论

以往认为非小细胞肺癌合并远处转移无法行根治性治疗，但目前认为部分寡转移肿瘤可通过手术或高剂量放疗获得较好的远期生存和生活质量。1~5个转移灶的肿瘤为局限性原发肿瘤与广泛性转移肿瘤之间的过渡阶段，根治性局部治疗可用于该类肿瘤治疗。1~3个寡转移灶的合适患者中，无进展生存期为12月，10%~15%的患者可获得3~5年的长期生存。但目前前瞻性报道较少，缺乏随机对照试验，因此对于寡转移肺癌患者的诊治仍有很多亟待解决的问题，如行根治性局部切除的合适适应证，根治性局部治疗联合全身治疗是否可提高患者生存。EGFR突变型肺癌有一较长的自然病程，提示其肿瘤惰性[20]，鉴于此，寡转移肺癌获得远期生存的原因可能也为其肿瘤本身偏惰性，而并非局部根治性治疗。MiR-NA200c参与了肿瘤寡转移生物学行为，这也说明肿瘤本身的惰性可能。全身性治疗的合适适应证也亟需研究确定，EGFR突变或ALK基因融合重排患者也需纳入这类研究，因为此类肿瘤往往为生长惰性，放疗敏感性肿瘤。

两项寡转移肺癌的临床Ⅱ期随机对照试验，NCT00887315，NCT00776100由于招募患者困难，已于近期关闭，另一项临床Ⅱ期随机对照试验SABR-COMET（NCT01446744）正在加拿大和荷兰进行中，将5个以下寡转移灶的肺癌患者随机分组到根治性立体定向射频消融治疗和姑息性化疗组中。相关随机对照试验招募患者困难，而回顾性报道较多，从侧面说明根治性局部治疗在缺乏明确证据支持的情况下正在成为寡转移肺癌患者的标准治疗方式，但无论如何，其价值仍需前瞻性的随机对照试验证明。

参考文献

1. Vansteenkiste J, De Ruysscher D, Eberhardt WE, ESMO Guidelines Working Group, et al. Early and locally advanced non-small-cell lung cancer (NSCLC): ESMO Clinical Practice Guidelines for diagnosis, treatment and follow-up. Ann Oncol. 2013;24 Suppl 6:vi89-98.
2. Oh Y, Taylor S, Bekele BN, et al. Number of metastatic sites is a strong predictor of survival in patients with non-small cell lung cancer with or without brain metastases. Cancer. 2009; 115:2930-8.
3. Khan AJ, Mehta PS, Zusag TW, et al. Long term disease-free survival resulting from combined modality management of patients presenting with oligometastatic, non-small cell lung carcinoma (NSCLC). Radiother Oncol. 2006;81:163-7.
4. Lo SS, Fakiris AJ, Chang EL, et al. Stereotactic body radiation therapy: a novel treatment modality. Nat Rev Clin Oncol. 2010;7:44-54.
5. Timmerman RD, Bizekis CS, Pass HI, et al. Local surgical, ablative, and radiation treatment of metastases. CA Cancer J Clin. 2009;59:145-70.
6. Siva S, MacManus M, Ball D. Stereotactic radiotherapy for pulmonary oligometastases: a systematic review. J Thorac Oncol. 2010;5:1091-9.
7. Rusthoven KE, Kavanagh BD, Burri SH, et al. Multi-institutional phase I/II trial of stereotactic body radiation therapy for lung metastases. J Clin Oncol. 2009;27:1579-84.
8. Rusthoven KE, Kavanagh BD, Cardenes H, et al. Multi-institutional phase I/II trial of ster-

eotactic body radiation therapy for liver metastases. J Clin Oncol. 2009;27:1572-8.
9. Lee MT, Kim JJ, Dinniwell R, et al. Phase I study of individualized stereotactic body radiotherapy of liver metastases. J Clin Oncol. 2009;27:1585-91.
10. Milano MT, Katz AW, Schell MC, et al. Descriptive analysis of oligometastatic lesions treated with curative-intent stereotactic body radiotherapy. Int J Radiat Oncol Biol Phys. 2008;72:1516-22.
11. Milano MT, Katz AW, Zhang H, et al. Oligometastases treated with stereotactic body radiotherapy: long-term follow-up of prospective study. Int J Radiat Oncol Biol Phys. 2012;83:878-86.
12. Cheruvu P, Metcalfe SK, Metcalfe J, et al. Comparison of outcomes in patients with stage III versus limited stage IV non-small cell lung cancer. Radiat Oncol. 2011;6:80.
13. Griffioen GH, Toguri D, Dahele M, et al. Radical treatment of synchronous oligometastatic non-small cell lung carcinoma (NSCLC): patient outcomes and prognostic factors. Lung Cancer. 2013;82:95-102.
14. Salama JK, Hasselle MD, Chmura SJ, et al. Stereotactic body radiotherapy for multisite extracranial oligometastases: final report of a dose escalation trial in patients with 1 to 5 sites of metastatic disease. Cancer. 2012;118:2962-70.
15. De Ruysscher D, Wanders R, van Baardwijk A, et al. Radical treatment of non-small-cell lung cancer patients with synchronous oligometastases: long-term results of a prospective phase II trial (NCT 01282450). J Thorac Oncol. 2012;7:1547-55.
16. Hellman S, Weichselbaum RR. Oligometastases. J Clin Oncol. 1995;13:8-10.
17. Weichselbaum RR, Hellman S. Oligometastases revisited. Nat Rev Clin Oncol. 2011;8:378-82.
18. Corbin KS, Hellman S, Weichselbaum RR. Extracranial oligometastases: a subset of metastases curable with stereotactic radiotherapy. J Clin Oncol. 2013;31:1384-90.
19. Ashworth A, Rodrigues G, Boldt G, Palma D. Is there an oligometastatic state in non-small cell lung cancer? A systematic review of the literature. Lung Cancer. 2013;82:197-203.
20. Mok TS, Wu YL, Thongprasert S, et al. Gefitinib or carboplatin-paclitaxel in pulmonary adenocarcinoma. N Engl J Med. 2009;361:947-57.
21. Lussier YA, Xing HR, Salama JK, et al. MicroRNA expression characterizes oligometastasis(es). PLoS One. 2011;6(12):e28650.
22. Johung KL, Yao X, Li F, et al. A clinical model for identifying radiosensitive tumor genotypes in non-small cell lung cancer. Clin Cancer Res. 2013;19:5523-32.

第 15 章
骨 转 移

作者:Vera Hirsh
译者:曾理平

介绍

骨骼是肺癌转移的好发部位,30%～40%的晚期肺癌患者出现骨转移[1]。骨转移可导致骨骼相关事件(SREs),如病理性骨折,脊髓压迫,往往需行放疗或手术治疗,以及高钙血症等。SREs是造成一系列人体衰弱的重要原因,显著降低患者生活质量(QOL)。骨转移是导致晚期恶心肿瘤患者癌性疼痛的最常见原因[2]。严重骨转移相关骨痛不仅需要强效麻醉药,还需要姑息放疗来控制疼痛。部分病理性骨折需要行手术治疗,而严重脊髓压迫和恶性高钙血症可危及生命。一项大样本前瞻性临床试验纳入460例原发实体肿瘤未乳腺癌,前列腺癌,肾癌和肺癌等骨转移患者,病理性骨折与患者的生存负相关[3]。骨骼系统并发症不仅会导致患者致残率增加和一般状况恶化,也会明显增加患者经济负担。数据表明,合并SRE患者的总医疗费用增加28 223美元(从1994年7月至2002年6月的评估)[4],与不合并SRE的患者相比,总医疗费用增加89%。直接归因于SRE医疗费用增加为9494美元/人(95%CI,7611～11 475美元)。相关的预防措施可降低患者SRE发病率,提高生活质量,减少医疗资源消耗。

随着各种新型疗法的出现,虽仍无法治愈转移性肺癌患者,但由于肺癌生存期的延长,需要对骨转移及后遗症提高关注。临床研究表明,大多数非小细胞肺癌(NSCLC)骨转移的患者在研究初期5个月内经历一次SRE[5]。

为防止SRE发生并提高患者的生活质量,良好的PS评分和生活独立能力,可提高患者接受进一步治疗的耐受性。

骨转移致残

骨转移的病理生理学

骨骼微环境特别有利于转移性病变发生发展,破骨细胞介导骨质溶解时可诱导骨基质中生长因子的释放[6]。肿瘤和骨骼之间相互作用可促进肿瘤生长,破坏骨骼完整性,导致骨骼疼痛和结构破坏。在溶骨性病变中,肿瘤细胞分泌的细胞因子可募集和激活破骨细胞,增加骨质溶解[7]。骨质溶解水平升高破坏骨骼的完整性,引起骨痛,并且可以通过骨基质释放矿物质破坏血清平衡,导致恶性高钙血症(HCM)[8]。骨再吸收也可释放出刺激肿瘤生长的生长因子并增加破骨细胞刺激因子的分泌[9]。相反,肿瘤细胞在成骨病变中分泌刺激负责形成新的骨组织(成骨)的成骨细胞的因子。成骨作用增加以及其他刺激,导致溶骨的水平提高,使骨基质中释放生长因子[7]。

尽管溶骨性病变中骨质破坏更加明显,但成骨性病变也含有很强的可以减少骨完整性的溶骨性成分[9,10]。此外,成骨性病变中异常新骨形成产生的新骨组织呈异常畸形,并不增加整体骨强度[9,11]。

骨转移的早期发现

非小细胞肺癌骨转移很容易被忽视。骨扫描可检测骨转移,但常在患者出现骨痛及骨转移相关症状及体征时,如骨特异性碱性磷酸酶(ALP)水平的升高时[10,12],才会行骨扫描等检查。有研究纳入 60 例初始评估可手术的非转移 NSCLC 患者进行了全身骨扫描[13]。11 例存在骨骼症状或检验提示骨骼病变可能的患者,3 例患者证实存在骨转移(27.3%)。而另 49 例患者虽没有骨转移相关临床症状,但 8 例(16.3%)患者证实存在骨转移,分期不准确导致治疗决策选择恰当,如对无根治性可能的患者行大手术或根治性放化疗。

美国临床肿瘤学会(ASCO)指南建议,对合并异常骨骼相关临床症状的 NSCLC 患者行骨扫描[14]。骨扫描识别的可疑病变需要 X 射线,计算机断层扫描(CT),磁共振成像(MRI),正电子发射断层扫描(PET)或活检等进一步检查明确[13-16]。最近,PET 扫描用于非小细胞肺癌的准确分期,包括Ⅳ期疾病,已被美国综合癌症网络(NCCN)认可[17]。与骨扫描相比,18-氟脱氧葡萄糖(FDG)-PET 检查对于检测 NSCLC 骨转移特异性更高(大约 90% vs 约 70%)[18,19],假阴性率更低(6% vs 39%)[20],而 FDG-PET 和骨扫描对于随访检测非小细胞肺癌骨转移的敏感性是相当的[18,19]。

骨转移的临床影响

大样本安慰剂对照双膦酸盐临床试验结果表明,经过 2 年时间,纳入骨转移患者,大部分患者均发生 SREs,多数患者每年发生多次 SREs[5,21-24],安慰剂组的 NSCLC 骨转移患者在研究初期 5 个月内经历了一次 SRE[25],生存期明显更短,结果与 Delea 等[26,27]的研究一致,即 NSCLC 患者在第一次 SRE 之后的中位生存期约为 4 个月。

除了频繁剧烈疼痛之外,SREs 可引起病理性骨折和脊髓压迫,导致患者的活动和功能自主性永久损害。已经发现,病理性骨折在多种肿瘤中与存活期缩短相关[28]。

一项大样本的回顾性研究纳入经历过 1 次 SREs 的前列腺癌患者 248 例,每种类型的 SRE 都和生活质量降低有关,导致患者生理、功能和情绪等显著受损[29]。因此延迟 SREs 的发作和减少 SREs 持续存在的风险,可使 NSCLC 骨转移患者获益。

SREs 与医疗费用的增加有关,这是因为发生骨骼损伤之后,额外支持治疗或者后续干预增加。因此 NSCLC 患者 SREs 的预防可以减少患者极大的经济负担[30]。

双膦酸盐

作用机制

双膦酸盐是沉积在骨重塑部位的焦磷酸盐类似物,可结合到骨矿物质表面,被破骨细胞摄入,抑制骨质溶解[31]。早期的双膦酸盐,即依替膦酸盐,氯膦酸盐,显示出治疗恶性高钙血症的疗效,为使用双膦酸盐减少骨转移导致的骨骼损伤提供了依据。但这些药物相对较弱对肿瘤的治疗效果有限[31]。目前,已开发出多种双膦酸盐[32]。双膦酸盐结构上一个氮基的引入导致药效提高,和早期一代双膦酸盐相比具有不同的细胞靶点,即法尼基焦磷酸合酶,甲羟戊酸途径中的关键酶。这些含氮双膦酸盐抑制蛋白质异戊二烯化和破骨细胞中的 RAS 信号发送,从而诱导细胞凋亡[33]。

在人类癌细胞系临床初期试验和肿瘤相关骨溶解动物模型中,证明新一代双膦酸盐唑来膦酸的活性在这些双膦酸盐中药效最强。在两种破骨细胞介导的骨再吸收模型中,唑来膦酸可始终维持最大的抗骨再吸收的效果[34,35]。在一个评估法尼基焦磷酸合酶活性的临床模型中,唑来膦酸在 $0.1\mu M$ 浓度就产生了对法尼基焦磷酸合酶活性接近完全的抑制作用,这个浓度 5~40 倍的低于其他双膦酸盐(例如,利塞膦酸盐,伊班膦酸钠,阿仑膦酸钠,帕米膦酸盐)需要的浓度[31]。

唑来膦酸:临床疗效

2002 年,唑来膦酸逐渐从多发性骨髓瘤或乳腺癌推广到其他实体肿瘤包括非小细胞肺癌的癌症患者。在美国,调整批准唑来膦酸用于有任何实体肿瘤的患者是基于一项Ⅲ期随机安慰剂对照的临床试验结果,该试验纳入 773 例非乳腺癌或前列腺癌的实体瘤发生骨转移患者接受唑来膦酸(4 或 8mg)或安慰剂的治疗,药物由 15 分钟的静脉输注给予,每 3 周一次,长达 21 个月[5]。随机分配到 4mg 唑来膦酸或安慰剂组的 507 例患者中,249 例为非小细胞肺癌,36 例为小细胞肺癌(SCLC),结果显示唑来膦酸显著减少经历至少一次 SRE 患者的数量,包括恶性高钙血症等,(39% vs 48%,$P=0.039$),也减少经历每一种类型 SRE 的患者比例(图 15.1)[5]。唑来膦酸可显著降低 SREs 的年发病率(1.74 次/年 vs 1.71 次/年,$P=0.012$),可显著推迟第一次 SRE 的时间(236 天 vs 155 天,$P=0.009$)[5]。该研究进一步通过 Andersen-Gill 模型对总人群多事件分析,不仅考虑 SREs 的数量,而且还包括多次 SREs 之间的时间间隔,可更敏感地比较两组患者之间 SREs 风险。结果表明,在所有试验人群中,与安慰剂相比,唑来膦酸减少了 31% 的 SREs 风险(相对危险度,$RR=0.693$,$P=0.003$),许多肺癌患者在第一次 SRE 之后才被确诊,先前存在的骨骼损伤的患者也能从唑来膦酸后续治疗中获益。已经经历一次 SRE 的患者出现后续事件的风险明显增高,通过对唑来膦酸治疗非小细胞肺癌和其他实体肿瘤患者的Ⅲ期临床试验的探索性分析发现,纳入研究之前有 SRE 病史的患者和无 SRE 病史的患者相比,研究过程中发生一次 SRE 的风险增加了 41%($P=0.036$)[36]。通过 Andersen-Gill 多事件分析发现,对于有 SRE 病史的患者,与安慰剂治疗组相比,唑来膦酸可使研究过程中出现一次 SRE 风险降低 31%($P=0.009$),骨骼伤残率也显著降低(1.96 次/年 vs 2.81 次/年,$P=0.030$)[36]。

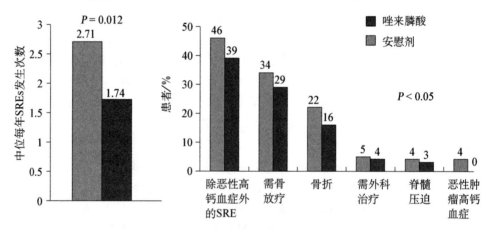

图 15.1 唑来膦酸减少患者各种 SRE 发生率

Ⅲ期临床试验,非小细胞肺癌或其他实体肿瘤发生骨转移的患者接受每 3 周 1 次的唑来膦酸或安慰剂治疗,治疗时间最长 21 个月;50% 的患者为非小细胞肺癌患者,7% 的患者为小细胞肺癌患者。SRE 骨骼相关事件,HCM 恶性肿瘤高钙血症(来自 Rosen 等[5])

此外,与安慰剂组相比,唑来膦酸使研究中出现首次 SRE 的中位时间显著延长了 4 个多月(215 天 vs 106 天,$P=0.011$)。唑来膦酸似乎也可使无 SRE 病史的亚组患者,但没有统计学意义。该研究表明,唑来膦酸可有效降低 SREs 发生率,包括对有 SREs 病史的患者。

唑来膦酸的耐受性和安全性

非小细胞肺癌临床研究表明唑来膦酸总体安全性与安慰剂相当,唑来膦酸和安慰剂最常见的不良反应是骨痛(分别为 48%、58%),恶心(分别为 47%、32%)和呼吸困难(分别为 45%、30%)[37]。唑来膦酸组骨痛发生相对较少可能是来自 SRE 减少的或该药的止痛效果,但两组之间镇痛药的用量没有差异。与安慰剂组相比,

4mg 唑来膦酸治疗组的骨姑息性放疗的发生率没有显著的降低[25]。在非小细胞肺癌患者中,目前还没有血清肌酐出现 4 级以上升高的相关报道。双膦酸盐治疗期间,目前推荐肾功能和口腔健康监测,以避免少见的潜在严重不良事件[38,39]。因为所有静脉给予的双膦酸盐通过肾脏清除,肾功能和含水量状态应该在每次输液前确定,以保证肾脏安全性。较少见的是,肾功能正常的患者可能会出现剂量和输注速度相关的损伤,但肾功能受损的患者出现进一步损伤的风险更大。因此,对肾功能受损的患者给予唑来膦酸治疗时,建议起始剂量减量[40]。

在接受双膦酸盐治疗的患者中,已报道可出现罕见的颌骨骨坏死(ONJ),其特征为在颌骨无转移性疾病或放疗的情况下,颌面部区域骨质外露,在经过 6 周合适的牙齿护理后没有愈合迹象[39]。通过回顾性分析和数据库报告显示,骨转移患者 ONJ 的发生率在 0.7% 和 12.6% 之间[41-43]。ONJ 发生率的宽幅度变化可能是由于双膦酸盐治疗之前和之中的牙预防措施的差异,双膦酸盐治疗期间的变化以及地域差异。已经确认,牙预防措施和适当的口腔卫生可显著降低双膦酸盐治疗期间 ONJ 的发生[39,44-46]。针对活动性 ONJ 病变患者一项研究发现,医用臭氧油混悬剂的局部应用可以使 ONJ 完全缓解[47]。

骨代谢生化标记物

唑来膦酸和生化标记物

有临床试验纳入非小细胞肺癌或其他实体瘤的患者 238 例,每 3 个月评估一次尿液 I 型胶原 N 末端肽(NTX)水平和血清骨形成标记物 BALP 水平[48],结果显示,与 NTX 低水平(<100 nmol/mmol 肌酐,图 15.2)的患者相比,高基线 NTX 水平($\geqslant 100$ nmol/mmol 肌酐)与第一次 SRE 风险增加($RR=1.85$, $P=0.076$)、骨疾病进展($RR=1.76$, $P=0.029$)有关[48]。NTX 高水平患者死亡风险增加了三倍以上($RR=3.03$, $P<0.001$),而中位生存期缩短了 5 个月(3.2 个月 vs 低基线 NTX 水平患者的 8.2 个月)[48]。与 BALP 低水平(<146 IU/L)的患者相比,高基线 BALP 水平($\geqslant 146$ IU/L)患者疾病进展($RR=1.77$, $P=0.005$)和死亡($RR=1.53$, $P=0.003$)风险都显著增加[48]。

唑来膦酸可显著抑制骨转移患者骨再吸收的生化标志物。在一项测量初诊骨转移、每 3~4 周接受唑来膦酸治疗患者($n=71$)的骨标志物水平的前瞻性研究中,在第一次(第 55 天)和第二次(第 115 天)治疗评估时,唑来膦酸显著降低 NTX 的水平(分别平均降低了 43%,45%),而且 NTX 水平在研究中自始至终都被抑制[50]。

研究显示,NTX 减少和骨疾病进展的较低发生率相关(分别为 18.8%,66.7%, $P=0.001$)[50],该结果与一项唑来膦酸Ⅲ期临床试验数据一致[51],该试验表明唑来膦酸在 3 个月内减少了非小细胞肺癌等实体瘤骨转移、有监测骨标记物

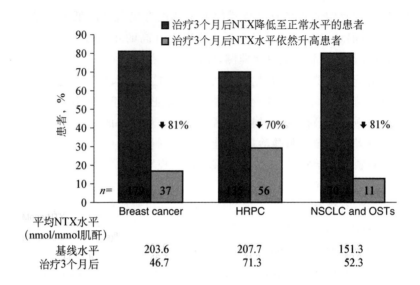

图 15.2 唑来膦酸可降低绝大部分患者的 NTX 水平

NTX Ⅰ型胶原 N 末端肽，HRPC 激素难治性前列腺癌，NSCLC 非小细胞肺癌，OST 其他实体肿瘤（数据来自 Lipton 等[49]）

的患者（$n=204$）的平均尿 NTX 水平[49]。和安慰剂相比，唑来膦酸也显著减少了高基线 NTX 水平（NTX$\geqslant$64 nmol/mmol 肌酐，$n=144$）的 NSCLC 患者 35% 的死亡相对危险度（RR=0.650，$P=0.024$）[52]。

在正常基线 NTX 亚组中，唑来膦酸组和安慰剂组的生存差异无统计学意义，和该亚组已报道的 SRE、死亡风险更低的结果是一致的[48,52]，唑来膦酸组患者获益可能是由于骨质溶解减少导致骨基质生长因子释放减少，从而降低 SRE 发生率，也可能由于唑来膦酸直接或间接的抗肿瘤作用，即凋亡增加，化疗药物的协同作用，抗血管生成和免疫系统刺激等。

唑来膦酸的抗肿瘤活性

临床数据库证据表明，唑来膦酸能抑制多种人类肿瘤细胞增殖，诱导凋亡[31,53]。体外实验表明唑来膦酸可抑制人原发肿瘤细胞系的生长，包括 12 种小细胞肺癌细胞系，IC50 范围为 13～30 mM[54]。在 16 种 NSCLC 细胞系中观察到其对细胞活力、增殖的抑制作用，IC50 范围约为 2～25 mM[55]。此外，10 mM 唑来膦酸可抑制上述高度活动性细胞系中的 3 种。

在 A549 肺癌细胞系中，唑来膦酸与化疗药物具有抗肿瘤协同作用[56]。和单独顺铂相比，唑来膦酸联合顺铂，100mM 的唑来膦酸可显著增强细胞毒性，达 70%（$P=0.007$）。与单一药物相比，唑来膦酸联合紫杉醇可协同抑制细胞增殖[57]。在鼠肺癌细胞系中，唑来膦酸可抑制肿瘤细胞生长，唑来膦酸[1mM/（kg·

周)]处理的小鼠的存活显著延长($P<0.05$)[58]。

临床模型研究表明多种机制参与唑来膦酸的抗肿瘤活性[59]。除了直接抗肿瘤作用外,含氮双膦酸盐具有免疫调节功能,如可调节在恶性肿瘤免疫监视中起重要作用 T 细胞亚群,γδT 细胞。唑来膦酸可诱导外周 γδT 细胞成熟和上调共刺激表面受体(如 CD 40,CD 80,CD 83)的表达[60]。此外,唑来膦酸可激活 γδT 细胞的细胞溶解活性,从而增强抗肿瘤免疫反应[61]。

目前正在进行相关的临床研究评估唑来膦酸对 NSCLC 患者骨转移预防和治疗作用。

狄诺塞麦和抗 RANKL 活性

狄诺塞麦:作用机制

狄诺塞麦是一种完全性人单克隆抗体,可与 RANKL(细胞核因子-κB 受体活化因子配体)结合,从而抑制破骨细胞功能并防止广泛的骨吸收和局部骨破坏。骨肿瘤细胞可导致破骨细胞及其前体的 RANKL 表达增加。RANKL 可调节破骨细胞功能、发生和存活[62-64]。RANKL 表达过多可诱导破骨细胞活性增加,引起骨吸收和局部骨质破坏,可表现为骨转换指标的升高,最终导致 SRE 的发生[48,51]。

两个晚期肿瘤骨转移患者的Ⅱ期临床试验和一个骨髓瘤的Ⅱ期临床试验对狄诺塞麦进行了研究[65-67]。结果显示,剂量范围为 30～180mg,每 4 周或 12 周给药的狄诺塞麦治疗和快速、持续的骨转换指标抑制作用有关,以及 SREs 发生的延迟,和静脉型双膦酸盐中观察到的结果相近。

狄诺塞麦 vs 唑来膦酸,Ⅲ期临床试验

一项随机双盲Ⅲ期试验纳入 1779 例期肿瘤骨转移(乳腺癌和前列腺癌除外)和多发性骨髓瘤患者,890 例患者使用唑来膦酸治疗,另 886 例使用狄诺塞麦组治疗[68]。两组患者间无明显选择性偏倚(表 15.1)。主要研究终点是研究中出现首次 SRE 的时间,次要研究终点,仅当非劣效性被证明才进行评估,是通过多重时间分析比较狄诺塞麦和唑来膦酸的研究中发生首次 SRE 的时间和第一次以及随后发生 SRE 时间的优越性检验。随后发生的 SRE 定义为前一次 SRE 发生之后 21 天以上发生的事件。

唑来膦酸剂量数的中位数为 7,狄诺塞麦也为 7;唑来膦酸累积药物暴露为 651.9 患者年,狄诺塞麦为 675.3 患者年。研究中位时间约为 7 个月。

疗效

研究中出现首次 SRE 的时间上($HR=0.84,P=0.0007$),狄诺塞麦不劣于唑来膦酸,减少 16% 危险(图 15.3)。研究中出现首次 SRE 的中位时间,狄诺塞麦为 20.6 个月,唑来膦酸为 16.3 个月。发生首次 SRE 的时间优越性检验显示 $P=0.06$,尚无统计学意义。发生首次以及随后发生 SREs 多重事件时间的分析显示,

狄诺塞麦比唑来膦酸的发生率比值为 0.9, $P=0.14$, 无显著统计学差异。总生存期(HR=0.95, $P=0.43$)和疾病进展(HR=1.00, $P=1.0$)在治疗组之间是相似的(图 15.4, 图 15.5)。

表 15.1 两组患者临床基本特征

因素 n(%)或者中位数	唑来膦酸($N=890$)	狄诺塞麦($N=886$)
男性	552(62)	588(66)
年龄	61	60
原发肿瘤	345(39)	345(39)
NSCLC	93(10)	86(10)
多发性骨髓瘤	452(51)	457(52)
ECOG 0-1 分	728(82)	748(84)
骨转移到随机化分组间隔	2	2
SRE 病史	446(50)	440(50)
内脏转移	448(50)	474(53)

引自 Henry 等[69]

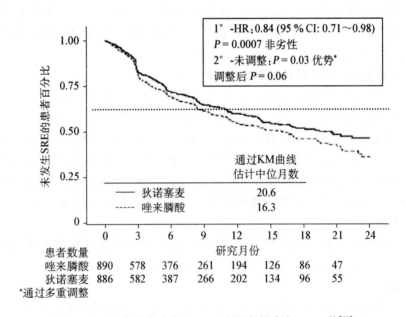

图 15.3 研究期间首次发生 SRE 时间(数据来自 Henry 等[69])

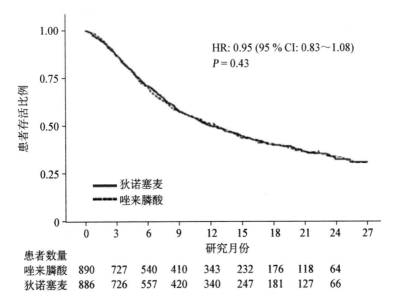

图 15.4　患者总体生存情况（数据来自 Henry 等[69]）

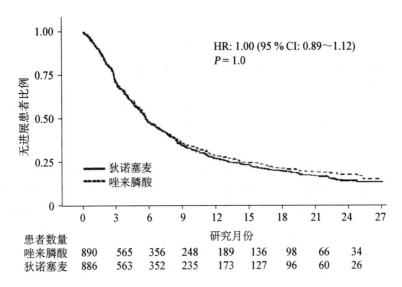

图 15.5　患者总体疾病进展情况（数据来自 Henry 等[69]）

依据肿瘤类别的疗效

相对于唑来膦酸，狄诺塞麦对发生首次 SRE 时间的影响，依据肿瘤类型，分别为：非小细胞肺癌的 HR=0.84，$P=0.20$；骨髓瘤为 1.03，$P=0.89$；其他实体瘤为 0.79 的，$P=0.04$。通过总体生存率分析显示，非小细胞肺癌的 $HR=0.79$，骨髓瘤为 2.26，其他实体瘤为 1.08。

安全性

两组患者不良事件（AEs）发生率相近（表 15.2）。唑来膦酸严重不良事件的发生率是 13.4%，而狄诺塞麦为 14.6%。3 例（0.3%）唑来膦酸患者出现新的原发恶性肿瘤，而狄诺塞麦治疗组有 5 例（0.6%）。狄诺塞麦组低钙血症发生率较高（狄诺塞麦组 10.8%，唑来膦酸组 5.8%），但未发现低血钙症导致的严重临床后遗症。

表 15.2 两组患者相关不良事件汇总

不良事件，n(%)	唑来膦酸($N=878$)	狄诺塞麦($N=878$)
感染	349(39.7)	358(40.8)
严重感染	118(13.4)	128(14.6)
急性期反应（治疗初期 3 天内）	127(14.5)	61(6.9)
肾毒性[a]	96(10.9)	73(8.3)
肾功能衰竭	25(2.8)	20(2.3)
急性肾功能衰竭	16(1.8)	11(1.3)
ONJ 累积发生率[b]	11(1.3)	10(1.1)
第一年	5(0.6)	4(0.5)
第二年	8(0.9)	10(1.1)
新的原发肿瘤	3(0.3)	5(0.6)

引自 Henry 等[69]

注：a. 包括血肌酐升高或异常、肾功能衰竭、急性肾功能衰竭、慢性肾功能衰竭、蛋白尿、血尿、肾功能不全、少尿、无尿、氮质血症、血清肌酐清除率下降；b. $P=1.0$

集中确定的白蛋白校准的钙水平的 3 级、4 级降低，唑来膦酸组出现 9 例（1%）钙水平的 3 级、4 级降低，狄诺塞麦组则为 20 例（2.3%）。2.7% 唑来膦酸组患者给予静脉钙剂，而狄诺塞麦组有 5.7%。ONJ 累积发生率，唑来膦酸组和狄诺塞麦组 1 年 ONJ 累积发生率为 0.6%、0.5%；2 年累积发生率为 0.9%、1.1%；3 年累积发生率为 1.3%、1.1%（$P=1.0$）。首次用药后 3 天内急性期反应，唑来膦酸组患者出现了 14.5%，狄诺塞麦组为 6.9%。最常见的反应为发热，关节痛和疲劳。唑来膦酸组 152 例（17.3%）患者需要调整剂量到低于 4mg；因为血清肌酐升高，78 例（8.9%）患者停止服药。而狄诺塞麦组没有出现需要剂量调整或者因肾功能停止服药。尽管唑来膦酸给药方案因肾功能进行适当调整，但是仍有证据显示唑来膦酸组有不少肾脏相关不良事件。狄诺塞麦是一种单克隆抗体，由吞噬细胞通过胞内消除分解代谢，没有证据表明对肾功能存在影响[70,71]。

骨转换生物标记物：狄诺塞麦 vs 唑来膦酸

与唑来膦酸相比,狄诺塞麦组患者的骨转换标记物抑制效果更明显。通过对比基线水平和治疗第 13 周之间的水平发现,狄诺塞麦($n=546$)尿 NTX/Cr 水平平均减少了 76%,唑来膦酸组($n=543$)为 65%,$P<0.001$;狄诺塞麦组($n=578$)骨特异性碱性磷酸酶下降了 37% 和唑来膦酸组($n=581$)为 29%,$P<0.001$。

肺癌中总生存期的探索性分析

811 例肺癌患者的亚组分析表明,与唑来膦酸相比,狄诺塞麦和总中位生存期的显著提高,有 1.2 个月的差异(KM 中位期 = 8.9 个月 vs 7.7 个月,HR = 0.80,$P=0.01$)(图 15.6)[72]。当总生存期依据相关基线协变量(年龄,性别,原发癌诊断到出现转移或首次骨转移、内脏转移的时间,和 ECOG 状态)进行调整,狄诺塞麦仍呈显著的生存优势,通过随机分层因素(先前的 SRE 和系统性抗癌治疗)分层时,HR = 0.81,$P=0.01$。对于内脏转移的患者(狄诺塞麦组 231 例和唑来膦酸组 233 例),狄诺塞麦可明显提高患者中位生存期,生存差异为 1.2 个月(KM 中位期 = 7.7 个月 vs 6.4 个月,HR = 0.79,$P=0.03$)。狄诺塞麦组患者生存期显著提高约 1.5 个月(KM 中位期 = 9.5 个月 vs 8.1 个月,HR = 0.78,$P=0.01$)(图 15.7)。

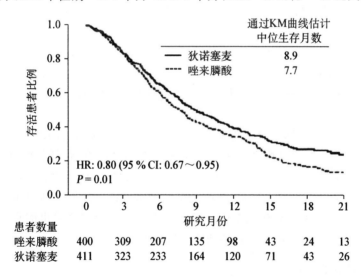

图 15.6 肺癌患者总体生存情况

狄诺塞麦治疗的肺癌患者生存期相对较长,其原因是其对肿瘤细胞的直接和间接作用。间接作用来自肿瘤细胞和促进骨破坏、肿瘤生长的骨髓微环境的共生关系。肿瘤细胞可分泌多种刺激产生 RANKL 的因子[62],肿瘤环境中 RANKL 表达增加可导致破骨细胞形成,活化和存活,并导致溶骨性病变[73],骨质溶解然后导致来源于骨的生长因子的释放[62,74]。

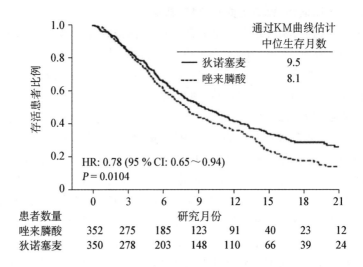

图 15.7　非小细胞肺癌患者总体生存情况

上述生长因子可增加甲状旁腺激素相关蛋白的产生，直接促进肿瘤的生长[62]。骨质破坏可增加局部细胞外钙的浓度，可促进肿瘤生长和甲状旁腺激素相关蛋白产生[74]。狄诺塞麦可通过破骨细胞以及破坏肿瘤细胞和骨微环境之间的相互作用来间接影响骨肿瘤的进展。RANKL 抑制作用可减少骨病变/骨溶解以及非小细胞肺癌模型中的骨肿瘤负荷[75]，并可提高其他治疗方案对骨肿瘤的抗肿瘤效果[76,77]。

狄诺塞麦也可能通过直接抑制表达 RANK 肿瘤细胞上的 RANKL 表达来提高生存期，这在乳腺癌细胞体内试验[78]和若干肿瘤细胞系（包括肺癌细胞）体外试验[79]中得到证明。RANKL 抑制可通过诱导凋亡和抗转移活性发挥直接抗肿瘤作用[80]。抑制 RANKL 或表达 RANK 的肿瘤细胞的抗癌活性机制的相关假说可参照 Solange Peters 和 Etienne Meylan 的综述文章[81]。狄诺塞麦可能有骨骼系统之外的抗肿瘤作用[82]，但需进一步的前瞻性临床研究证明。

新型骨靶向药物

较早在肺癌中开展临床研究的骨靶向药物有达沙替尼（抗 Src 活性）[83]，ACE-011(Sotatercept-Activin TRAP)[84,85]，Cabozantinib（抗 RET 药物）[86]，和镭 223（靶向 α 发射器）[87]。

结论

骨疾病可影响患者生活质量，功能状态和严重致残。随着新型化疗和生物靶向药物的研发，患者生存期明显提高，但 SRE 出现可能也随之增加。骨转移的早期发现及 SREs 的管理是维持生活质量以及控制医疗费用的关键。早期治疗有助于维持患者的正常生理功能，使患者更好耐受后续治疗，如新型靶向治疗等，从而改善患者生存预后[36]。NSCLC 患者发生骨转移危险因素的识别、优化筛查、早期治疗，可防止或延缓 SREs 的发生。

唑来膦酸和狄诺塞麦治疗 ONJ 安全性较高，患者耐受较好。

对实体瘤患者进行回顾性Ⅲ期临床研究亚组分析显示，狄诺塞麦具有总生存期优势，可延缓首次 SRE 的发生。狄诺塞麦皮下给药优于静脉给药，可减少急性不良反应，不需要肾功能监测，但低血钙症发生率较高。两种药物都是骨靶向治疗的较好选择。正在进行的临床试验有助于了解这些药物是否可预防骨转移和内脏转移，从而延长 NSCLC 患者的无疾病进展和总生存期。

参考文献

1. Coleman RE. Skeletal complications of malignancy. Cancer. 1997;80(suppl):1588-94.
2. Mercadante S. Malignant bone pain:pathophysiology and treatment. Pain. 1997;69:1-18.
3. Hansen BH, Keller J, Laitinen M, et al. The Scandinavian Sarcoma Group Skeletal Metastasis Register. Survival after surgery for bone metastases in the pelvis and extremities. Acta Orthop Scand Suppl. 2004;75:11-5.
4. Delea TE, McKiernan JM, Liss M, et al. Impact of skeletal complications on total medical care costs in lung cancer patients with bone metastases. Proc Am Soc Clin Oncol. 2004;23:533 [Abstract 6064].
5. Rosen LS, Gordon D, Tchekmedyian NS, et al. Long-term efficacy and safety of zoledronic acid in the treatment of skeletal metastases in patients with non-small cell lung carcinoma and other solid tumors:a randomized, phase Ⅲ, double-blind, placebo-controlled trial. Cancer. 2004;100:2613-21.
6. Mundy GR. Mechanisms of bone metastasis. Cancer. 1997;80(suppl):1546-56.
7. Saad F, Schulman CC. Role of bisphosphonates in prostate cancer. Eur Urol. 2004;45:26-34.
8. Coleman RE. Metastatic bone disease:clinical features, pathophysiology, and treatment strategies. Cancer Treat Rev. 2001;27:165-76.
9. Kakonen SM, Mundy GR. Mechanisms of osteolytic bone metastases in breast carcinoma. Cancer. 2003;97(suppl):834-9.
10. Coleman RE. Bisphosphonates:clinical experience. Oncologist. 2004;9 suppl 4:14-27.
11. Lipton A. Pathophysiology of bone metastases:how this knowledge may lead to therapeutic intervention. J Support Oncol. 2004;2:205-13.
12. Sabino MA, Mantyh PW. Pathophysiology of bone cancer pain. J Support Oncol. 2005;3:15-24.
13. Iordanidou L, Trivizaki E, Saranti S, et al. Is there a role of whole body bone scan in early stages of non-small cell lung cancer patients? J BUON. 2006;11:491-7.
14. Pfister DG, Johnson DH, Azzoli CG, et al. American Society of Clinical Oncology treatment of un-

resectable non-small cell lung cancer guideline:update 2003. J Clin Oncol. 2004; 22:330-53.
15. Baum RP,Hellwig D, Mezzetti M. Position of nuclear medicine modalities in the diagnostic workup of cancer patients:lung cancer. Q J Nucl Med Mol Imaging. 2004;48:119-42.
16. Silvestri GA, Tanoue LT, Margolis ML, et al. The non-invasive staging of non-small cell lung cancer:the guidelines. Chest. 2003;123(suppl):147S-56.
17. National Comprehensive Cancer Network. NCCN clinical practice guidelines in oncology:non-small cell lung cancer. 2008. http://www.nccn.org/professionals/physician_gls/PDF/nsclc.pdf.
18. Bury T,Barreto A, Daenen F, et al. Fluorine-18 deoxyglucose positron emission tomography for the detection of bone metastases in patients with non-small cell lung cancer. Eur J Nucl Med. 1998;25:1244-7.
19. Gayed I, Vu T, Johnson M, et al. Comparison of bone and 2-deoxy-2-[18F] fluoro-D-glucose positron emission tomography in the evaluation of bony metastases in lung cancer. Mol Imaging Biol. 2003;5:26-31.
20. Hetzel M,Arslandemir C, Konig HH, et al. F-18 NaF PET for detection of bone metastases in lung cancer:accuracy, cost-effectiveness, and impact on patient management. J Bone Miner Res. 2003;18:2206-14.
21. Lipton A,Theriault RL, Hortobagyi GN, et al. Pamidronate prevents skeletal complications and is effective palliative treatment in women with breast carcinoma and osteolytic bone metastases:long term follow-up of two randomized, placebo-controlled trials. Cancer. 2000;88:1082-90.
22. Berenson JR, Lichtenstein A, Porter L, et al. Long term Pamidronate treatment of advanced multiple myeloma patients reduces skeletal events. Myeloma Aredia Study Group. J Clin Oncol. 1998;16:593-602.
23. Saad F. Clinical benefit of zoledronic acid for the prevention of skeletal complications in advanced prostate cancer. Clin Prostate Cancer. 2005;4:31-7.
24. Lipton A. Bisphosphonate therapy in the oncology setting. Expert Opin Emerg Drugs. 2003;8(2):469-88.
25. Rosen LS, Gordon D,Tchekmedyian S, et al. Zoledronic acid versus placebo in the treatment of skeletal metastases in patients with lung cancer and other solid tumors:a phase Ⅲ, double-blind, randomized trial - the Zoledronic Acid Lung Cancer and other Solid Tumors Study Group. J Clin Oncol. 2003;21:3150-7.
26. Delea T, McKiernan J, Liss M, et al. Cost of skeletal complications in patients with bone metastases of lung cancer [abstract]. Lung Cancer. 2003;41 suppl 2:S7 [Abstract O9].
27. Delea T, Langer C, McKiernan J, et al. The cost of treatment of skeletal-related events in patients with bone metastases from lung cancer. Oncology. 2004;67:390-6.
28. Saad F, Lipton A, Cook R, et al. Pathologic fractures correlate with reduced survival in patients with malignant bone disease. Cancer. 2007;110:1860-7.
29. Weinfurt KP, Li Y, Castel LD, et al. The significance of skeletal-related events for the

healthrelated quality of life of patients with metastatic prostate cancer. Ann Oncol. 2005;16: 579-84.
30. Saba N, Khuri F. The role of bisphosphonates in the management of advanced cancer with a focus on non-small cell lung cancer. Part 2: clinical studies and economic analyses. Oncology. 2005;68:18-22.
31. Green JR. Preclinical profile and anticancer potential of zoledronic acid. In: Birch EV, editor. Trends in bone cancer research, vol. 24. New York: Nova Science Publishers Inc; 2006. p. 217-45.
32. Fleisch H. Development of bisphosphonates. Breast Cancer Res. 2002;4:30-4.
33. Green JR. Bisphosphonates: preclinical review. Oncologist. 2004;9 suppl 4:3-13.
34. Green J. Zoledronate: the preclinical pharmacology. Br J Clin Pract Suppl. 1996;87:16-8.
35. Green JR, Muller K, Jaeggi KA. Preclinical pharmacology of CGP 42'446, a new, potent, heterocyclic bisphosphonate compound. J Bone Miner Res. 1994;9:745-51.
36. Hirsh V, Tchekmedyian NS, Rosen LS, et al. Clinical benefit of zoledronic acid in patients with lung cancer and other solid tumors: analysis based on history of skeletal complications. Clin Lung Cancer. 2004;6(3):170-4.
37. Bukowski R, Rosen L, Gordon D, et al. Long-term therapy with zoledronic acid is effective and safe in reducing the risk of skeletal complications in patients with bone metastases from non-small cell lung cancer (NSCLC) [poster]. In: 10th world conference on Lung Cancer (WCLC), Vancouver; 10-14 Aug 2003 [Abstract 150].
38. Conte P, Guarneri V. Safety of intravenous and oral bisphosphonates and compliance with dosing regimens. Oncologist. 2004;9 suppl 4:28-37.
39. Weitzman R, Sauter N, Eriksen EF, et al. Critical review: updated recommendations for the prevention, diagnosis, and treatment of osteonecrosis of the jaw in cancer patients - May 2006. Crit Rev Oncol Hematol. 2007;62:148-52.
40. Zometa [package insert]. East Hanover: Novartis Pharmaceuticals Corporation; 2005.
41. Durie BG, Katz M, Crowley J. Osteonecrosis of the jaw and bisphosphonates. N Engl J Med. 2005;353:99-102.
42. Hoff AO, Toth BB, Altundag K, et al. Frequency and risk factors associated with osteonecrosis of the jaw in cancer patients treated with intravenous bisphosphonates. J Bone Miner Res. 2008;23:826-36.
43. Pozzi S, Marcheselli R, Sacchi S, et al. Bisphosphonate-associated osteonecrosis of the jaw: a review of 35 cases and an evaluation of its frequency in multiple myeloma patients. Leuk Lymphoma. 2007;48:56-64.
44. Dimopoulos MA, Kastritis E, Bamia C, et al. Reduction of osteonecrosis of the jaw (ONJ) after implementation of preventive measures in patients with multiple myeloma treated with zoledronic acid. Ann Oncol. 2009;20:117-20.
45. Montefusco V, Gay F, Spina F, et al. Antibiotic prophylaxis before dental procedures may reduce the incidence of osteonecrosis of the jaw in patients with multiple myeloma treated

with bisphosphonates. Leuk Lymphoma. 2008;49:2156-62.

46. Ripamonti CI, Maniezzo M, Campa T, et al. Decreased occurrence of osteonecrosis of the jaw after implementation of dental preventive measures in solid tumour patients with bone metastases treated with bisphosphonates. The experience of the National Cancer Institute of Milan. Ann Oncol. 2009;20:137-45.

47. Ripamonti C, Maniezzo M, Ghiringhelli R, et al. Medical oil suspension applications heal osteonecrosis of the jaw (ONJ) in patients treated with bisphosphonates (BPs):preliminary results of a single institution protocol [poster]. In:Primary therapy of early breast cancer, 11th international conference [Poster 194], St. Gallen, Switzerland; 2009.

48. Brown JE, Cook RJ, Major P, et al. Bone turnover markers as predictors of skeletal complications in prostate cancer, lung cancer, and other solid tumors. J Natl Cancer Inst. 2005;97:59-69.

49. Lipton A, Cook R, Saad F, et al. Normalization of bone markers is associated with improved survival in patients with bone metastases from solid tumors and elevated bone resorption receiving zoledronic acid. Cancer. 2008;113:193-201.

50. Pectasides D, Nikolaou M, Farmakis D, et al. Clinical value of bone remodeling markers in patients with bone metastases treated with zoledronic acid. Anticancer Res. 2005;25:1457-63.

51. Coleman RE, Major P, Lipton A, et al. Predictive value of bone resorption and formation markers in cancer patients with bone metastases receiving the bisphosphonate zoledronic acid. J Clin Oncol. 2005;23:4925-35.

52. Hirsh V, Major PP, Lipton A, et al. Zoledronic acid and survival in patients with metastatic bone disease from lung cancer and elevated markers of osteoclast activity. J Thorac Oncol. 2008;3:228-36.

53. Green JR. Antitumor effects of bisphosphonates. Cancer. 2003;97(suppl):840-7.

54. Matsumoto S, Kimura S, Segawa H, et al. Efficacy of combining the third generation bisphosphonate, zoledronate with imatinib mesylate in suppressing small cell lung cancer cell line proliferation [abstract]. Proc Am Soc Clin Oncol. 2003;22(suppl):684 [Abstract 2750].

55. Berger W, Kubista B, Elbling L, et al. The N-containing bisphosphonate zoledronic acid exerts potent anticancer activity against non-small cell lung cancer cells by inhibition of protein geranylgeranylation [abstract]. Proc Am Assoc Cancer Res. 2005;46 [Abstract 4981].

56. Ozturk OH, Bozcuk H, Burgucu D, et al. Cisplatin cytotoxicity is enhanced with zoledronic acid in A549 lung cancer cell line:preliminary results of an in vitro study. Cell Biol Int. 2007;31:1069-71.

57. Gjyrezi A, O'Brate A, Chanel-Vos C, et al. Zoledronic acid synergizes with Taxol in an HDAC6-dependant manner:novel mechanistic implications for combination anticancer therapy with taxanes [abstract]. Proc Am Assoc Cancer Res. 2007; [Abstract 1425].

58. Li YY, Chang JW, Chou WC, et al. Zoledronic acid is unable to induce apoptosis but slows tumor growth and prolongs survival for non-small cell lung cancers. Lung Cancer. 2008;59:180-91.

59. Matsumoto S, Kimura S, Segawa H, et al. Efficacy of the third-generation bisphosphonate, zoledronic acid alone and combined with anti-cancer agents against small cell lung cancer cell lines. Lung Cancer. 2005;47:31-9.
60. Landmeier S, Altvater B, Pscherer S, et al. Presentation of Epstein Barr virus (EBV) epitopes by activated human γδ T cells induces peptide-specific cytolytic CD8+ T cell expansion [abstract]. Blood. 2006;108 [Abstract 1738].
61. Fournier PG, Chirgwin JM, Guise TA. New insights into the role of T cells in the vicious cycle of bone metastases. Curr Opin Rheumatol. 2006;18:396-404.
62. Roodman GD. Mechanisms of bone metastasis. N Engl J Med. 2004;350:1655-64.
63. Hofbauer LC, Neubauer A, Heufelder AE. Receptor activator of nuclear factor-kappa B ligand and osteoprotegerin: potential implications for the pathogenesis and treatment of malignant bone diseases. Cancer. 2001;92:460-70.
64. Selvaggi G, Scagliotti GV. Management of bone metastases in cancer: a review. Crit Rev Oncol Hematol. 2005;56:365-78.
65. Body JJ, Facon T, Coleman RE, et al. A study of the biological receptor activator of nuclear factor-kappa B ligand inhibitor, denosumab, in patients with multiple myeloma or bone metastases from breast cancer. Clin Cancer Res. 2006;12:1221-8.
66. Fizazi K, Lipton A, Mariette X, et al. Randomized phase II trial of denosumab in patients with bone metastases from prostate cancer, breast cancer, or other neoplasms after intravenous bisphosphonates. J Clin Oncol. 2009;27:1564-71.
67. Lipton A, Steger GG, Figueroa J, et al. Randomized active-controlled phase II study of denosumab efficacy and safety in patients with breast cancer-related bone metastases. J Clin Oncol. 2007;25:4431-7.
68. Henry D, Costa L, Goldwasser F, et al. Randomized, double-blind study of denosumab versus zoledronic acid in the treatment of bone metastases in patients with advanced cancer (excluding breast and prostate cancer) or multiple myeloma. J Clin Oncol. 2011;29(9):1125-32.
69. Henry D, et al. Randomized Study of Denosumab versus Zoledronic Acid for the Treatment of Bone metastases in Patients with Advanced Cancer (Excluding Breast and Prostate Cancer) or Multiple Myeloma. Eur J Cancer Suppl. 2009;7(3):11. Abstract 20LBA and Oral Presentation.
70. Tabrizi MA, Tseng CM, Roskos LK. Elimination mechanisms of therapeutic monoclonal antibodies. Drug Discov Today. 2006;11:81-8.
71. Wang W, Wang EQ, Balthasar JP. Monoclonal antibody pharmacokinetics and pharmacodynamics. Clin Pharmacol Ther. 2008;84:548-58.
72. Scagliotti G, Hirsh V, Siena S, et al. Overall survival improvement in patients with lung cancer and bone metastases treated with denosumab versus zoledronic acid: subgroup analysis from a randomized, phase 3 study. J Thorac Oncol. 2012;7(12):1823-9.
73. Kitazawa S, Kitazawa R. RANK ligand is a prerequisite for cancer-associated osteolytic lesions. J Pathol. 2002;198:228-36.

74. Mundy GR. Metastasis to bone:causes, consequences, and therapeutic opportunities. Nat Rev Cancer. 2002;2:584-93.
75. Feeley BT, Liu NQ, Conduah AH, et al. Mixed metastatic lung cancer lesions in bone are inhibited by noggin overexpression and Rank:Fc administration. J Bone Miner Res. 2006;21:1571-80.
76. Miller R, Jones J, Roudier M, et al. The RANKL inhibitor OPG-Fc either alone, or in combination with docetaxel, blocks lung cancer-induced osteolytic lesions or reduces skeletal tumor burden in a murine model of non-small cell lung cancer in bone. Presented at the 9th international conference on Cancer-Induced Bone Disease, Arlington; 28-31 Oct 2009.
77. Miller RE, Roudier M, Jones J, et al. RANK ligand inhibition plus docetaxel improves survival and reduces tumor burden in a murine model of prostate cancer bone metastasis. Mol Cancer Ther. 2008;7:2160-9.
78. Gonzalez-Suarez E, Jacob AP, Jones J, et al. RANK ligand mediates progestin-induced mammary epithelial proliferation and carcinogenesis. Nature. 2010;468:103-7.
79. Chen LM, Kuo CH, Lai TY, et al. RANKL increases migration of human lung cancer cells through intercellular adhesion molecule-1 up-regulation. J Cell Biochem. 2011;112:933-41.
80. Jones DH, Nakashima T, Sanchez OH, et al. Regulation of cancer cell migration and bone metastasis by RANKL. Nature. 2006;440:692-6.
81. Peters S, Meylan E. Targeting receptor activator of nuclear factor-kappa B as a new therapy for bone metastasis in non-small cell lung cancer. Curr Opin Oncol. 2013;25(2):137-44.
82. Hirsh V. Bisphosphonates in lung cancer:can they provide benefits beyond prevention of skeletal morbidity? Anticancer Agents Med Chem. 2012;12(2):137-43.
83. Luo FR, Camuso A, McGlinchey K, et al. Evaluation of anti-osteoclastic activity of the novel, oral multi-targeted kinase inhibitor Dasatinib (BMS-354825). AACR-NCI-EORTC international conference:Molecular Targets and Cancer Therapeutics, Philadelphia; 14-18 Nov 2005, p 173 [Abstract B178].
84. Fields SZ, Parshad S, Anne M, et al. Activin receptor antagonists for cancer-related anemia and bone disease. Expert Opin Investig Drugs. 2013;22(1):87-101.
85. Borgstein NG, Yang Y, Condon CH, et al. ACE-011, a soluble activin receptor type IIA IgG-Fc fusion protein decreases follicle stimulating hormone and increases bone-specific alkaline phosphatase, a marker of bone formation, in postmenopausal healthy women. Cancer Res. 2008;69(2 Suppl):Abstract 1160.
86. Hellerstedt BA, Edelman G, Vogelzang NJ, et al. Activity of cabozantinib (XL 184) in metastatic NSCLC:results from a phase II randomized discontinuation trial (RDT). J Clin Oncol. 2012;30(suppl):Abstract 7514.
87. Parker C, Nilsson S, Heinrich D, et al. Alpha emitter radium-223 and survival in metastatic prostate cancer. N Engl J Med. 2013;369(3):213-23.

第 16 章
脑转移肿瘤

作者：Antonin Levy, Frederic Dhermain
译者：程　钧

背景

恶性肿瘤发生脑转移常见，肺癌患者脑转移发生率可以高达20%。而由于肿瘤诊断和全身治疗的发展，脑转移肿瘤的发生率持续上升[1]。美国脑转移肿瘤的发生率为7/100 000~14/100 000[2]。由于脑转移肿瘤存在神经毒害作用，因此常认为是预后不良因素。根据分级诊断预后评估(DS-GPA)中的重要的预后因素(年龄，Karnofsky评分，远处转移，脑转移数量)，肺癌合并脑转移患者的生存期为3~14.8个月(表16.1)[3]。DS-GPA评分可为局部和全身治疗提供指导性建议，对于根据评分预后良好的患者应积极干预。放疗及手术治疗是脑转移肿瘤的标准治疗方式。全身治疗也可行，但是效果往往有限，可能是因为药物难以通过血脑屏障(BBB)。肿瘤转移过程及分子生物学研究发展，为脑转移瘤的治疗提供了新的方法。影像学、外科、放疗、化疗、靶向治疗等多方面的进展为肺癌合并脑转移患者延长生存提供了可能。

表16.1　肺癌合并脑转移患者DS-GPA评分

预后因素	评分标准		
	0	0.5	1
年龄(岁)	>60	50~60	<50
KS评分	<70	70~80	90~100
颅外转移	存在	—	不存在
颅内转移灶数量	>3	2~3	1

根据DS-GPA评分预测中位生存期：≤1=3个月；1.5~2=5.5个月；2.5~3=9.4个月；≥3.5=14.8个月

脑转移瘤生物学认识进展

包括脑血管内皮细胞及间质细胞(小胶质细胞和星形胶质细胞)在内的脑部微环境为肿瘤细胞的生长、转移提供了基础。星形胶质细胞可通过对神经元输送营养物质及易化神经信号转导来参与维持脑微环境的稳定,但该机制也可通过减少凋亡发生或上调生长基因,使肿瘤细胞在化疗药物的毒性作用下依旧存活[4],转移性脑肿瘤的生长也依赖于血管生成和血管内皮生长因子(VEGF)的表达。无序的血管生长导致肿瘤相关的血管的结构及功能异常,其特征在于有缺陷的血管内皮细胞,周细胞的覆盖及基底膜。这些异常可直接限制氧气的输送,导致肿瘤内低氧,增加对全身性药物和电离辐射治疗的抵抗能力。肿瘤细胞的另一种保护机制是血脑屏障,血脑屏障是体循环和脑脊液之间脑微血管内皮细胞、周细胞和星形胶质细胞形成一个选择性屏障,该屏障可将化学治疗和分子靶向药物等亲水性分子排除在中枢神经系统以外,除非它们可以通过主动转运受体介导的转运过程进入。血脑屏障表达高水平的药物外排泵如 P-糖蛋白(PGP)/多药抗性蛋白质,可将某些化疗药物移除出颅内[5,6]。目前,正在研究可选择性通过血脑屏障发挥抗肿瘤作用的药物。肿瘤细胞的表型改变可促进肿瘤进展。如表皮生长因子受体(EGFR)通路(通过基因扩增,过表达或基因突变),或 EML4-ALK 易位表达通路等多种分子信号通路激活可在肺部原发病灶和颅内转移灶同时检测到。

脑部影像学新技术

目前认为,增强磁共振成像(MRI)是检测脑转移瘤较好的方法,特别是新的成像方法,如动态对比增强成像(灌注加权的 MRI:PWI)和磁共振波谱(MRS)可更好的用于脑转移瘤的影像学检测。PWI 成像可通过测量脑血量(CBV)评估微血管环境,MRS 成像可检测脑肿瘤中 N-乙酰胆碱水平的改变,这些标志物可用于鉴别放射性坏死和脑转移或复发[8,9]。初步研究表明 11C 蛋氨酸正电子发射断层扫描(MET-PET)也可很好的鉴别脑转移肿瘤与放射性坏死[10]。其他 MRI 成像技术发展,如磁化传递和三剂钆成像正在研究,可以进一步提高病变的检出[11]。

外科新进展

患者 DS-GPA 评分是评估患者是否适合手术的重要指标。20 世纪 90 年代以来,手术切除加术后辅助放疗认为患者预后相对较好,已作为位置较好的孤立性脑转移肿瘤的标准方案。两项随机临床试验表明,手术加全脑放疗(WBRT)相对于单独进行全脑放疗增加患者的生存获益[12,13]。Patchell 等报道,25 例行手术治疗加放疗的患者,患者局部复发率明显下降,(20% vs 52%),生存率提高(40 vs 15 周),生活质量良好。目前,有学者建议对肿瘤部位行放射外科(SRS)治疗以取代手术后全脑放射治疗。回顾性研究显示该方法的局部控制率与术后全脑放疗相近。目前正在开展一项随机Ⅲ期临床试验,比较术后全脑放疗与术后 SRS 治疗脑转移肿瘤患者的临床效果。[http://clinicaltrials.gov:NCT01372774]。

多项技术的发展对肿瘤的完整切除,避免正常组织的损伤提供了极大的帮助。随机对照研究表明,术中磁共振技术可用于评估原发性恶性脑肿瘤的残留病灶[17],另有类似的非随机对照临床试验也证明了其价值[18]。清醒状态下开颅手术肿瘤切除及术中神经电生理的功能监测目前已经发展。因此,对于位于初级运动皮层中的转移性肿瘤行完整的显微手术切除在技术上可行有效[19,20]。其他包括光学和分子可视化技术,如手术中的 5-氨基乙酰丙酸(5-ALA)荧光或者荧光素染色恶性肿瘤等方法也将为实现外科精准切除脑转移瘤提供帮助。

放疗优化

SRS 使用线性加速器产生的高能量 X 射线,目前已成为一种预后良好的数量有限的脑转移瘤的常用治疗方法。SRS 的治疗原则为集中高剂量辐射杀伤肿瘤,同时避免损伤健康组织,从而最大限度地避免可能导致的神经认知下降。转移瘤由于病灶小(<3cm),病灶局限,因此多为 SRS 合适治疗适应证,SRS 与外科手术相比,可治疗手术无法到达的部位,还可同时治疗多个病灶,并且创伤小,价格低。目前外科和 SRS 随机临床对照试验较少,但越来越多的非对照临床研究表明,SRS 对于治疗肺癌合并脑转移瘤患者效果良好,肺癌的颅内局部控制率可达到 81%～98%[22,23]。仅有的一项随机对照研究试验,纳入 64 例肺癌合并脑转移患者,研究结果表明伽马刀与手术切除后加全脑放疗临床效果相似[24]。

除了对 SRS 支持的证据,也有反对 SRS 的研究证据,如两项临床随机对照研究表明,与单独全脑放疗相比,SRS 加全脑放疗并不能使患者更多获益[25,26]。其中一项较大的随机临床试验(RTOG:放射治疗肿瘤学组 9508),纳入 333 例患者,其中 167 例患者接受 SRS 治疗,术后 6 个月的 PS 评分较差,而生存期并无明显提高,但孤立脑转移结节行 SRS 及预计预后较好的患者生存期明显较长[25]。也有前瞻性临床试验研究 SRS 加全脑放疗的临床疗效,其中较大的一项是由欧洲癌症研究及治疗组织(EORTC22952-26001)牵头开展的,该研究纳入 359 例 1～3 个脑转移灶的患者,随机分配到彻底治疗(SRS 或手术)加全脑放疗或不加全脑放疗,其主要研究终点为肿瘤进展到使患者 PS 评分大于 2 分,结果发现两组患者主要终点研究结果相似,但全脑放疗可显著降低原发病灶和颅内病灶的局部复发率,而总体生存期无显著差异,联合治疗组的中位生存期为 10.9 个月,而单纯治疗组中位生存期为 10.7 个月[27]。另外两项前瞻性研究与该研究结果相似,使用放疗联合 SRS 并不能改善数量较少脑转移灶患者的生存,但未接受全脑放疗的患者,有相当一部分发生了颅内复发[28,29]。另一方面,有研究认为 SRS(或手术)后的全脑放射治疗的效果可降低患者认知功能[30,31]。另一项由北部中央癌症治疗组织（NCCTG）进行的大型随机试验目前正在开展拟评估放疗联合 SRS 的临床效果（NCT00377156）。

不久，SRS 可能用于治疗多达十个以上病灶的脑转移瘤患者。Yamamoto 等最近发现，SRS 后不进行全脑放疗可以用于治疗 5～10 个转移灶的脑转移肿瘤。该前瞻性研究结果显示，有 5～10 个脑转移灶的患者在总体生存率，颅内肿瘤控制率，神经功能损伤和死亡等方面与只有 2～4 个脑转移灶的患者没有明显区别[32]。另有一项随机对照临床研究（NCT01731704），可以帮助我们确定 SRS 和全脑放射治疗 5 个以上转移灶的脑转移瘤的价值。

单独全脑放疗目前多用于不适合手术、SRS 或预防性脑放疗，而 DS-GPA 评分预测预后不良的患者。小细胞肺癌行单纯 SRS 治疗效果欠佳，易出现非治疗部位的转移复发。全脑放疗与支持治疗比较，可以提高数个月的生存[33-35]。目前仅有一项来自医学研究理事会（MRC）研究比较放疗与支持治疗的优劣，该研究拟纳入 500 例非小细胞肺癌合并脑转移患者，目前包含 151 例患者的中期研究报告显示，放疗联合支持治疗与单纯支持治疗在患者生存和生活质量等方面均无明显差异[36]。

目前正在研制新技术或药物，以减少全脑放疗后神经认知功能衰退。RTOG0933 Ⅱ 期研究（NCT01227954）拟评估海马区外低剂量辐射，纳入 42 例证实为非小细胞肺癌的患者，初步结果显示，与历史对照组（传统治疗）比较，海马区外放疗患者 4 个月后反应迟缓程度显著下降。仅 3 例患者在海马区域内肿瘤复发[37]。一种口服 N-甲基-D-天冬氨酸（NMDA）受体拮抗剂，美金刚，已在接受全脑放疗的患者中进行随机试验评估，其主要研究终点为治疗 24 周时记忆力减退状况，149 例患者中仅 29% 的患者可评估记忆力，结果显示，美金刚可延迟认知记忆能力的下降，但差异缺乏显著性[38]。有 Ⅲ 期临床试验研究放疗增敏剂，如莫特沙芬钆和乙丙昔罗，是否可以增强全脑放疗的治疗效果，结果显示与安慰剂对比，放疗增敏剂并无明显优势[33-35]。全脑放疗也可同期与全身化疗或靶向治疗联合治疗。

个体化全身治疗

脑转移瘤的主要治疗方法为手术或放疗。肺癌多为化疗敏感性肿瘤，因此化疗可能对于合并脑转移的患者有一定效果[39-42]。尽管患者对化疗有部分反应，全脑放疗的价值仍不能忽视[43]。全身治疗如替莫唑胺可用于补救性治疗[44]。一项由 EORTC 开展的 Ⅲ 期临床试验，将 120 例患者随机分配到全脑放疗联合替尼泊苷化疗联合治疗组或者单独替尼泊苷化疗组，结果发现联合治疗组患者缓解率明显较高，但总体生存期并无明显改善[45]。而另一些化疗药物与全脑放射治疗非小细胞肺癌患者则并不理想[46-48]。全脑放疗联合替莫唑胺治疗非小细胞肺癌目前尚有争议。部分研究认为该方法治疗肿瘤缓解率高而不良反应较少[49-51],而另一些研究(包括提前终止RTOG0302 Ⅲ期临床试验)则表明该方法不良反应较多,而并不改善患者生存状况[52-53]。

原发性非小细胞肺癌多存在各种分子生物学改变,表16.2总结了靶向药物应用于肺癌合并脑转移患者的前瞻性临床研究结果。同原发肿瘤相似,脑转移瘤也可发生EGFR突变[54,55],抗EGFR酪氨酸激酶抑制剂(EGFR-TKI),如厄洛替尼和吉非替尼,在非小细胞肺癌脑转移患者具有抗肿瘤活性[56-60]。较野生型EGFR肿瘤患者相比,EGFR-TKI治疗存在EGFR突变患者的肿瘤缓解率和生存状况相对较好[61]。前瞻性研究显示,同期厄洛替尼联合全脑放疗治疗肺癌合并脑转移患者,总体缓解率为86%,中位生存期达到了12个月[62]。然而,随机对照试验RTOG0302,比较使用厄洛替尼(或替莫唑胺或没有全身治疗)联合全脑放射以及SRS,与单独使用全脑放疗或者SRS治疗的临床效果,结果相比联合治疗组总体生存较差,不良反应也较多[3,52]。但RTOG0302研究广受批评,该研究并不是根据分子基因类型来分配治疗方案,统计价值较差,而且单纯治疗组的结果明显优于前期其他临床研究结果。目前缺乏前瞻性随机对照试验明确EGFR靶向药物治疗肺癌合并脑转移的合适适应证,因此EGFR靶向药物可用于放疗后治疗,或者在放射治疗因故延迟(非神经症状的全身性颅外疾病)[63]。

表16.2 非小细胞肺癌脑转移靶向治疗的前瞻性研究

研究者	药物	患者数量(例)	试验类型	联合治疗	ORR/SD	局部复发率	PFS(月)	OS(月)
Sperduto 等,[52]	厄洛替尼	126	Ⅲ期试验	全脑放疗+SRS+	未报道	未报道		
				观察			8.1	13.4
				替莫唑胺			4.6	6.3
				厄洛替尼			4.8	6.1
Welsh 等,[62]	厄洛替尼	40	Ⅱ期试验	全脑放疗	83%/3%	27.5%	8	11.8
Wu 等,[63]	厄洛替尼	48	Ⅱ期试验	无	58.3%/16.7%	88%	10.1	18.4
Ma 等,[56]	厄洛替尼	21	Ⅱ期试验	全脑放疗	81%/14%	未报道	10	13
Wu 等,[58]	吉非替尼	40	Ⅱ期试验	无	36%/45%	未报道	9	15
Chiu 等,[57]	吉非替尼	76	Ⅱ期试验	无	33.3%/35%	未报道		9.9
Ceresoli 等,[59]	吉非替尼	41	Ⅱ期试验	无	10%/17%	未报道	3	5

注:ORR.客观缓解率;PFS.无疾病生存期;OS.总生存期

其他靶向治疗也在肺癌合并脑转移患者中进行了研究评估。有研究表明ALK 靶向药物克唑替尼的穿透力差,难以进入脑脊液[64],但也有个案报道认为克唑替尼可缓解肿瘤[65,66]。其他 ALK 抑制剂(ceritinib,alectinib)在 ALK 重排的非小细胞肺癌中正在进行临床研究。血管生成抑制靶向药物也进行了在回顾性研究,6 例脑转移瘤患者中,贝伐单抗治疗 6 例脑转移患者,2 例患者部分缓解(PR),3 例患者病灶稳定(SD)[67]。目前认为贝伐单抗联合化疗药物或厄洛替尼是安全的,可降低中枢神经系统的出血率[68]。另外,胰岛素样生长因子 1 受体,CXC 基序趋化因子受体 4(CXCR4)等分子途径将来有可能成为脑转移瘤靶向治疗新途径[69,70]。

总结

过去 10 年中,肺癌合并脑转移的诊断治疗在多方面均大幅改进,对转移发展过程中的分子生物学的认识进一步提高,为 EGFR 或 ALK 靶向治疗提供新的发展机遇。影像学技术的进步,能早期检测出肿瘤并且提供全面的治疗相关信息。重复使用 SRS 或海马区外低剂量全脑放疗,可提高肿瘤的控制率及减少放射性脑损伤。脑转移瘤的前瞻性研究应包括成本效益分析,以为病人提高最大限度的生存率和生活质量为目标。

参考文献

1. Barnholtz-Sloan JS, Sloan AE, Davis FG, et al. Incidence proportions of brain metastases in patients diagnosed (1973 to 2001) in the Metropolitan Detroit Cancer Surveillance System. J Clin Oncol. 2004;22:2865-72.
2. US Census Bureau. Census. gov. 2010. http://www.census.gov/prod/cen2010/briefs/c2010br-01.pdf.
3. Sperduto PW, Kased N, Roberge D, et al. Summary report on the graded prognostic assessment:an accurate and facile diagnosis-specific tool to estimate survival for patients with brain metastases. J Clin Oncol. 2012;30:419-25.
4. Fidler IJ, Yano S, Zhang RD, et al. The seed and soil hypothesis:vascularisation and brain metastases. Lancet Oncol. 2002;3:53-7.
5. Abbott NJ, Rönnbäck L, Hansson E. Astrocyte-endothelial interactions at the blood-brain barrier. Nat Rev Neurosci. 2006;7:41-53.
6. Neuwelt EA. Mechanisms of disease:the blood-brain barrier. Neurosurgery. 2004;54:131-40.
7. Connell JJ, Chatain G, Cornelissen B, et al. Selective permeabilization of the blood-brain barrier at sites of metastasis. J Natl Cancer Inst. 2013;105(21):1634-43.
8. Barajas RF, Chang JS, Sneed PK, et al. Distinguishing recurrent intra-axial metastatic tumor from radiation necrosis following gamma knife radiosurgery using dynamic susceptibility-weighted contrast-enhanced perfusion MR imaging. AJNR Am J Neuroradiol. 2009;30:367-

72.

9. Mitsuya K, Nakasu Y, Horiguchi S, et al. Perfusion weighted magnetic resonance imaging to distinguish the recurrence of metastatic brain tumors from radiation necrosis after stereotactic radiosurgery. J Neurooncol. 2010;99:81-8.
10. Terakawa Y, Tsuyuguchi N, Iwai Y, et al. Diagnostic accuracy of 11C-methionine PET for differentiation of recurrent brain tumors from radiation necrosis after radiotherapy. J Nucl Med. 2008;49:694-9.
11. Liu G, Gao J, Ai H, et al. Applications and potential toxicity of magnetic iron oxide nanoparticles. Small. 2013;9:1533-45.
12. Patchell RA, et al. A randomized trial of surgery in the treatment of single metastases to the brain. N Engl J Med. 1990;322:494-500.
13. Vecht CJ, Haaxma-Reiche H, Noordijk EM, et al. Treatment of single brain metastasis:radiotherapy alone or combined with neurosurgery? Ann Neurol. 1993;33:583-90.
14. Hartford AC, Paravati AJ, Spire WJ, et al. Postoperative stereotactic radiosurgery without whole-brain radiation therapy for brain metastases:potential role of preoperative tumor size. Int J Radiat Oncol Biol Phys. 2013;85:650-5.
15. Brennan C, Yang TJ, Hilden P, et al. A phase 2 trial of stereotactic radiosurgery boost after surgical resection for brain metastases. Int J Radiat Oncol Biol Phys. 2014;88:130-6.
16. Robbins JR, Ryu S, Kalkanis S, et al. Radiosurgery to the surgical cavity as adjuvant therapy for resected brain metastasis. Neurosurgery. 2012;71:937-43.
17. Senft C, Bink A, Franz K, et al. Intraoperative MRI guidance and extent of resection in glioma surgery:a randomised, controlled trial. Lancet Oncol. 2011;12:997-1003.
18. Senft C, Ulrich CT, Seifert V, et al. Intraoperative magnetic resonance imaging in the surgical treatment of cerebral metastases. J Surg Oncol. 2010;101:436-41.
19. Weil RJ, Lonser RR. Selective excision of metastatic brain tumors originating in the motor cortex with preservation of function. J Clin Oncol. 2005;23:1209-17.
20. Shinoura N, Yoshida M, Yamada R, et al. Awake surgery with continuous motor testing for resection of brain tumors in the primary motor area. J Clin Neurosci. 2009;16:188-94.
21. Marbacher S, Klinger E, Schwyzer L, et al. Use of fluorescence to guide resection or biopsy of primary brain tumors and brain metastases. Neurosurg Focus. 2014;36:E10.
22. Motta M, del Vecchio A, Attuati L, et al. Gamma knife radiosurgery for treatment of cerebral metastases from non-small-cell lung cancer. Int J Radiat Oncol Biol Phys. 2011;81:e463-8.
23. Gerosa M, Nicolato A, Foroni R, et al. Analysis of long-term outcomes and prognostic factors in patients with non-small cell lung cancer brain metastases treated by gamma knife radiosurgery. J Neurosurg. 2005;102S:75-80.
24. Muacevic A, Wowra B, Siefert A, et al. Microsurgery plus whole brain irradiation versus Gamma Knife surgery alone for treatment of single metastases to the brain:a randomized controlled multicentre phase Ⅲ trial. J Neurooncol. 2008;87:299-307.

25. Andrews DW, Scott CB, Sperduto PW, et al. Whole brain radiation therapy with or without stereotactic radiosurgery boost for patients with one to three brain metastases: phase Ⅲ results of the RTOG 9508 randomised trial. Lancet. 2004;363:1665-72.
26. Kondziolka D, Patel A, Lunsford LD, et al. Stereotactic radiosurgery plus whole brain radiotherapy versus radiotherapy alone for patients with multiple brain metastases. Int J Radiat Oncol Biol Phys. 1999;45:427-34.
27. Kocher M, Soffietti R, Abacioglu U, et al. Adjuvant whole-brain radiotherapy versus observation after radiosurgery or surgical resection of one to three cerebral metastases: results of the EORTC 22952-26001 study. J Clin Oncol. 2011;29:134-41.
28. Aoyama H, Shirato H, Tago M, et al. Stereotactic radiosurgery plus whole-brain radiation therapy vs stereotactic radiosurgery alone for treatment of brain metastases: a randomized controlled trial. JAMA. 2006;295:2483-91.
29. Sneed PK, Suh JH, Goetsch SJ, et al. A multi-institutional review of radiosurgery alone vs. radiosurgery with whole brain radiotherapy as the initial management of brain metastases. Int J Radiat Oncol Biol Phys. 2002;53:519-26.
30. Chang EL, Wefel JS, Hess KR, et al. Neurocognition in patients with brain metastases treated with radiosurgery or radiosurgery plus whole-brain irradiation: a randomised controlled trial. Lancet Oncol. 2009;10:1037-44.
31. Soffietti R, Kocher M, Abacioglu UM, et al. A European Organisation for Research and Treatment of Cancer phase Ⅲ trial of adjuvant whole-brain radiotherapy versus observation in patients with one to three brain metastases from solid tumors after surgical resection or radiosurgery: quality-of-life results. J Clin Oncol. 2013;31:65-72.
32. Yamamoto M, Serizawa T, Shuto T, et al. Stereotactic radiosurgery for patients with multiple brain metastases (JLGK0901): a multi-institutional prospective observational study. Lancet Oncol. 2014;15:387-95.
33. Mehta MP, Rodrigus P, Terhaard CH, et al. Survival and neurologic outcomes in a randomized trial of motexafin gadolinium and whole-brain radiation therapy in brain metastases. J Clin Oncol. 2003;21:2529-36.
34. Suh JH, Stea B, Nabid A, et al. Phase Ⅲ study of efaproxiral as an adjunct to whole-brain radiation therapy for brain metastases. J Clin Oncol. 2006;24:106-14.
35. Meyers CA, Smith JA, Bezjak A, et al. Neurocognitive function and progression in patients with brain metastases treated with whole-brain radiation and motexafin gadolinium: results of a randomized phase Ⅲ trial. J Clin Oncol. 2004;22:157-65.
36. Langley RE, Stephens RJ, Nankivell M, et al. QUARTZ Investigators Interim data from the Medical Research Council QUARTZ Trial: does whole brain radiotherapy affect the survival and quality of life of patients with brain metastases from non-small cell lung cancer? Clin Oncol (R Coll Radiol). 2013;25:e23-30.
37. Gondi V, Mehta MP, Pugh S, et al. Memory preservation with conformal avoidance of the hippocampus during whole-brain radiation therapy for patients with brain metastases: primary

endpoint results of RTOG 0933. Int J Radiat Oncol Biol Phys. 2013;87S.
38. Brown PD, Pugh S, Laack NN, Radiation Therapy Oncology Group (RTOG), et al. Memantine for the prevention of cognitive dysfunction in patients receiving whole-brain radiotherapy: a randomized, double-blind, placebo-controlled trial. Neuro Oncol. 2013;15:1429-37.
39. Lee JS, Murphy WK, Glisson BS, et al. Primary chemotherapy of brain metastasis insmall-cell lung cancer. J Clin Oncol. 1989;7:916-22.
40. Lee DH, Han JY, Kim HT, et al. Primary chemotherapy for newly diagnosed nonsmall cell lung cancer patients with synchronous brain metastases compared with whole-brain radiotherapy administered first: result of a randomized pilot study. Cancer. 2008;113:143-9.
41. Chen G, Huynh M, Fehrenbacher L, et al. Phase II trial of irinotecan and carboplatin for extensive or relapsed small-cell lung cancer. J Clin Oncol. 2009;27:1401-4.
42. Bailon O, Chouahnia K, Augier A, et al. Upfront association of carboplatin plus pemetrexed in patients with brain metastases of lung adenocarcinoma. Neuro Oncol. 2012;14:491-5.
43. Wagenius G, Brodin O, Nyman J, et al. Radiotherapy vs. temozolomide in the treatment of patients with lung cancer and brain metastases: a randomized phase II study (abstract). J Clin Oncol. 2006;24:398s.
44. Pietanza MC, et al. Phase II trial of temozolomide in patients with relapsed sensitive or refractory small cell lung cancer, with assessment of methylguanine-DNA methyltransferase as a potential biomarker. Clin Cancer Res. 2012;18:1138-45.
45. Postmus PE, Haaxma-Reiche H, Smit EF, et al. Treatment of brain metastases of small-cell lung cancer: comparing teniposide and teniposide with whole-brain radiotherapy - a phase III study of the European Organization for the Research and Treatment of Cancer Lung Cancer Cooperative Group. J Clin Oncol. 2000;18:3400-8.
46. Guerrieri M, Wong K, Ryan G, et al. A randomised phase III study of palliative radiation with concomitant carboplatin for brain metastases from non-small cell carcinoma of the lung. Lung Cancer. 2004;46:107-11.
47. Neuhaus T, Ko Y, Muller RP, et al. A phase III trial of topotecan and whole brain radiation therapy for patients with CNS-metastases due to lung cancer. Br J Cancer. 2009;100:291.
48. Robinet G, Thomas P, Breton JL, et al. Results of a phase III study of early versus delayed whole brain radiotherapy with concurrent cisplatin and vinorelbine combination in inoperable brain metastasis of non-small-cell lung cancer: Groupe Français de Pneumo-Cancérologie (GFPC) Protocol 95-1. Ann Oncol. 2001;12:59-67.
49. Addeo R, De Rosa C, Faiola V, et al. Phase 2 trial of temozolomide using protracted low-dose and whole-brain radiotherapy for nonsmall cell lung cancer and breast cancer patients with brain metastases. Cancer. 2008;113:2524-31.
50. Antonadou D, Paraskevaidis M, Sarris G, et al. Phase II randomized trial of temozolomide and concurrent radiotherapy in patients with brain metastases. J Clin Oncol. 2002;20:3644-50.
51. Verger E, Gil M, Yaya R, et al. Temozolomide and concomitant whole brain radiotherapy in patients with brain metastases: a phase II randomized trial. Int J Radiat Oncol Biol Phys.

2005;61:185-91.

52. Sperduto PW, Wang M, Robins HI, et al. A phase 3 trial of whole brain radiation therapy and stereotactic radiosurgery alone versus WBRT and SRS with temozolomide or erlotinib for non-small cell lung cancer and 1 to 3 brain metastases: Radiation Therapy Oncology Group 0320. Int J Radiat Oncol Biol Phys. 2013;85:1312-8.

53. Chua D, Krzakowski M, Chouaid C, et al. Whole-brain radiation therapy plus concomitant temozolomide for the treatment of brain metastases from non-small-cell lung cancer: a randomized, open-label phase II study. Clin Lung Cancer. 2010;11:176-81.

54. Sun M, et al. HER family receptor abnormalities in lung cancer brain metastases and corresponding primary tumors. Clin Cancer Res. 2009;15:4829-37.

55. Breindel JL, et al. EGF receptor activates MET through MAPK to enhance non-small cell lung carcinoma invasion and brain metastasis. Cancer Res. 2013;73:5053-65.

56. Ma S, Xu Y, Deng Q, Yu X. Treatment of brain metastasis from non-small cell lung cancer with whole brain radiotherapy and Gefitinib in a Chinese population. Lung Cancer. 2009;65:198-203.

57. Chiu CH, Tsai CM, Chen YM, et al. Gefitinib is active in patients with brain metastases from non-small cell lung cancer and response is related to skin toxicity. Lung Cancer. 2005;47:129-38.

58. Wu C, et al. Gefitinib as palliative therapy for lung adenocarcinoma metastatic to the brain. Lung Cancer. 2007;57:359-64.

59. Ceresoli GL, et al. Gefitinib in patients with brain metastases from non-small-cell lung cancer: a prospective trial. Ann Oncol. 2004;15:1042-7.

60. Kim JE, et al. Epidermal growth factor receptor tyrosine kinase inhibitors as a first-line therapy for never-smokers with adenocarcinoma of the lung having asymptomatic synchronous brain metastasis. Lung Cancer. 2009;65:351-4.

61. Porta R, Sánchez-Torres JM, Paz-Ares L, et al. Brain metastases from lung cancer responding to erlotinib: the importance of EGFR mutation. Eur Respir J. 2011;37:624-31.

62. Welsh JW, Komaki R, Amini A, et al. Phase II trial of erlotinib plus concurrent whole-brain radiation therapy for patients with brain metastases from non-small-cell lung cancer. J Clin Oncol. 2013;31:895-902.

63. Wu YL, Zhou C, Cheng Y, et al. Erlotinib as second-line treatment in patients with advanced non-small-cell lung cancer and asymptomatic brain metastases: a phase II study (CTONG-0803). Ann Oncol. 2013;24:993-9.

64. Costa DB, Kobayashi S, Pandya SS, et al. CSF concentration of the anaplastic lymphoma kinase inhibitor crizotinib. J Clin Oncol. 2011;29:e443-5.

65. Takeda M, Okamoto I, Nakagawa K. Clinical impact of continued crizotinib administration after isolated central nervous system progression in patients with lung cancer positive for ALK rearrangement. J Thorac Oncol. 2013;8:654-7.

66. Kaneda H, Okamoto I, Nakagawa K. Rapid response of brain metastasis to crizotinib in a pa-

tient with ALK rearrangement-positive non-small-cell lung cancer. J Thorac Oncol. 2013;8: e32-3.
67. De Braganca KC, Janjigian YY, Azzoli CG, et al. Efficacy and safety of bevacizumab in active brain metastases from non-small cell lung cancer. J Neurooncol. 2010;100:443-7.
68. Socinski MA, Langer CJ, Huang JE, et al. Safety of bevacizumab in patients with non-small cell lung cancer and brain metastases. J Clin Oncol. 2009;27:5255-61.
69. Wu PF, et al. Phosphorylated insulin-like growth factor-1 receptor (pIGF1R) is a poor prognostic factor in brain metastases from lung adenocarcinomas. J Neurooncol. 2013;115:61-70.
70. Chen G, Wang Z, Liu XY, et al. High-level CXCR4 expression correlates with brain-specific metastasis of non-small cell lung cancer. World J Surg. 2011;35:56-61.

附录　彩　图

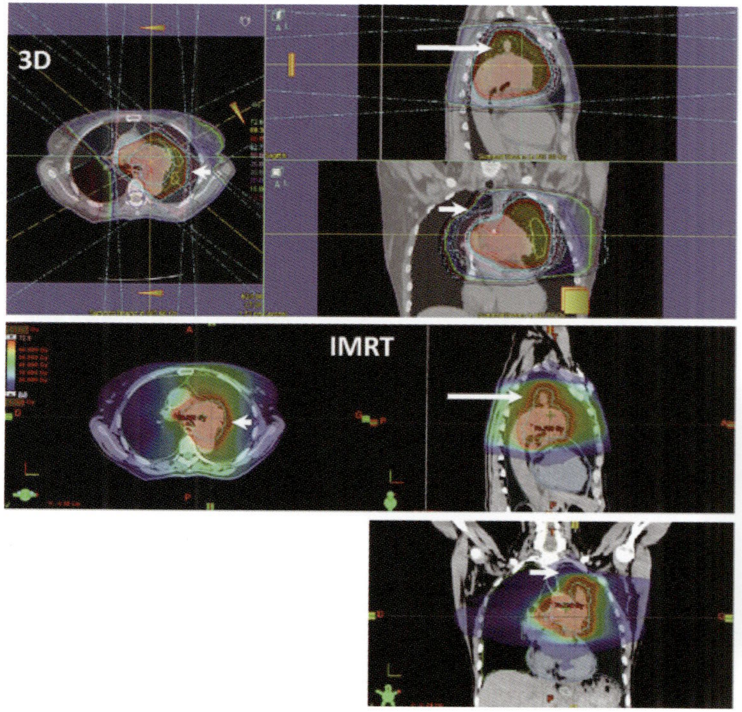

DVH比较

3D	V5	V10	V20	V30	V35	V50	V66
心脏	32 %	26.70 %	21 %	16.60 %	13.80 %	8.50 %	0.90 %
肺（－PTV）	56.20 %	47.20 %	32.70 %	23.70 %	13.80 %	8.50 %	4.40 %
食管	63.80 %	59.90 %	55 %	50.70 %	47.70 %	36.90 %	3 %
脊髓	27 %	25.40 %	16.40 %	13.40 %	12.20 %	0	0
IMRT RAPIDARC	V5	V10	V20	V30	V35	V50	V66
心脏	37 %	20.30 %	14 %	9.10 %	7.30 %	3.70 %	1.10 %
肺（－PTV）	60.50 %	43.80 %	27.40 %	16.70 %	14.40 %	7.20 %	0
食管	68.10 %	56.80 %	45 %	38.50 %	36.60 %	31.40 %	5 %
脊髓	27 %	23.40 %	20.30 %	16.00 %	13.00 %	0	0

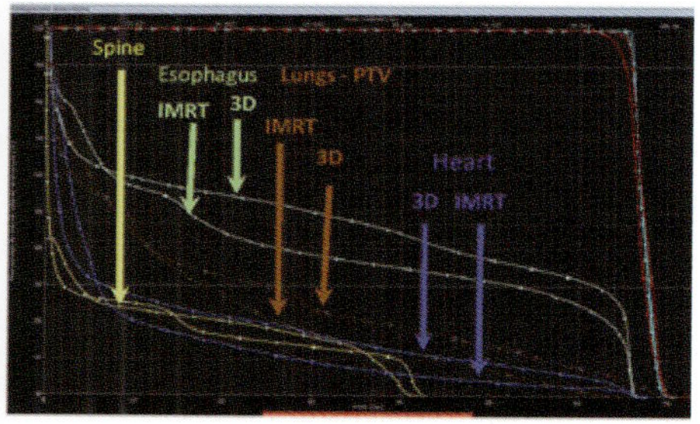

图6.1　局部晚期不可手术非小细胞肺癌IMRT计划的剂量分布

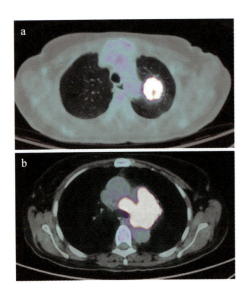

图 6.2　PET/CT 应用于放射治疗方案设计

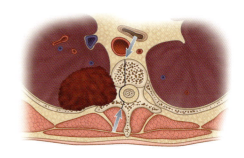

图 7.1　左上沟支气管肺癌侵犯胸廓入口，包括锁骨下动脉。箭头示达到 R0 切除的切除范围

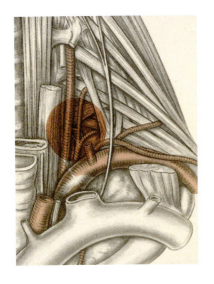

图 7.2　右胸顶肿瘤侵犯肋横突间隙、椎间孔和部分同侧椎体；先行前路切口分离肿瘤，然后经后中线切口行半椎体切除

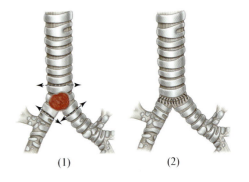

图 7.3　隆突切除后"新隆突"重建(1)，隆突病灶小范围侵犯主气管(1)。虚线为拟切割线(1)。左右主支气管内侧壁用 4-0 PDS 缝线行间断缝合成"新隆突"(2)

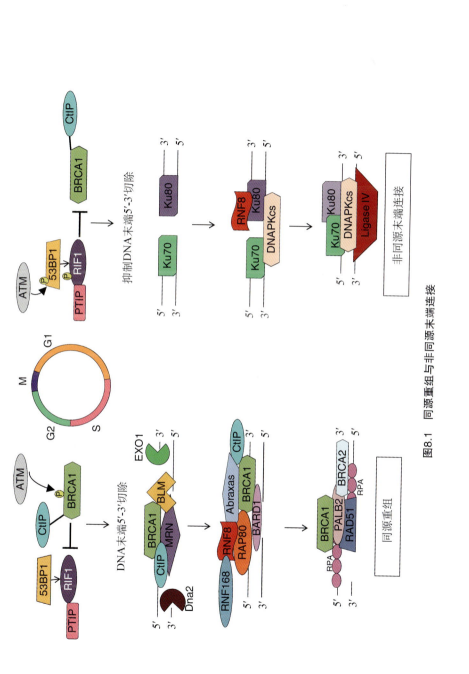

图8.1 同源重组与非同源末端连接

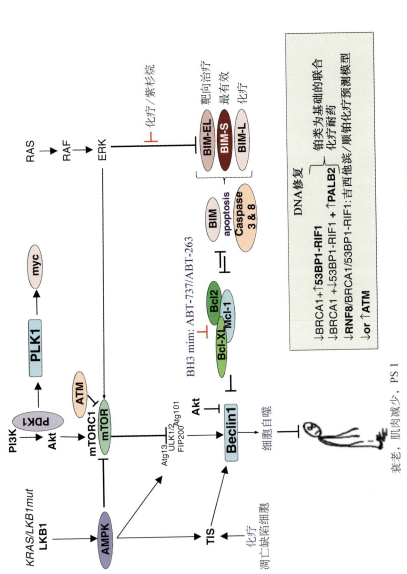

图8.2 凋亡、细胞自噬、细胞衰老交叉调节导致化疗耐药

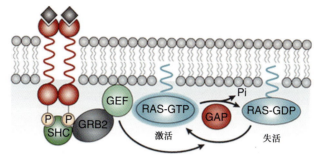

图 11.1 RAS 蛋白 GTP 酶激活与失活[7]

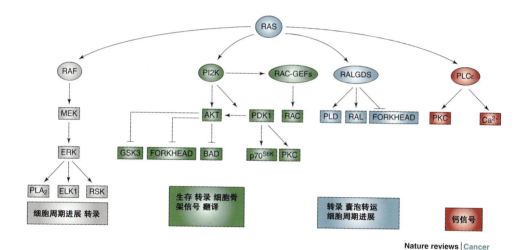

图 11.2 RAS 下游信号通路

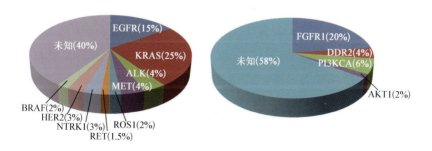

图 12.1 NSCLC 驱动基因：(a)腺癌；(b)鳞癌